Pediatric Endocrinology

Pediatric Endocrinology

Editor: Jeffery Desmond

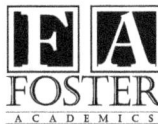

FOSTER
ACADEMICS

www.fosteracademics.com

www.fosteracademics.com

FA
FOSTER
ACADEMICS

Cataloging-in-Publication Data

Pediatric endocrinology / edited by Jeffery Desmond.
    p. cm.
Includes bibliographical references and index.
ISBN 978-1-63242-780-9
    1. Pediatric endocrinology. 2. Endocrine glands--Diseases. 3. Pediatric endocrinology--Diagnosis.
4. Pediatric endocrinology--Treatment. I. Desmond, Jeffery.
RJ418 .P43 2019
618.924--dc23

Foster Academics,
118-35 Queens Blvd., Suite 400,
Forest Hills, NY 11375, USA

ISBN 978-1-63242-780-9 (Hardback)

Contents

Preface

The study, diagnosis and treatment of the disorders of the endocrine glands that affect the physical growth and sexual development in children is under the scope of pediatric endocrinology. Some common disorders dealt within this field are type 1 diabetes and growth disorders. Adrenal, thyroid and pituitary problems in children, hypoglycemia, puberty-related conditions and hyperglycemia are also addressed within pediatric endocrinology. Pediatric endocrinologists also specialize in the areas of lipid metabolism, bone metabolism, inborn errors of metabolism and adolescent gynecology. Children with intersex disorders are also referred to a pediatric endocrinologist. This book covers in detail some existing theories and innovative concepts revolving around pediatric endocrinology. The various studies that are constantly contributing towards advancing clinical practices and theoretical understanding of this field are examined in detail. It is an essential guide for both academicians and those who wish to pursue this discipline further.

The information shared in this book is based on empirical researches made by veterans in this field of study. The elaborative information provided in this book will help the readers further their scope of knowledge leading to advancements in this field.

Finally, I would like to thank my fellow researchers who gave constructive feedback and my family members who supported me at every step of my research.

Editor

Evolutionary fitness as a function of pubertal age in 22 subsistence-based traditional societies

Ze'ev Hochberg[1*], Aneta Gawlik[1,2] and Robert S Walker[3]

Abstract

Context: The age of puberty has fallen over the past 130 years in industrialized, western countries, and this fall is widely referred to as the secular trend for earlier puberty. The current study was undertaken to test two evolutionary theories: (a) the reproductive system maximizes the number of offspring in response to positive environmental cues in terms of energy balance, and (b) early puberty is a trade-off response for high mortality rate and reduced resource availability.

Methods: Using a sample of 22 natural-fertility societies of mostly tropical foragers, horticulturalists, and pastoralists from Africa, South America, Australia, and Southeastern Asia, this study compares indices of adolescence growth and menarche with those of fertility fitness in these non-industrial, traditional societies.

Results: The average age at menarche correlated with the first reproduction, but did not correlate with the total fertility rate TFR or reproductive fitness. The age at menarche correlated negatively with their average adult body mass, and the average adult body weight positively correlated with reproductive fitness. Survivorship did not correlate with the age at menarche or age indices of the adolescent growth spurt. The population density correlated positively with the age at first reproduction, but not with menarche age, TFR, or reproductive fitness.

Conclusions: Based on our analyses, we reject the working hypotheses that reproductive fitness is enhanced in societies with early puberty or that early menarche is an adaptive response to greater mortality risk. Whereas body mass is a measure of resources is tightly associated with fitness, the age of menarche is not.

Introduction

The age of puberty has fallen over the past 130 years in industrialized, western countries, where menarche age has receded from 16.5 years in 1880 to the current 12.5 years in western societies; this decline has occurred concomitantly with an improvement in child health [1]. The progressively declining age of thelarche and menarche may have multiple explanations. Primates' studies suggest a role for prenatal androgens and social factors (like the social rank) [2,3]. In the last decade, a popular notion among investigators is that early puberty may result from environmental exposure to endocrine disrupting chemicals (EDC), thus accelerating hypothalamic maturation [4]. Whereas EDC may have a bearing on the earlier age of thelarche, evolutionary forces may add a new angel to explain the secular trend in the age of menarche over the last 130 years. Even though the age at menarche is strongly linked to genetic variations [5], the time course of the secular trend suggests strong environmental influence.

This secular trend for early onset of puberty is a topic of much research interest. This trend was recently examined from a life-history evolutionary perspective, and we previously suggested that transition from juvenility to adolescence is a period of adaptive plasticity [6,7]. Two models have been proposed to explain this adaptation. Gluckman and Hanson suggested that life-history strategies for greater reproductive fitness (a product of the fertility rate and survivorship) could account for the current early onset of puberty [8]. The declining age of pubertal development have both been proposed as an adaptive response to positive environmental cues in terms of energy balance [7]. The assumption is that the reproductive system maximizes the number of offspring by balancing the benefit of more births against the costs of maternal mortality. With

* Correspondence: z_hochberg@rambam.health.gov.il
[1]Division of Pediatric Endocrinology, Meyer Children's Hospital, Rambam Medical Center, and Rappaport Faculty of Medicine and Research Institute, Technion-Israel Institute of Technology, Haifa, Israel
Full list of author information is available at the end of the article

respect to puberty, women face a trade-off between spending a long time accumulating resources through childhood growth and weight gain in order to improve the likelihood for successful pregnancy, against an early-age reproduction in order to increase the number of reproductive cycles. Indeed, heavy women in pre-industrial societies are more fertile, and both increased body weight and fertility are correlated with high birth rates [9]. This trade-off model has been used to predict that 18 years is the optimal age for first birth, which is near the observed average 17.5 years in such societies [10].

A different evolutionary trade-off was suggested by Migliano *et al* [11]. Based on analysis of the stature, growth, and reproductive fitness for the Aeta and the Batak pygmy from the Philippines, they argued that that the small body size of pygmy populations is an adaptation that evolved as the result of a life history tradeoff between the fertility benefits of a large body size against the costs of late growth cessation, under the circumstances of significant young and adult mortality. They showed that the small pygmy body size evolved through the early onset age of juvenility and adolescence [12], and suggested early cessation of growth is a trade-off for high mortality rate and reduced resource availability. Thus, short life expectancy may be initially a determinant of early puberty but subsequently, early puberty as

an adaptive response may determine longer lifespan due to reduced adult size and resource need.

The present study was designed to explore these two hypotheses. To this end, it takes an inter-population approach that compares indices of adolescence (menarche, and the growth spurt) with those of fertility fitness in non-industrial, traditional societies. Using a sample of 22 natural-fertility societies of mostly tropical foragers, horticulturalists, and pastoralists from Africa, South America, Australia, and Southeastern Asia, we hypothesized that (a) early adolescence would be associated with greater reproductive fitness or (b) with mortality risk, and predicted that the age at menarche and indices of pubertal growth will (a) negatively correlate with fertility rate or (b) positively correlate with survivorship. Although the reproductive and life history strategies of males and females are quite distinct in these societies, similar considerations might apply to the males, for which we included indices of adolescent growth spurt in our study.

Methods
Natural-fertility human societies
The sample used here is 22 subsistence-based societies and the demographic characteristics of each society, collected at different times during 1967-1988; these have been previously described [13] (Table 1). Information on

Table 1 Ecology and economy type of the twenty tribes comprising the study populations

Name	Country	Ecology	Economy	Subjects
Aeta	Philippines	tropical forest	mixed	365
Baka (West Pygmy)	Cameroon	tropical forest	forager	217
Batak	Philippines	tropical forest	mixed	36
Arnhem land	Australia	coastal/desert	farming-foraging	> 700
Guaja	Brazil	neotropical forest	forager	103
Hadza	Tanzania	savanna/woodland	forager	> 700
Hiwi	Venezuela	savanna/gallery	forager	59
Ju'/hoansi	Botswana/Namibia	desert/savanna	forager	278
Maku-Nadeb	Brazil	neotropical forest	farming-foraging	97
Tsimane	Bolivia	neotropical forest	farming-foraging	603
Yanomamo	Venezuela	neotropical forest	farming-foraging	116
Ache	Paraguay	neotropical forest	farming-foraging	484
Casiguran Agta	Philippines	tropical forest	forager	155
Aka	Congo/C.A.R.	tropical forest	forager	186
Efe (East Pygmy)	Congo (Ituri)	tropical forest	forager	145
Gainj & Asai	New Guinea	highlanders	farming-foraging	153
Turkana	Kenya	savanna	pastoral/mixed	417
Warao	Venezuela	tropical forest	forager	116
Gambia	Gambia	savanna/forest gallery	farming-foraging	> 700
Toba	Argentina	savanna/dry forest	mixed	411
Wichi	Argentina	savanna/dry forest	mixed	328
Maya	Mexico	forest/savanna	mixed	182

the life history and population density of these societies and their average height, body weight, and BMI is available at http://anthropology.missouri.edu/people/walker. html as compiled by one of us (RSW) from previous reports [14-16] and sources therein. In these societies, the age of menarche ranged from 12.6-18.4, and the age at growth spurt takeoff ranged from 10-13.5 years.

The stages of puberty were determined in girls of each society by the mean age of menarche, by the adolescent takeoff height velocity, peak height velocity, and for the end of puberty - the return to weight and height takeoff velocities. Indices of fertility in each society were determined from the average age at first reproduction, the interbirth interval (IBI, by self report), and total fertility rate (TFR). Reproductive fitness was calculated per society from the population average survivorship to age 15 (L15, range 0.33-0.80) and the TFR (range 2.6-9.0), TFR*L15, as previously suggested [17]. Mortality risk was determined from the survivorship to age 15 and life expectancy at birth (range 24.3-47.5) and age 15 (range 29.6-47.0).

At the time of data collection, ethical approval was considered not required, and the authors had no access to individuals' data.

Statistical analyses

Linear regression analyses with 95% confidence intervals of outcome as a function of IBI were performed using *Statistica 6.0*. For these analyses, the average of each study parameter for each society was a single point in the regression analysis. One-way analysis of variance (ANOVA) was used to determine whether statistical differences exist between the study parameters in the 22 studied societies. Statistical significance was set at $p < 0.05$.

Results

Adolescent age and reproductive fitness

The age at menarche correlated positively with the age at first reproduction ($r = 0.762$, $p < 0.001$), and the average duration between the two events was four years (Figure 1). When we tested the hypothesis that early adolescence is associated with increased reproductive fitness, the age at menarche and the growth indices (age at takeoff, peak velocity, and the return to weight and height takeoff velocity) did not correlate with the IBI (Table 2). The age at menarche did not correlate with TFR or reproductive fitness (NS: $r = -0.208$, $p = 0.440$; $r = -0.008$, $p = 0.983$, respectively), whereas the age at first reproduction correlated positively with the age at height spurt takeoff ($r = 0.794$, $p = 0.003$; Figure 2), peak height velocity ($r = 0.791$, $p = 0.011$), and return to takeoff height velocity ($r = 0.765$, $p = 0.027$), but TFR and reproductive fitness did not correlate with any of these variables (Table 2).

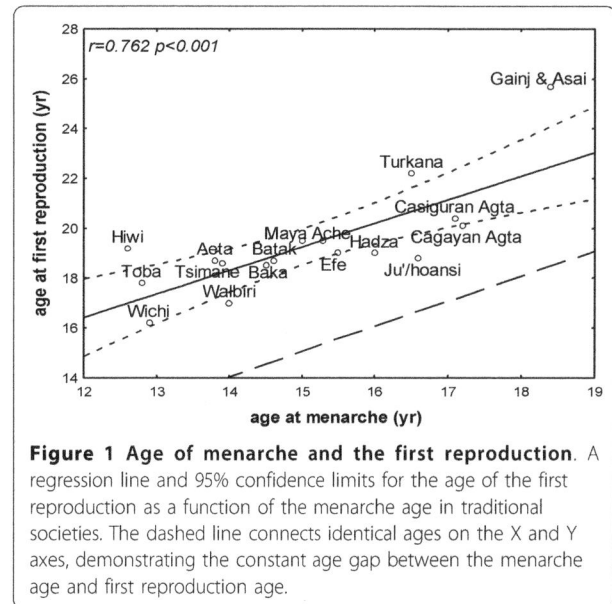

Figure 1 Age of menarche and the first reproduction. A regression line and 95% confidence limits for the age of the first reproduction as a function of the menarche age in traditional societies. The dashed line connects identical ages on the X and Y axes, demonstrating the constant age gap between the menarche age and first reproduction age.

Body size

The average age at menarche correlated negatively with the average adult body weight (kg) ($r = -0.599$, $p = 0.014$; Figure 3) and body mass index (BMI) ($r = -0.632$, $p = 0.009$; Figure 3), but not with the average adult height

Table 2 Insignificant correlations

	Correlations	r	p
Fitness	Age at menarche vs IBI	0.248	0.354
	Age at takeoff velocity vs IBI	0.501	0.117
	Age at menarche vs TFR	-0.208	0.440
	Age at menarche vs reproductive fitness	-0.008	0.983
	TFR vs age at takeoff velocity	-0.565	0.089
	Reproductive fitness vs age at takeoff velocity	-0.356	0.489
	Reproductive fitness vs age at peak velocity	-0.457	0.543
Body size	Age at menarche vs average adult height	-0.109	0.687
	Average adult height vs age at first reproduction	-0.042	0.856
	Average adult height vs TFR	0.355	0.148
	Average adult height vs reproductive fitness	0.480	0.135
	BMI vs TFR	0.296	0.232
	BMI vs reproductive fitness	0.347	0.295
Density	Population density vs age at menarche	0.235	0.486
	Population density vs TFR	0.202	0.530
	Population density vs reproductive fitness	0.141	0.698
Survivorship	Survivorship to age 15 vs age at menarche	0.207	0.541
	Life expectancy at birth vs age at menarche	0.146	0.688
	Life expectancy at age 15 vs age at menarche	0.139	0.701

BMI - body mass index, IBI - interbirth interval, TFR - total fertility rate,

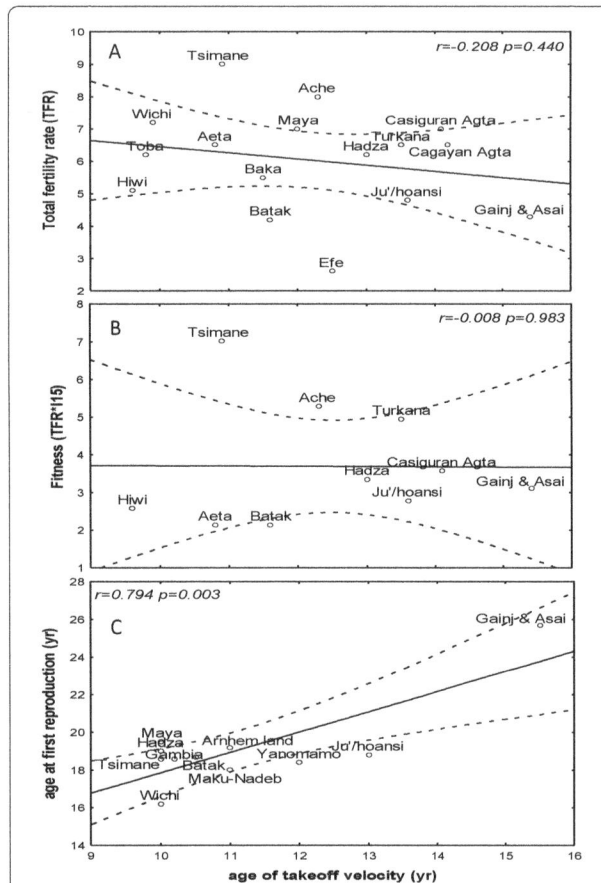

Figure 2 Puberty and reproductive fitness. A regression and 95% confidence limits for the age at first reproduction as a function of the height spurt takeoff in girls of traditional societies.

(Table 2). The average adult body weight (kg) correlated negatively with the age at first reproduction (r = -0.450, p = 0.041), and the average adult body weight (kg) positively correlated with the respective society's reproductive fitness (r = 0.660, p = 0.027; r = 0.717, p = 0.013, respectively; Figure 3). The average adult heights did not correlate with the age at first reproduction, TFR, or reproductive fitness (Table 2). The BMI correlated with the age at first reproduction (r = -0.466, p = 0.033), but not with the TFR or reproductive fitness.

Adolescent age and the physical environment
The average age at menarche and parameters of the growth spurt for each society did not correlate with their respective population density. The population density correlated positively with the women's age at first reproduction (r = 0.680, p < 0.005), but not with menarche age, TFR, or reproductive fitness (Table 2).

Adolescent age and survivorship expectancy
When we tested the hypothesis that early adolescence and small body size is a trade-off for high mortality risk,

we found that the survivorship to age 15 and life expectancy at birth or age 15 did not correlate with the age at menarche or age indices of the adolescent growth spurt (Table 2). Adding survivorship to a multivariate analysis for age at menarche or age at first reproduction as a function of BMI and population density added no statistical significance.

Ecological and economic correlates
When the societies were categorizing societies by their ecology, dwellers of the tropical forest, the neotropical forest, and the savanna had comparable ages at menarche and reproductive fitness. Of the studied societies, the TFR was highest among dwellers of neotropical forests (8.3 ± 0.6), as compared to those in the savanna (6.5 ± 0.7) and the tropical forests (5.4 ± 1.7, p = 0.015; Table 3). When the societies were categorized by their economy type, the age at menarche, TFR, and reproductive fitness were not significantly different between the farmers-foragers, the foragers, and the mixed-economy groups (results not shown).

Discussion
In considering human adolescence in the context of evolutionary fitness, we considered key traits that were available from data collected in 1967-1988. These include the age of menarche, the pattern and timing of the adolescent growth spurt, the body size, and the determinants of reproductive fitness, namely the age of the first reproduction, the IBI, the number of progeny, and mortality risk [18]. The database contains no information on birth size, which may influence the age at menarche. Extended growth and large body size in humans prompt fertility gains and reduced offspring mortality [19]. Consequently there is a pressure for delayed reproductive onset, whereas early reproduction minimizes the likelihood of death before reproduction.

Several limitations of this approach require consideration. i. By nature of this approach, comparing population level averages and attributing differences to ecological differences may not be straightforward. It assumes that the relationships observed would be the same if examined at an individual level [20]. In their report, Greenland and Robin construct several epidemiological examples that show that data at the ecologic level can be misinterpreted if nonlinear effects at the individual level, and other confounds, are not accounted for. Such data for the individual level were not available to us. ii. Comparative studies across societies may also suffer from problems of phylogenetic non-independence. This was addressed for these data previously by adjusting for geographical location (Africa, South America, Australia and Southeast Asia), but the effect was very weak and not significant in any of the multiple regressions [13].

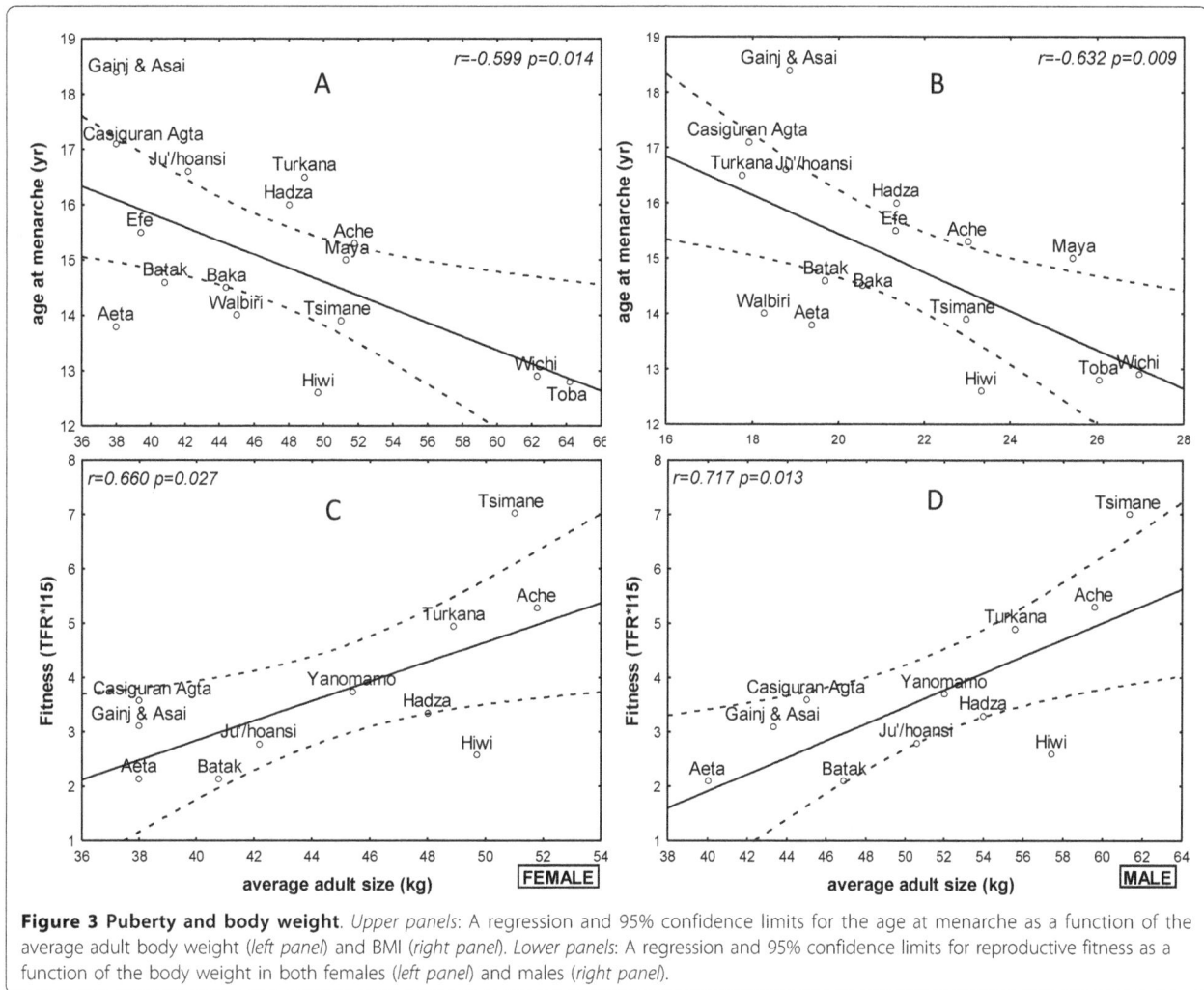

Figure 3 Puberty and body weight. *Upper panels*: A regression and 95% confidence limits for the age at menarche as a function of the average adult body weight (*left panel*) and BMI (*right panel*). *Lower panels*: A regression and 95% confidence limits for reproductive fitness as a function of the body weight in both females (*left panel*) and males (*right panel*).

Pubertal timing is not a univocal parameter; secular changes may occur differently for some pubertal events. Whereas the age of thelarche has reduced in the last decades, changes in menarche have been more subtle and mental maturation - deferred. Also, it is not clear that menarche is a good proxy for fecundity. The age at first reproduction in the present study strongly correlated with menarche, but the potential role of anovulatory menstrual cycles after menarche and potential nonlinearity of this trend remain options. For example, it is possible that girls who differ on age at menarche may be similar with regard to age of fecundity; earlier menarche may relate to a greater number of anovulatory cycles [21], and indeed, regular (ovulatory) cycling was shown to follow a secular trend towards delay as opposed to early menarche [22].

The data show that at natural fertility, early adolescence in girls, as assessed by the age of menarche and the growth pattern, corresponds to a young age with the first reproduction occurring about four years later, as

Table 3 Ecology type of the societies comprising the study populations

VARIABLES	Tropical forest	Neotropical forest	Savanna/other	p Value
Age at menarche (n)	(n = 6)	(n = 2)	(n = 6)	0.45
	15.5 ± 1.4	14.6 ± 1.0	14.3 ± 1.8	
TFR (n)	(n = 6)	(n = 3)	(n = 7)	**0.015**
	5.4 ± 1.7	8.3 ± 0.6	6.5 ± 0.7	
Reproductive fitness (n)	(n = 3)	(n = 3)	(n = 4)	0.09
	2.6 ± 0.9	5.3 ± 1.7	3.9 ± 1.2	

TFR - total fertility rate, mean ± SD

previously suggested [23]. However, based on our analyses, we reject the two working hypotheses: reproductive fitness is enhanced in societies with early puberty [8] and early menarche is an adaptive response to greater mortality risk [11].

We focus here on subsistence-based societies because most resources are invested as somatic capital in terms of growth, body size and fertility (reproductive fitness), as opposed to stored and inherited wealth [15]. The relative contribution of biological and behavioral factors in determining natural fertility change with the environment. Environmental factors to consider in an interpopulation study include the physical environment (e.g., population density), the biological environment (e.g., food availability, disease, and other mortality risks) and social behaviors (e.g., age at marriage) [15]. We defined reproductive fitness as a function of TFR and L15, as previously suggested [17]; these two variables were selected among other because information on these two parameters was available for almost all of the societies in the database. The age at menarche did not correlate with TFR or reproductive fitness. Whereas reproduction starts early in societies in which puberty occurs early, in the context of high population density [19], their reproductive fitness does not increase. The dwellers of the neotropical forests have a high TFR, but given their mortality risk, they have comparable reproductive fitness to the other ecology groups.

We confirm a previous assertion for greater reproductive fitness among heavier, better-nourished traditional societies [9,24]. When considered as a whole, we found that the average adult body weight, but not height, correlated negatively with age at menarche and the age at first reproduction, and positively with reproductive fitness. The BMI may not work as well in the extremes of size; in very small or very tall populations the BMI is not as accurate as it is in average size populations. Even though, these findings provide indirect support to the hypothesis that early puberty among girls who live in affluent and developed countries is a response to a positive energy balance. Indeed, among contemporary girls in developing countries, the age at menarche among the prosperous is earlier than that of the underpriviledged [1].

Based on the high mortality rates of the Philippine pygmy, Migliano et al suggested that early fertility is part of the "fast" extreme of life history strategies to which the pygmy adapt [25], with both longevity and resource availability as limiting factors [11]. Indeed, early life stress is associated with premature juvenility and adolescence [1,12,26]. The results of the present study do not confirm the fast life history theory; we found no correlation between adult height and the age of menarche with survivorship. Yet, population density correlated with the age of first reproduction, in addition to our previous assertion that body size in a traditional society was dependent upon the population density [19]. We have previously suggested that population density acts through two pathways - nutritional constraints and juvenile mortality - at varying intensities, and can contribute to a nearly twofold range in body size across human societies [19]. The sample of the present study includes two African pygmy groups - the Baka (West pygmy) and the Efe (East pygmy), both of whom are not consistent with the Migliano risk/early fertility model. The average age of menarche and age at first reproduction in these two societies, 14.5 and 15.5, respectively 18.5 and 19, respectively, were close to those of all of the other studied societies [13].

The secular trend for an early age of menarche has been rapid over the past 130 years in developed countries [27]. This trend is rightly interpreted as a reflection of improved nutrition and health in childhood [18]. Life history theory postulates tradeoffs of current versus future reproduction and fertility versus mortality risk. Life-history modeling predicted that a reduction in juvenile mortality reduces the age of menarche [8] or that low survivorship accelerates the life history [11]. Given the close interaction between resource availability and reproduction, we anticipated that those environmental factors that determine late metabolic homeostasis, attainment of adult size and cessation of growth would interface with those influencing the timing of sexual maturation. The data do not support these predictions. Whereas body mass as a measure of resources is tightly associated with fitness in these traditional societies, the age of menarche is not. Thus, it may be that women's physiology tracks its own condition in such a way as to maximize their individual fitness.

Abbreviations
BMI: Body mass index; IBI: Interbirth interval; EDC: endocrine disrupting chemicals; L15: survivorship to age 15; TFR: Total fertility rate

Author details
[1]Division of Pediatric Endocrinology, Meyer Children's Hospital, Rambam Medical Center, and Rappaport Faculty of Medicine and Research Institute, Technion-Israel Institute of Technology, Haifa, Israel. [2]Department of Pediatric Endocrinology and Diabetes, Medical University of Silesia, Katowice, Poland. [3]Department of Anthropology, University of Missouri, Columbia MO 65211, USA.

Authors' contributions
ZH contributed to the concept and design, analysis and interpretation of data, writing the article. AC contributed to the design, analysis and interpretation of data. RSW contributed to the concept and design, acquisition and interpretation of data. All authors read and approved the final manuscript.

Competing interests
The authors declare that they have no competing interests.

References

1. Parent AS, et al: The timing of normal puberty and the age limits of sexual precocity: variations around the world, secular trends, and changes after migration. *Endocr Rev* 2003, **24**(5):668-93.

2. Zehr JL, Van Meter PE, Wallen K: Factors regulating the timing of puberty onset in female rhesus monkeys (Macaca mulatta): role of prenatal androgens, social rank, and adolescent body weight. *Biol Reprod* 2005, **72**(5):1087-94.

3. Wilson ME, et al: Timing of sexual maturity in female rhesus monkeys (Macaca mulatta) housed outdoors. *J Reprod Fertil* 1984, **70**(2):625-33.

4. Toppari J, Juul A: Trends in puberty timing in humans and environmental modifiers. *Mol Cell Endocrinol* 2010, **324**(1-2):39-44.

5. Ong KK, et al: Associations between the Pubertal Timing-Related Variant in LIN28B and BMI Vary Across the Life Course. *J Clin Endocrinol Metab* 2010.

6. Hochberg Z: Juvenility in the context of life history theory. *Arch Dis Child* 2008, **93**(6):534-9.

7. Hochberg Z: Evo-devo of child growth II: human life history and transition between its phases. *Eur J Endocrinol* 2009, **160**(2):135-41.

8. Gluckman PD, Hanson MA: Evolution, development and timing of puberty. *Trends Endocrinol Metab* 2006, **17**(1):7-12.

9. Pawlowski B: Prevalence of menstrual pain in relation to the reproductive life history of women from the Mayan rural community. *Ann Hum Biol* 2004, **31**(1):1-8.

10. Simondon KB, Simondon F: Mothers prolong breastfeeding of undernourished children in rural Senegal. *Int J Epidemiol* 1998, **27**(3):490-4.

11. Migliano AB, Vinicius L, Lahr MM: Life history trade-offs explain the evolution of human pygmies. *Proc Natl Acad Sci USA* 2007, **104**(51):20216-9.

12. Hochberg Z: Evo-Devo of child growth III: premature juvenility as an evolutionary trade-off. *Horm Res Paediatr* 2010, **73**(6):430-7.

13. Walker RS, et al: The trade-off between number and size of offspring in humans and other primates. *Proc Biol Sci* 2008, **275**(1636):827-33.

14. Binford L: Constructing frames of reference: An analytical method for archaeological theory building using ethnographic and environmental data sets. Berkeley: University of California Press; 2001.

15. Walker R, et al: Growth rates and life histories in twenty-two small-scale societies. *Am J Hum Biol* 2006, **18**(3):295-311.

16. Hill KR, et al: Co-residence patterns in hunter-gatherer societies show unique human social structure. *Science* 2011, **331**(6022):1286-9.

17. Gurven M, Kaplan H: Longevity among hunter-gatherers: a cross-cultural examination. *Population Develop Rev* 2007, , **33**: 321-365.

18. Hochberg Z, Albertsson-Wikland K: Evo-devo of infantile and childhood growth. *Pediatr Res* 2008, **64**(1):2-7.

19. Walker R, Hamilton MJ: Life-history consequences of density dependence and the evolution of human body size. *Curr Anthropol* 2008, **49**:115-122.

20. Greenland S, Robins J: Invited commentary: ecologic studies–biases, misconceptions, and counterexamples. *Am J Epidemiol* 1994, **139**(8):747-60.

21. Apter D, Vihko R: Early menarche, a risk factor for breast cancer, indicates early onset of ovulatory cycles. *J Clin Endocrinol Metab* 1983, **57**(1):82-6.

22. Clavel-Chapelon F: Evolution of age at menarche and at onset of regular cycling in a large cohort of French women. *Hum Reprod* 2002, **17**(1):228-32.

23. Kramer KL: Early sexual maturity among Pume foragers of Venezuela: fitness implications of teen motherhood. *Am J Phys Anthropol* 2008, **136**(3):338-50.

24. Ellison PT: Morbidity, morality, and menarche. *Hum Biol* 1981, **53**(4):635-43.

25. Harvey P, Clutton-Brock T: Life history variation in primates. *Evolution* 1985, **39**:559-581.

26. Cizza G, et al: Circulating plasma leptin and IGF-1 levels in girls with premature adrenarche: potential implications of a preliminary study. *Horm Metab Res* 2001, **33**(3):138-43.

27. Garn SM: The secular trend in size and maturational timing and its implications for nutritional assessment. *J Nutr* 1987, **117**(5):817-23.

Prospective memory and glycemic control in children with type 1 diabetes mellitus: a cross-sectional study

Jennifer N Osipoff[1*], Denise Dixon[2], Thomas A Wilson[1] and Thomas Preston[3]

Abstract

Background: Prospective memory is that memory which is required to carry out intended actions and is therefore essential in carrying out the daily activities required in the self-management of type 1 diabetes mellitus (T1DM). This study aimed to identify the relationships between prospective memory and diabetic control in children with T1DM.

Method: 94 children aged 6–18 years with T1DM completed an innovative prospective memory screen, PROMS, and a series of cognitive tests. Parents answered questionnaires about their children's diabetic histories and cognitive skills.

Results: No association between total PROMS score and glycemic control was found. Lower HbA1C was associated with higher (better) scores on the 20 minute event-based task on the PROMS. Parental concerns about working memory and metacognition in their children were mirrored by higher HbA1C.

Conclusions: This study suggests that there may be an association between glycemic control and prospective memory for event based tasks. Additional studies need to be done to determine reproducibility, causality, and if prospective memory based interventions can improve diabetic control.

Keywords: Hemoglobin A1C, Pediatrics, Adolescents, Psychological testing, Diabetes mellitus, Memory

Background

Cognitive and executive functioning in type one diabetes mellitus (T1DM) has slowly gained attention in the literature over the past two decades. Studies in this area, particularly within pediatrics, are still scarce. Two recent meta-analyses incorporating studies from 1985–2005 and from 1980–2005 found only 19 and 24 studies respectively that focused on executive function in children with T1DM [1,2]. Both conclude these children have poorer performance on tests of visuo-spatial ability, motor speed, writing, sustained attention, reading, full IQ, performance IQ, and verbal IQ [1,2]. Most of the studies reviewed in these meta-analyses focused on cognition. Research specifically examining pediatric T1DM and memory is even more limited [3-10]. In two reports children with T1DM scored lower on tests of short term

memory compared to their healthy peers [4,8]. Hershey *et. al* suggested that severe hypoglycemia had a negative impact on declarative and long-term spatial memory with no such effect seen with procedural memory [3,5-7].

Only two publications have looked at the role that memory plays in diabetic management rather than investigating if T1DM impairs different components of memory [9,10]. Holmes *et. al.* utilized The Wide Range Assessment of Memory and Learning (WRAML), a test designed to assess immediate and delayed recall of verbal and visual memory. This study [9], evaluating youth 9 to 17 years old, concluded that rote verbal memory accounted for 5.5% of the variance in the frequency of blood glucose (BG) testing in children 12.5 years and older and quantitative memory accounted for 9.9% of variance in carbohydrate consumption in adolescents 14.8 years and older. However, these behaviors did not predict mean hemoglobin A1C (HbA1C) values over the prior 6 months. The second paper [10] developed a biopsychosocial model of predictors of

* Correspondence: Jennifer.osipoff@stonybrookmedicine.edu
[1]Division of Pediatric Endocrinology, Department of Pediatrics, Stony Brook Children's Hospital, HSC Level 11 Room 080, Stony Brook, NY 11794-8111, USA
Full list of author information is available at the end of the article

youth diabetes care behaviors and metabolic control after studying more than 200 children 9 to 16 years old. A significant inverse correlation of modest magnitude was obtained between higher scores on the memory index of the WRAML and lower HbA1C.

These studies build a foundation for further research involving memory and T1DM. One important gap in our knowledge is the role of prospective memory, an essential component of executing intended actions at an appropriate time in the future, in children with T1DM. Prospective memory is particularly important in T1DM because the medical regimen is complex. Patients must remember to check their BG and count the amount of carbohydrates in foods each time they eat, take insulin a minimum of two times per day, and adjust insulin doses based on their health status, activity, carbohydrate intake and current BG. Adult care takers initially play a large role in this intensive care plan, but as children get older and more independent, more responsibility is placed upon them. Despite its importance in diabetic care, only one study about prospective memory in diabetic subjects has been published. That study looked at prospective memory in adult patients with diabetes under both euglycemic and hypoglycemic conditions and ultimately concluded that acute hypoglycemia impaired prospective memory [11]. The approach used to measure prospective memory in that study was not appropriate for pediatric populations. Research in prospective memory is hindered by the lack of a gold standard for testing. The prospective memory test used in our study, PROMS (see Table 1), was designed with a pediatric population in mind and consists of developmentally appropriate tasks, allowing us to investigate prospective memory in a pediatric T1DM population.

Our primary study aim was to determine if poorer glycemic control (as measured by higher HbA1C values) is associated with lower prospective memory scores in children with T1DM. Our second aim was to determine if greater parental concerns regarding their child's cognitive functioning are associated with lower prospective memory scores.

Methods

One hundred twenty children were recruited during outpatient appointments, hospitalizations, diabetes camp, and via advertising in the local Juvenile Diabetes Research Foundation chapter from July 2009 to November 2010. Eligibility criteria were age 6–18 years, diagnosed with T1DM for at least three months, and fluency in English. Exclusion criteria were neurologic, psychiatric, or medical disorders known to effect cognition and attendance in special education programs prior to the diagnosis of T1DM.

The protocol was approved by the institutional review board and the General Clinical Research Center (GCRC); the latter provided grant support (GCRC grant #MO1RR10710) to purchase $40 gift cards for each family to serve as an incentive to participate. Consent and assent were obtained from all parent–child pairs. At the start of the study visit, the child's BG (Accucheck glucometer) and HbA1C (Siemens DCA analyzer) were measured. Hypoglycemia (BG < 70 mg/d), if present, was to be treated prior to testing and the child given a minimum of 20 minutes of recovery time from the hypoglycemic nadir to the onset of memory testing. Cognitive impairment secondary to an acute episode of hypoglycemia has been demonstrated to be fully reversed in this period of time [12]. If the BG was more than 240 mg/dL, urine ketones were checked. No participants had hypoglycemia or moderate or large ketones at the onset of the study.

One GCRC staff member received intensive training from our neuropsychologist (TP) to administer the PROMS and other cognitive tests. This person had no prior interactions with any of the children and remained blinded to the BG and HbA1C results. If hypoglycemia was suspected during testing, the child's BG was retested and treatment was provided as needed. Only one child experienced low BG during testing.

Prospective memory was assessed using a revised version of the Prospective Memory Screening [13,14] utilizing a combination of eight event-based prospective memory tasks (EBT) and time-based prospective memory tasks (TBT). The PROMS was conducted concurrently with academic testing in order to provide an index of prospective memory that is both sensitive and ecologically valid [15]. The 2-subtest version of the Wechsler Abbreviated Scale of Intelligence (WASI) evaluated general intellect [16]. Academic skills were measured using the Wechsler Individual Achievement Test – Second Edition (WIAT 2) [17]. The California Verbal Learning Test – Children's Version (CVLT C) assessed declarative memory [18]. Working memory was investigated by the Digit Span subtest of the Wechsler Intelligence Scale for Children – Fourth Edition (WISC 4) [19]. At completion, a repeat BG level was obtained.

The accompanying parent answered questions regarding the child's diabetic history and the family's socioeconomic status. Information collected about the child's diabetic history included age at diagnosis, current insulin regimen, frequency of diabetic ketoacidosis and number of episodes of severe hypoglycemia, defined for our study as loss of consciousness, seizure activity, and/or necessitating glucagon administration. The Behavior Rating Inventory of Executive Functions (BRIEF) was also completed to capture parents' observations of their child's capacities across several sub-domains of executive

Table 1 Description of PROMS

PROMS Task #	Time (min)	Instructions to Subject	Instructor's Prompt	Subject's Action
1	0	1. When I tap on table, get that book for me (EBT)	Gives first two tasks to carry out	
2		2. In exactly two minutes, write your grade in school (TBT)		
3	2	When I show you a manila folder state your phone number (EBT to occur in 5 minutes)		Writes grade in school
4	7	In exactly 5 minutes, get me that CD (TBT)	Shows manila folder	States phone number
5	12	When I show you a stapler tell me to organize my papers (EBT to occur in 10 minutes)		Gets CD
6	20	In exactly 10 minutes put a penny in the envelope (TBT)	Taps on table	Gets book
7	22	When I show you a green paper, write a problem you are having in school (EBT to occur in 15 minutes)	Shows stapler	Says to organize papers
8	30	In exactly 20 minutes ask me what we are going to do next (TBT)		Puts penny in envelope
	37		Shows green paper	Writes down school problem
	50			Asks what are we doing next?

A digital clock is placed on the table between the instructor and the child. The instructor ensures that the child is able to determine what time it will be at different time intervals. Then the instructor gives the child the first two tasks to remember to carry out which starts the test. The instructor gives the next task to remember at the predetermined times regardless of whether or not the child has correctly completed the prior tasks. For scoring purposes tasks are divided into event based tasks (EBT) and time based tasks (TBT).

function, including self-regulation, planning/organization, and working memory [20].

Statistical Analysis
Power Analyses
A projected sample size of 100 participants provided 88% power for detecting significant correlations (e.g., for $r = .30$), and a two-tailed significance level set at $p < .05$. The *a priori* power analyses for each regression model (IBM SPSS SamplePower 2.0), included 7 control variables entered in Step 1 of the equation (chronological age at time of PROMS ; age at diabetes diagnosis; age at first severe episode of hypoglycemia; number of episodes of hypoglycemia; duration of T1DM; gender; socioeconomic status), yielding an R-square of .25. The second step of the regression (entering PROMS score) yielded a unique increment of .06 (total R-square for each equation = .31), providing a power of 0.80 for the final increment (and 0.95 for all 8 variables entered into the regression models) with the given sample size of 100 and alpha set at .05. The test was based on Model 2 error, such that variables entered into the regression subsequent to the set of interest served to reduce the error term in the significance test, and therefore were included in the power analysis. This effect was selected as the smallest effect that would be important to detect, in the sense that any smaller effect would not have been of clinical or substantive significance. It was assumed that this effect size was reasonable, in the sense that the effects of this magnitude have been demonstrated by prior research in this field of research [3-6,21,22]. Thus, the analyses provided adequate power for testing the assumptions underlying the statistical models.

Data Analysis
All variables were examined for accuracy of data entry, missing values, and fit between their distributions and the assumptions of multivariate analysis. The ratio of cases to independent variables appeared satisfactory for each of the regression analyses. The majority of the variables met the assumptions of normality, linearity, and homoscedasticity of residuals, with the exception of HbA1C and number of severe hypoglycemic episodes. Therefore, these two variables were log transformed prior to entry in the regression analyses.

No significant outliers were identified among the residuals. Co-linearity diagnostics performed for each regression analysis determined that the majority of the independent variables appeared sufficiently independent to enter into the regression analyses, with the exception of age, age at diagnosis and duration of illness, and number of episodes of diabetic ketoacidosis and low BG episodes. As a result, age and number of low BG episodes were selected as empirically based variables for the parsimonious regression equations. The levels of association among the background and control, explanatory, and outcome variables were computed with Pearson product moment correlations. Control variables were entered into hierarchical regression analyses at Step 1, followed by the explanatory variable to determine if the explanatory variable contributed additional unique variance to the multivariate models. Hierarchical regression analyses were deemed appropriate, as they provided primarily descriptive and exploratory information related to cognitive and psychosocial factors as predictors of HbA1C values in a reasonably novel study population. Also, this analysis provided the relative contributions of the delineated independent factors to the outcome variables of HbA1C values. All data were analyzed using IBM SPSS for Mac (Version 18.0).

Results

One hundred child–parent pairs completed the study. Despite agreeing to participate, twenty families ultimately failed to schedule an appointment with the GCRC. Six children were excluded due to medical co-morbidities or special education needs not disclosed prior to participation. Data from 94 participants was analyzed. Demographic and clinical characteristics are shown in Table 2.

Associations of control variables

No association between total PROMS score and glycemic control was found (see Figure 1). Lower HbA1C values were associated with higher (better) scores on the 20 minute EBT on PROMS ($r = -0.2$, $p < .05$). Parental concerns about their child's working memory & metacognition were related to higher HbA1C ($r = 0.21$, $p < 0.05$ for each). No relationship between PROMS scores and parental ratings of the child's cognition on the BRIEF was found. PROMS scores did not correlate with the child's performance on the standardized cognitive tests, gender, nor BG level at the start of the PROMS.

PROMS as a predictor of HBA1c values

A hierarchical regression was performed to determine if the PROMS 20 minute EBT would improve predictions of HbA1C values after controlling for participant age, gender, race, socioeconomic status, IQ, and number of severe hypoglycemic episodes. The equation was significant with all of the independent variables entered ($R^2 = .14$, $p < .05$). Increased age predicted higher HbA1C. None of the other control variables were significantly associated with HbA1C values when entered in the same block of the regression equation. The addition of the PROMS 20 minute EBT scores predicted additional variance in HbA1C values, with the beta weight indicating that lower PROMS 20 minute EBT scores predicted higher HbA1C values ($\beta = -0.22$, $p < 0.05$). Altogether, 14% (7% adjusted) of HbA1C values were predicted by

knowing scores on the independent variable of PROMS 20 minute EBT.

Discussion

This study represents the first of its kind investigating prospective memory and glycemic control in children with type 1 diabetes mellitus. While as a whole this was a largely negative study, the association between glycemic control and the PROMS 20 minute EBT warrants further exploration. Deficits in EBT could help explain why children, even those with a long standing history of T1DM, have difficulty remembering to check BG and take insulin at meal times, as these events require event-based prospective memory. It is not clear why the only significant correlation between HbA1C and PROMS was the 20 minute EBT and not the shorter EBT. Multiple inputs at the outset of the PROMS and the length of time from request to cue for the task may have contributed to tendency to forget the task. However, this might best mimic expectations outside of the laboratory setting and could impact upon daily diabetic care. Positron emission tomography scans have demonstrated that EBT and TBT activate different areas of the rostral prefrontal cortex [23] and at least one study has shown that deficits in EBT and TBT are not always congruent [24].

Our study also found a modest correlation between HbA1C and parental concerns about the children's working memory and metacognition as assessed by the BRIEF. This finding is consistent with that reported by McNally et. al who concluded that higher levels of executive functioning (i.e. lower reports of parental concern on the BRIEF) was associated with increased treatment adherence which predicted improved HbA1C levels [25].

Most studies involving pediatric T1DM and cognition concluded severely low BG increases the risk of learning difficulties and need for special education [26]; decreased spatial ability and slower motor speeds [6]; impairments in memory, learning, and executive functioning [26]; weaker visual and verbal delayed recall [7,26]; poorer verbal short term memory [2]; inferior analytic skills [21]; and problems with attention [27]. Two studies argue that severe hypoglycemia has no impact on cognition [28,29]. Another concluded that subtle hypoglycemia actually led to an increase in test scores in academic achievement, memory, verbal comprehension and general cognition [30]. Although not one of our primary aims, our study only found a significant correlation between increased hypoglycemic events and increased episodes of diabetic ketoacidosis ($r = 0.45$, $p < 0.001$). While the relationship between increased episodes of hypoglycemia and lower full-scale IQs trended towards significance ($r = -0.185$, $p = 0.076$), more frequent

Table 2 Demographic and Clinical Characteristics

	n=94
Age (years)	12.5 ± 3.4 (range 6.17 -17.95)
Gender (% Female)	49
Ethnicity (% white, not of Hispanic origin)	87.2
Full Scale IQ	106.8 ± 10.5 (range 79–142)
Academic Achievement (%)	
As	53.8
As & Bs	7.7
Bs	28.6
Bs & Cs	5.5
Cs	2.2
Cs & Ds	1.1
As, Bs, & Cs	1.1
Education Level of Mother (%)	
Some High School	1.1
High School Graduate	16
Some College	16
Associate's Degree	13.8
Bachelor's Degree	31.9
Master's Degree	16
Doctorate	3.2
Other	2.1
Education Level of Father (%)	
Some High School	0
High School Graduate	25.5
Some College	19.1
Associate's Degree	8.5
Bachelor's Degree	27.7
Master's Degree	7.4
Doctorate	5.3
Other	6.4
Total household income (%)	
<$25,000	3.2
$25-49,999	7.4
$50-74,999	13.8
$75-99,999	24.5
$100-124,999	23.4
>$125,000	23.4
Didn't answer	4.3
Caregiver completing study questionnaires (% mother)	81.9
Hemoglobin A1C (%)	7.9 ± 1.2 (range 5.8 – 14.1)
Type 1 diabetes duration (years)	4.9 ± 3.5 (range 0.2 - 12.3)
Age at diagnosis of type 1 diabetes (years)	7.6 ± 3.8 (range 0.9 - 14.9)
Blood glucose at start of study (mg/dL)	209.7 ± 84.5 (range 87 – 452)

Table 2 Demographic and Clinical Characteristics
(Continued)

Method of Insulin Delivery	
Multiple daily injections (%)	20
CS II (%)	65.6
History of severe low blood glucose reaction (%)	20.4
History of diabetic ketoacidosis (%)	40.4

episodes of severe low BG did not impact performance on the PROMS or academic achievement.

Hyperglycemia, gender, and SES have also been investigated as causal factors of cognitive dysfunction in pediatric T1DM. Conflicting results about the effect of acute hyperglycemia have been published. One study concluded that acute hyperglycemia, defined as >360 mg/dL, had no effect on cognitive functioning [31]. A later study demonstrated that when BG was acutely raised between 360–540 mg/dL in 12 children with T1DM, 8 of the children had a decrease in their performance IQ [32]. Receptive language scores among thirty-six preschoolers with a mean BG of 174mg/dL were found to be inversely correlated with higher blood glucoses; ambient blood glucose did not correlate with other measures of cognitive or motor testing [29]. In the current study, no correlations were seen between ambient BG and PROMS scores, performance on digit span testing, or full scale IQ. Studies testing prospective memory under both euglycemic and hyperglycemic conditions in the same child need to be conducted before conclusions regarding the effect of elevated BG on this component of memory can be made. Several studies have found that boys with T1DM have a higher incidence of learning problems compared to girls with T1DM [33-36]. Our data did not support these findings as gender did not impact prospective memory or cognitive test scores nor did parents of sons report more concerns on the BRIEF. Although lower SES has also been implicated as an additional risk factor for cognitive incongruities [35] this was not found amongst our children.

There are several limitations of this study. While the prospective memory screen used in our study was specifically developed with a pediatric population in mind and has face validity, it is not a standard tool used in psychometric evaluation. However, no other "gold standard" exists. One could argue the shorter tasks measured working memory and not prospective memory, thereby limiting our findings.

The demographic characteristics of our participants were not representative of a broader T1DM population. Our final study population consisted primarily of academically high-achieving children from well-educated,

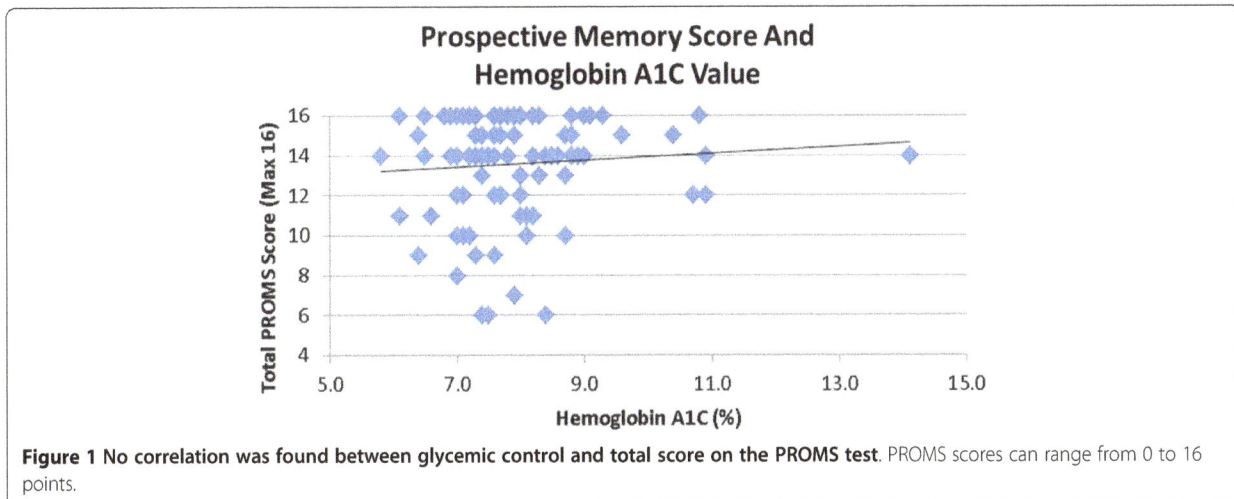

Figure 1 No correlation was found between glycemic control and total score on the PROMS test. PROMS scores can range from 0 to 16 points.

middle to upper class families. As prospective memory is an integral component of daily functioning and success, this self-selected group likely has higher prospective memory skills compared to a more general population of families with children with T1DM. Second, the majority of the participants used intensive insulin regimens and maintained desirable HbA1Cs. It is possible that the prescribing physicians unknowingly assessed aspects of prospective memory skills of these children and their parents and deemed them capable of remembering to carry out the tasks needed for success with an intensive insulin regimen. Third, patients with lower HbA1C, and arguably better prospective memory, may have been more willing to volunteer for the study. Patients with poor glycemic control often failed to come to appointments, theoretically due to deficits in prospective memory, and thus had fewer opportunities to be asked to participate. Generally these patients and their families are seen as "unmotivated" to care for T1DM by health care providers; this lack of motivation may actually represent poor prospective memory skills which make diabetic care that much more challenging for these families.

Mean HbA1C of the 20 consented children who ultimately did not participate in the study despite reminder phone calls and opportunities to reschedule was 9% compared to 7.9% of those who completed the study. As the reminder phone calls were directed to the parents, one must question the adults' prospective memory and its role in the children's glycemic control. Future examination of this relationship is warranted, particularly in younger patients in whom adults generally assume responsibility for providing the child's diabetic care.

The lack of significant relationships between frequency of hypoglycemia and prospective memory, academic achievement, and full-scale IQ may not be generalizable to a more diverse sample of children with higher rates of hypoglycemia. Only 20% of the families reported one or more episode of severe hypoglycemia. The accuracy of this occurrence rate is limited by parental recall and individual interpretation of severe hypoglycemia. The lack of association between lower SES and cognitive functioning may also be due to the homogeneity of our sample, with virtually all of the families earning well above our national poverty threshold.

Conclusions

Our study introduces the idea that prospective memory and glycemic control may be interrelated in children with T1DM. The association between the 20 minute EBT score and hemoglobin A1C and not the 20 minute TBT raises the possibility that diabetic control only affects event based prospective memory. Further studies need to be conducted to determine causal linkage and direction, as it is equally plausible that either a high HbA1C negatively impacts one's prospective memory or poor prospective memory predicts difficulty adhering to a diabetic regimen. Additional studies are warranted to determine if deficits in EBT prospective memory are reproducible and to determine how disease duration and fluctuations in HbA1C serially influence this aspect of prospective memory.

Abbreviations
T1DM: Type One Diabetes Mellitus; HbA1C: Hemoglobin A1C; GCRC: General Clinical Research Center; BG: Blood glucose; BRIEF: Behavior Rating Inventory of Executive Functions; SES: Socio-economic status; EBT: Event based task; TBT: Time based task.

Competing interests
The authors declare that they have no competing interests.

Authors' contributions
JNO conceived of the study, participated in its design, authored the protocol and consent/assent forms submitted for review by the institutional review board, recruited subjects, helped scored the data collected, participated in data analysis, and drafted the manuscript with the exception of the section on statistical analysis. DD participated in the design of the study, completed

the statistical analyses, and authored the section on statistical analysis. TAW participated in the study design, edited all material submitted to the institutional review board, recruited subjects, and played a large role in editing the manuscript. TP participated in study design, authored PROMS and trained the GCRC nurse staff in its administration as well as the other cognitive tests, helped in scoring the data collected, and helped draft the manuscript. All authors read and approved the final manuscript.

Acknowledgements

The authors would like to thank Drs. Janet Fischel and Catherine Messina for their invaluable contributions in editing the final manuscript, Patricia Noren, LPN for her time and dedication in learning how to administer the PROMS and other cognitive tests, and the GCRC for their generous grant and providing the physical space and nursing staff to carry out our study.

Author details

[1]Division of Pediatric Endocrinology, Department of Pediatrics, Stony Brook Children's Hospital, HSC Level 11 Room 080, Stony Brook, NY 11794-8111, USA. [2]Suffolk Health Psychology Services, PLLC, 646 Main Street, 2nd floor Suite 203, Port Jefferson, NY 11777, USA. [3]Department of Neuropsychology, Stony Brook Medicine, Health Sciences Center, Stony Brook, NY 11794-8511, USA.

References

1. Gaudieri PA, Chen R, Greer TF, Holmes CS: **Cognitive function in children with type 1 diabetes: a meta-analysis.** *Diabetes Care* 2008, **31**(9):1892–1897.
2. Naguib JM, Kulinskaya E, Lomax CL, Garralda ME: **Neuro-cognitive Performance in Children with Type 1 Diabetes--A Meta-analysis.** *J Pediatr Psychol* 2008, **34**(3):271–282.
3. Hershey T, Lillie R, Sadler M, White NH: **A prospective study of severe hypoglycemia and long-term spatial memory in children with type 1 diabetes.** *Pediatr Diabetes* 2004, **5**(2):63–71.
4. Kovacs M, Ryan C, Obrosky DS: **Verbal intellectual and verbal memory performance of youths with childhood-onset insulin-dependent diabetes mellitus.** *J Pediatr Psychol* 1994, **19**(4):475–483.
5. Hershey T, Lillie R, Sadler M, White NH: **Severe hypoglycemia and long-term spatial memory in children with type 1 diabetes mellitus: a retrospective study.** *J Int Neuropsychol Soc* 2003, **9**(5):740–750.
6. Hershey T, Bhargava N, Sadler M, White NH, Craft S: **Conventional versus intensive diabetes therapy in children with type 1 diabetes: effects on memory and motor speed.** *Diabetes Care* 1999, **22**(8):1318–1324.
7. Hershey T, Craft S, Bhargava N, White NH: **Memory and insulin dependent diabetes mellitus (IDDM): Effects of childhood onset and severe hypoglycemia.** *J Int Neuropsychol Soc* 1997, **3**:509–520.
8. Wolters CA, Yu SL, Hagen JW, Kail R: **Short-term memory and strategy use in children with insulin-dependent diabetes mellitus.** *J Consult Clin Psychol* 1996, **64**(6):1397–1405.
9. Soutor SA, Chen R, Streisand R, Kaplowitz P, Holmes CS: **Memory matters: developmental differences in predictors of diabetes care behaviors.** *J Pediatr Psychol* 2004, **29**(7):493–505.
10. Holmes CS, Chen R, Streisand R, Marschall DE, Souter S, Swift EE, Peterson CC: **Predictors of youth diabetes care behaviors and metabolic control: a structural equation modeling approach.** *J Pediatr Psychol* 2006, **31**(8):770–784.
11. Warren RE, Zammitt NN, Deary IJ, Frier BM: **The effects of acute hypoglycaemia on memory acquisition and recall and prospective memory in type 1 diabetes.** *Diabetologia* 2007, **50**(1):178–185.
12. Evans ML, Pernet A, Lomas J, Jones J, Amiel SA: **Delay in onset of awareness of acute hypoglycemia and of restoration of cognitive performance during recovery.** *Diabetes Care* 2000, **23**(7):893–897.
13. Sohlberg MM, Mateer CA, Geyer S: *Prospective Memory Survey.* Puyallup: Assocation for Neuropsychological Research and Development; 1985.
14. Sohlberg M, Mateer C, Geyer S, Preston T: *Prospective Memory Screening Test- Revised Unpublished Test Manual.* Stony Brook, NY: Developed at Stony Brook University Medical Center; 2009.
15. Preston T, Eisenberg P: *Prospective Memory in Clinically Referred and Nonreferred Children.* Boston, MA: Presented at 39th Annual Meeting of the International Neuropsychological Society; 2011.
16. Wechsler D: *Wechsler Abbreviated Scale of Intelligence (WASI).* San Antonio Texas: Psychological Corporation; 1999.
17. Harcourt Assessment, Inc: *Wechsler Individual Achievement Test- Second Edition (WIAT 2).* San Antonio Texas: Psychological Corporation; 2002.
18. Delis D, Kramer JH, Kaplan E, Ober BA: *California Verbal Learning Test- Children's Version (CVLT-C).* San Antonio, Texas: Psychological Corporation; 1994.
19. Wechsler D: *Wechsler Intelligence Scale for Children- Fourth Edition (WISC 4).* San Antonio, Texas: Psychological Corporation; 2004.
20. Gioia GA, Isquith PK, Guy SC, Kenworthy L: *Behavior Rating Inventory of Executive Function.* Lutz, Florida: Psychological Assessment Resources; 2000.
21. Perantie DC, Lim A, Wu J, Weaver P, Warren SL, Sadler M, White NH, Hershey T: **Effects of prior hypoglycemia and hyperglycemia on cognition in children with type 1 diabetes mellitus.** *Pediatr Diabetes* 2008, **9**(2):87–95.
22. Kovacs M, Goldston D, Iyengar S: **Intellectual Development and Academic Performance of Children with Insulin-Dependent Diabetes Mellitus: A Longitudinal Study.** *Dev Psychol* 1992, **28**(4):676–684.
23. Okuda J, Fujii T, Ohtake H, Tsukiura T, Yamadori A, Frith CD, Burgess PW: **Differential involvement of regions of rostral prefrontal cortex (Brodmann area 10) in time- and event-based prospective memory.** *Int J Psychophysiol* 2007, **64**(3):233–246.
24. Katai S, Maruyama T, Hashimoto T, Ikeda S: **Event based and time based prospective memory in Parkinson's disease.** *J Neurol Neurosurg Psychiatry* 2003, **74**(6):704–709.
25. McNally K, Rohan J, Pendley JS, Delamater A, Drotar D: **Executive functioning, treatment adherence, and glycemic control in children with type 1 diabetes.** *Diabetes Care* 2010, **33**(6):1159–1162.
26. Hannonen R, Tupola S, Ahonen T, Riikonen R: **Neurocognitive functioning in children with type-1 diabetes with and without episodes of severe hypoglycaemia.** *Dev Med Child Neurol* 2003, **45**(4):262–268.
27. Ryan C, Vega A, Drash A: **Cognitive deficits in adolescents who developed diabetes early in life.** *Pediatrics* 1985, **75**(5):921–927.
28. Wysocki T, Harris MA, Mauras N, Fox L, Taylor A, Jackson SC, White NH: **Absence of adverse effects of severe hypoglycemia on cognitive function in school-aged children with diabetes over 18 months.** *Diabetes Care* 2003, **26**(4):1100–1105.
29. Patino-Fernandez A, Delamater AM, Applegate EB, Brady E, Eidson M, Nemery R, Gonzalez-Mendoza L, Richton S: **Neurocognitive Functioning in Preschool-age Children with Type 1 Diabetes Mellitus.** *Pediatr Diabetes* 2010, **11**(6):424–430.
30. Kaufman FR, Epport K, Engilman R, Halvorson M: **Neurocognitive functioning in children diagnosed with diabetes before age 10 years.** *J Diabetes Complications* 1999, **13**(1):31–38.
31. Gschwend S, Ryan C, Atchison J, Arslanian S, Becker D: **Effects of acute hyperglycemia on mental efficiency and counterregulatory hormones in adolescents with insulin-dependent diabetes mellitus.** *J Pediatr* 1995, **126**(2):178–184.
32. Davis EA, Soong SA, Byrne GC, Jones TW: **Acute hyperglycaemia impairs cognitive function in children with IDDM.** *J Pediatr Endocrinol Metab* 1996, **9**(4):455–461.
33. Fox MA, Chen RS, Holmes CS: **Gender differences in memory and learning in children with insulin-dependent diabetes mellitus (IDDM) over a 4-year follow-up interval.** *J Pediatr Psychol* 2003, **28**(8):569–578.
34. Holmes CS, Dunlap WP, Chen RS, Cornwell JM: **Gender differences in the learning status of diabetic children.** *J Consult Clin Psychol* 1992, **60**(5):698–704.
35. Holmes CS, Cant MC, Fox MA, Lampert NL, Greer T: **Disease and Demorgraphic Risk Factors for Disrupted Cognitive Functioning in Children with Insulin-Dependent Diabetes Mellitus.** *Sch Psychol Rev* 1999, **28**:215–227.
36. Holmes CS, O'Brien B, Greer T: **Cognitive functioning and academic achievement in children with insulin-dependent diabetes mellitus (IDDM).** *Prof Sch Psychol* 1995, **10**(4):329–344.

Risk factors for cardiovascular disease and type 2 diabetes retained from childhood to adulthood predict adult outcomes: the Princeton LRC Follow-up Study

John A Morrison[1], Charles J Glueck[2,3*], Jessica G Woo[1] and Ping Wang[2]

Abstract

Background: Pediatric risk factors predict adult cardiovascular disease (CVD) and type 2 diabetes (T2DM), but whether they predict events independently of adult risk factors is not fully known.

Objective: Assess whether risk factors for CVD and T2DM retained from childhood to adulthood predict CVD and T2DM in young adulthood.

Study design: 770 schoolchildren, ages 5–20 (mean age 12), 26-yr prospective follow-up. We categorized childhood and adult risk factors and 26-year changes (triglycerides [TG], LDL cholesterol, BMI, blood pressure [BP] and glucose ≥, and HDL cholesterol < pediatric and young adult cutoffs). These risk factors and race, cigarette smoking, and family history of CVD and T2DM were assessed as predictors of CVD and T2DM at mean age 38.

Results: Children who had high TG and retained high TG as adults had increased CVD events as adults ($p = .0005$). Children who had normal BMI and retained normal BMI as adults had reduced CVD events as adults ($p = .02$). Children who had high BP or high TG and retained these as adults had increased T2DM as adults ($p = .0006$, $p = .003$).

Conclusions: Risk factors for CVD and T2DM retained from childhood to adulthood predict CVD and T2DM in young adulthood and support universal childhood screening.

Keywords: Risk factors, Cardiovascular disease, Type 2 diabetes mellitus, Obesity, High blood pressure, Tracking

Background

Recently, an expert panel recommended screening all American children for risk factors for cardiovascular disease (CVD) [1], not just children of parents with known CVD or high risk factors. Pediatric risk factors for atherosclerosis have been shown to associate with young adult atherosclerotic lesions [2], carotid intima-media thickening (CIMT) [3-7], and cardiovascular disease (CVD) events [8]. Moreover, adolescent CVD risk factor status predicts increased adult CIMT, independent of adult risk factors [9,10], and children with metabolic syndrome (MetS) have

2–3 times greater risk of high CIMT and type 2 diabetes mellitus (T2DM) as adults versus children free of MetS [11]. Obese children who remained obese as adults have increased type 2 diabetes (T2DM), hypertension, dyslipidemia, and increased CIMT, but risks for these outcomes are attenuated in obese children who became non-obese adults, with outcomes similar to those non-obese in both childhood and adulthood [12].

It is not well understood whether childhood risk factors cause adult CVD directly, independent of adult risk factors, or only in those individuals whose risk factors tracked into adulthood, thereby increasing the length of exposure to high risk factors [10,13]. The best predictor of high blood pressure (HBP) in adulthood has been reported to be adult obesity or change in obesity; pediatric obesity does not predict adult HBP when adult obesity is

* Correspondence: cjglueck@health-partners.org
[2]From the Cholesterol and Metabolism Center, Jewish Hospital of Cincinnati, Cincinnati, USA
[3]Cholesterol Center, UC Health Business Center, 3200 Burnet Avenue, Cincinnati, OH 45229, USA
Full list of author information is available at the end of the article

in the model [13]. However, HBP is itself a risk factor, not a CVD event. Positive associations between childhood BMI and adult CIMT are generally attenuated once adjusted for adult BMI [14]. Child-adult relationships may be dependent on tracking of BMI from childhood to adulthood [14], since risk of events increases with the length of exposure [15,16]. There is a stepwise increase in the incidence of T2DM with the duration of obesity [15].

In the current study, our specific aim was to assess whether risk factors for CVD and T2DM retained from childhood to adulthood predict CVD and T2DM in young adulthood or whether childhood risk factors are attenuated [12] by changes in risk factors from childhood to young adulthood.

Methods
We used data from the NHLBI Princeton Follow-up Study (PFS, 1999–2003), a 22–30 year follow-up of black and white former schoolchildren first studied in the NHLBI Lipid Research Clinics (LRC, 1973–1976) [8,17]. PFS collected data following a protocol approved by the Children's Hospital Institutional Review Board, with signed informed consent [17].

Princeton LRC and PFS studies
The Princeton LRC [18] study was a multistage survey of lipids and other CVD risk factors in students in grades 1–12 and a 50% random sample of their parents by household. The student population in LRC was 72% white and 28% black, with a mean age of 12.3 ± 3.4 years. Participation rates did not differ significantly between races.

The PFS [8] was conducted in adults, 22 to 30 years after their initial pediatric LRC sampling to assess relationships of pediatric risk factors to subsequent adult health events. The subjects' CVD, T2DM and high blood pressure (HBP) status and use of prescribed medications for lipids, diabetes mellitus, and blood pressure were obtained by questionnaire with an interviewer [8].

After an overnight fast, blood was drawn for measurements of plasma triglyceride (TG), high density lipoprotein cholesterol (HDLC), low density lipoprotein cholesterol (LDLC), systolic blood pressure (SBP), diastolic blood pressure (DBP), BMI, and glucose in children and their parents at the LRC assessment and at the subsequent PFS study 26 years later. There was no contact with the former schoolchildren or their parents during the 26-year interval between the LRC and PFS studies.

Diagnosis of CVD, type 2 diabetes and impaired fasting glucose
At PFS, CVD was defined as myocardial infarction, coronary artery bypass graft, angioplasty, ischemic stroke, and carotid or peripheral artery bypass surgery [8]. Diagnosis of diabetes (T2DM) was based on World Organization of Health criteria, fasting glucose ≥ 7 mmol/l (126 mg/dl) and/or self-report of diabetes with treatment by a physician [19]. We excluded from these analyses 10 subjects who had reported type 1 diabetes mellitus as children at LRC. However, in PFS we did not have a measurement of C-peptides or diabetes autoantibody levels, the gold standard methods of distinguishing type 1 from type 2 diabetes [19]. Diagnosis of impaired fasting glucose (IFG) was made when fasting blood glucose was ≥ 100 but <126 mg/dl.

Pediatric and young adult risk factor cutoffs
Pediatric risk factor cutoffs included high LDLC (≥ 110 mg/dl [2.82 mmol/l]) [20], high BMI ($\geq 85^{th}$ CDC 2000 age-gender specific percentile), high BP (SBP and/or DBP $>90^{th}$ age-height specific percentiles in current cohort), and cutoffs published for pediatric metabolic syndrome [21]: high TG (≥ 110 mg/dl [1.24 mmol/l]), low HDLC (≤ 50 mg/dl [1.28 mmol/l] in girls, ≤ 40 [1.03 mmol/l] in boys), and high glucose (≥ 100 mg/dl [5.6 mmol/l]).

Risk factor cutoffs at the PFS were those of the NCEP/AHA Metabolic syndrome (waist ≥ 102 cm men, ≥ 88 cm women, SBP ≥ 130 mmHg and/or DBP ≥ 85, TG ≥ 150 mg/dl [1.69 mmol/l], HDLC <40 mg/dl [1.03 mmol/l] men, <50 mg/dl [1.28 mmol/l] women, glucose ≥ 100 mg/dl [5.6 mmol/l]) [22]. BMI and LDLC cutpoints at the PFS respectively were ≥ 30 kg/m^2 (CDC, US Obesity Trends, Trends by State 1985–2009), and the current cohort's gender-race-specific 90th percentile levels.

Statistical methods
CVD risk factor measures in the cohort in childhood (LRC) and adulthood (PFS) were summarized.

To assess for possible selection bias, comparisons were made between the 770 subjects with complete CVD risk factor measures at both the LRC visit and the PFS visit 26 years later, and 695 subjects without complete measures. Comparisons were made by Wilcoxon test or by chi-square test.

Risk factor measures at LRC and PFS were categorized as high vs. not high (for TG, LDLC, BMI, SBP-DBP, and glucose) or low vs. not low (for HDLC) using the above-mentioned cutoffs. The change in status for each risk factor from LRC to PFS was indicated by 4 dummy variables (normal to normal vs. others; abnormal to normal vs. others; normal to abnormal vs. others; abnormal to abnormal vs. others).

Stepwise logistic regression analysis was used to identify significant independent risk factors for young adult CVD, T2DM and IFG at PFS in multivariate analyses. Explanatory variables included age at follow-up and categorical variables: race, pediatric and young adult risk factor status group (high vs. not high) for TG, LDLC,

BMI, glucose, blood pressure, HDLC (low vs. not low), cigarette smoking (yes vs. no), and parental history (yes vs. no) of CVD or T2DM, as well as changes in risk factor status from childhood to young adulthood. Including only significant explanatory variables from stepwise selection, logistic regression models were re-evaluated allowing more observations to be used.

From the logistic regression model, the changes in TG, BMI or BP from LRC to PFS were significant predictors for the CVD or T2DM at PFS. The associations of these risk factor changes with CVD or T2DM status were graphed. Pediatric to adult changes in risk factors were ordered to represent increasing risk, with lowest risk being normal to normal, then abnormal to normal, normal to abnormal and highest being abnormal to abnormal. The Mantel-Haenszel test was used to measure the significance of associations between the risk factor status groups in childhood and adulthood and the adult development of CVD or T2DM.

Results

In the LRC study, there were 1465 subjects eligible for the PFS, and 909 subjects were studied in PFS 26 years later (follow-up rate 62%). Of these 909 subjects, complete data (required for the resultant logistic model) was available in 770 (85%), Table 1. Compared with the 695 eligible subjects not included in the current report, BMI was higher in the sampled group (20.1 ± 4.3 vs 19.2 ± 4.2 kg/m^2, $p < .0001$), but there were no differences (p $>$ 0.05) in TG, HDLC, LDLC, SBP and DBP at the LRC visit. In the sampled group, percent white was higher 73% vs 66% ($p = .008$), and percent male was lower 46% vs 57% ($p < .0001$).

Pediatric and adult CVD risk factor measures 26 years later were highly correlated, Table 1. Twenty-six of the 770

subjects (3.4%) were taking cholesterol-lowering medications at their PFS visit, Table 1. Excluding their LDLC values from the analyses of correlations between LRC and PFS did not appreciably affect the correlation coefficients, Table 1. After adjusting for BMI at mean ages 12 and 38, age 12 and age 38 risk factors remained closely correlated, Table 1.

High TG in childhood retained into adulthood characterized the 19 subjects who had CVD in adulthood, while normal TG at both visits characterized the 751 subjects free of CVD at the PFS visit, Figure 1. There were 55 subjects with high TG at both visits, of whom 8 (14.6%) had CVD compared to 5 of 490 with normal TG at both visits (1%) for a risk ratio of 14.6 to 1, Figure 1, Table 2. The incidence of CVD was 1.9% in subjects with high TG at LRC but normal TG at PFS, and 2.9% in subjects with normal TG at LRC but high TG at PFS. Thus, there was a linear trend for CVD across the four TG classification groups ($p < .0001$), Table 2.

Normal BMI in childhood retained into adulthood characterized the 751 subjects free of CVD at the PFS visit, while high BMI in childhood retained into adulthood characterized the 19 subjects who had adult CVD, Figure 2. There were 113 subjects with high BMI at both visits, of whom 7 (6.2%) had CVD and 427 with normal BMI at both visits of whom 4 had CVD (0.9%) for a risk ratio of 6.9 to 1. The incidence of CVD was 2.5% in subjects with high BMI at LRC but normal BMI at PFS, and 4.0% in subjects with normal BMI at LRC but high TG at PFS. Thus, there was a linear trend for CVD across the four BMI classification groups ($p = .0005$), Table 2.

High blood pressure retained from childhood to adulthood was much more common in the 29 subjects who had adult T2DM (28%) than in the 417 free of adult T2DM (5%), while normal childhood blood pressure

Table 1 Risk factors for cardiovascular disease and type 2 diabetes mellitus, measured during childhood (LRC) and 26 years later in young adulthood (PFS) in 770 subjects

Race	W 561 (73%), B 209 (27%)				
Gender	M 351 (46%), F 419 (54%)				
	At LRC	**At PFS**		**Spearman correlation Between LRC and PFS**	
	Mean ± SD	**Mean ± SD**			
Age (yr)	12.4 ±3.3 range [5–20.5]	38.5 ±3.6 range [29–48]	**Adjusted for BMI at LRC**	**Adjusted for BMI at PFS**	**Adjusted for BMIat LRC and at PFS**
BMI (kg/m2)	20.1 ±4.3	28.6 ±6.7			
TG (mg/dl)	77 ±38	136 ±133	r = 0.33, p < .0001	r = 0.34, p < .0001	r = 0.38, p < .0001
HDLC (mg/dl)	55 ±12	46 ±15	r = 0.44, p < .0001	r = 0.44, p < .0001	r = 0.46, p < .0001
LDLC (mg/dl)	107 ±30 106 ±29*	121 ±36 121 ±36*	r = 0.48, p < .0001 r = 0.49, p < .0001*	r = 0.48, p < .0001 r = 0.50, p < .0001*	r = 0.48, p < .0001 r = 0.50, p < .0001*
LDLC/HDLC	2.05 ±0.76 2.03 ±0.75*	2.94 ±1.34 2.94 ±1.33*	r = 0.44, p < .0001 r = 0.44, p < .0001*	r = 0.45, p < .0001 r = 0.45, p < .0001*	r = 0.46, p < .0001 r = 0.46, p < .0001*
Glucose (mg/dl)	86 ±8	90 ±23	r = 0.18, p < .0001	r = 0.18, p < .0001	r = 0.18, p < .0001

*After removal of 26 subjects taking cholesterol lowering medications at PFS.

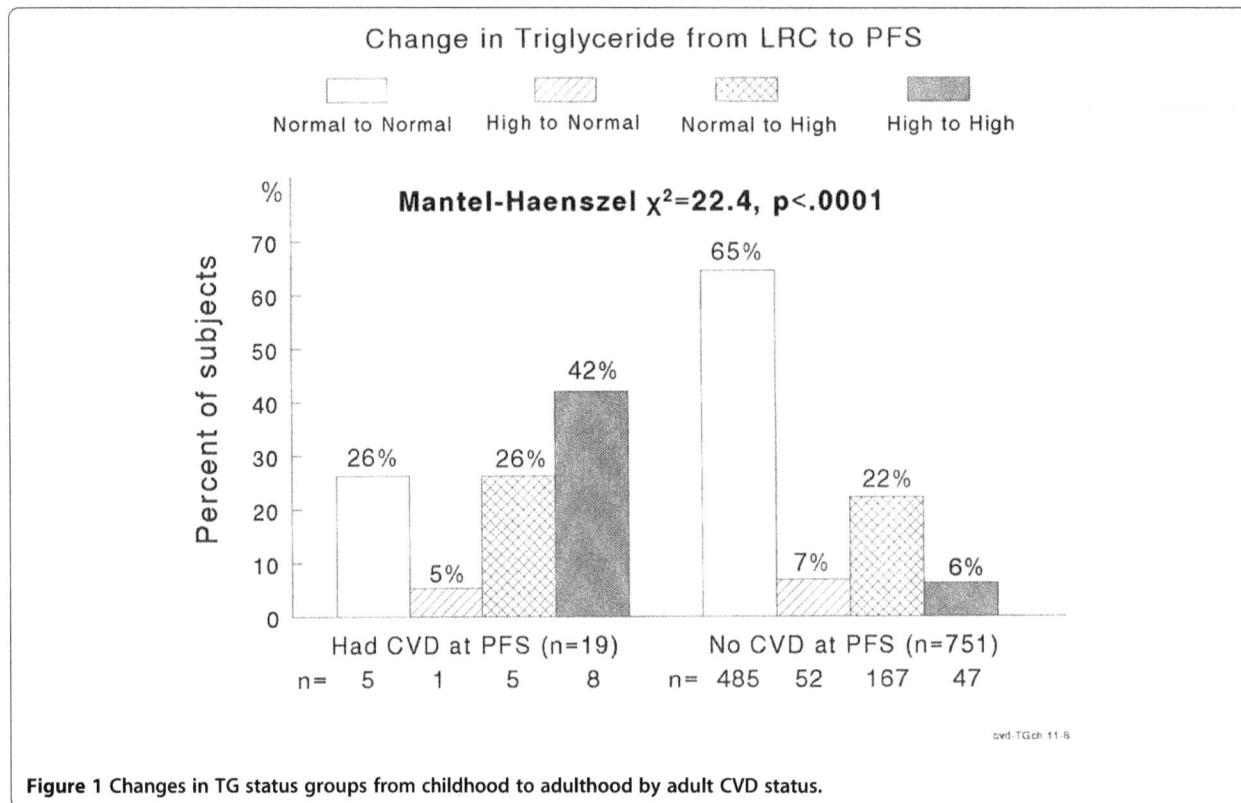

Figure 1 Changes in TG status groups from childhood to adulthood by adult CVD status.

retained into adulthood characterized the 417 subjects free of T2DM at the PFS visit (65%), Figure 3. The incidence of T2DM was 28.6% in subjects with high BP at LRC and PFS compared to 3.6% in subjects with normal BP at both LRC and PFS, for a relative risk of 8 to 1. The one of 22 subjects with high BP at LRC but normal BP at PFS did have T2DM so the incidence rate was 4.6%. In subjects with normal BP at LRC but high BP at PFS the incidence of T2DM was 8.6%. Thus, there was a linear trend for T2DM across the four BP classification groups ($p < .0001$), Table 2.

High TG retained from childhood to adulthood was much more common in subjects who developed T2DM as adults (31%) than in those free of T2DM (6%), Figure 4. The incidence of T2DM was 27.3% in subjects with high TG at LRC and PFS compared to 3.8% in subjects with

normal TG at both LRC and PFS, for a relative risk of 7.1. No person with high TG at LRC but normal TG at PFS had T2DM, incidence rate = 0.0%. In subjects with normal TG at LRC but high TG at PFS the incidence of T2DM was 9.6%. Thus, there was a linear trend for T2DM across the four TG change classification groups ($p < .0001$), Table 2.

By stepwise logistic regression, adult CVD (19 yes, 751 no) was independently and significantly associated with high childhood TG retained adulthood ($p = .0005$) and with age at follow-up ($p = .0009$), and was inversely associated with normal BMI from childhood retained into adulthood, $p = .02$, Table 3.

Adult T2DM (29 yes, 417 no) was associated with BP and TG high in childhood and retained into adulthood ($p = .0006$, .003), with childhood glucose ($p = .006$), with adult age ($p = .002$), and with black race ($p = .04$), Table 3.

Table 2 Incidence rate (%) of cardiovascular disease (CVD) by triglyceride (TG) and BMI classification in childhood and adulthood and of type 2 diabetes mellitus (T2DM) by blood pressure and triglyceride classification in childhood and adulthood

Incidence rate	Normal - Normal	High - Normal	Normal - High	High - High	Trend of incidence rate by Mantel-Haenszel χ2 test
CVD (TG)	1.0	1.9	2.9	14.6	$\chi^2 = 22.4, p < .0001$
CVD (BMI)	0.9	2.5	4.0	6.2	$\chi^2 = 12.1, p = .0005$
T2DM (BP)	3.6	4.6	8.6	28.6	$\chi^2 = 17.8, p < .0001$
T2DM (TG)	3.8	0	9.6	27.3	$\chi^2 = 20.3, p < .0001$

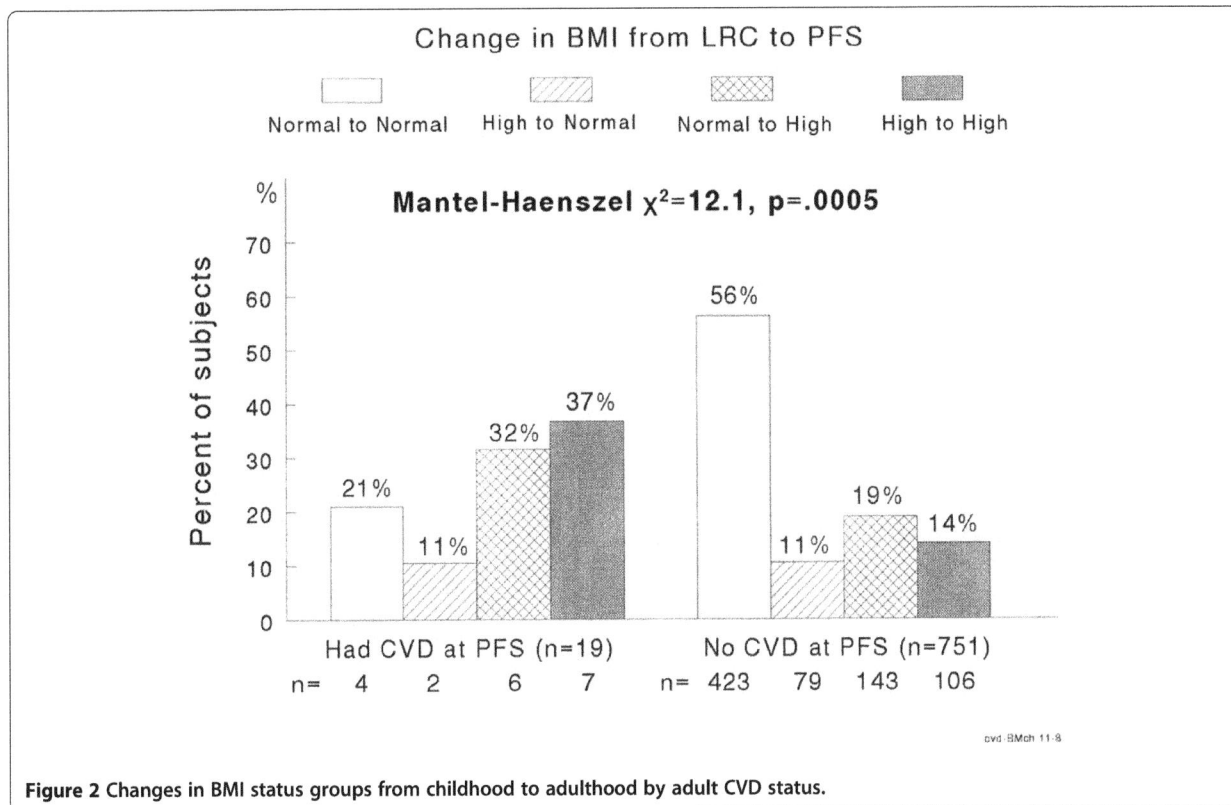

Figure 2 Changes in BMI status groups from childhood to adulthood by adult CVD status.

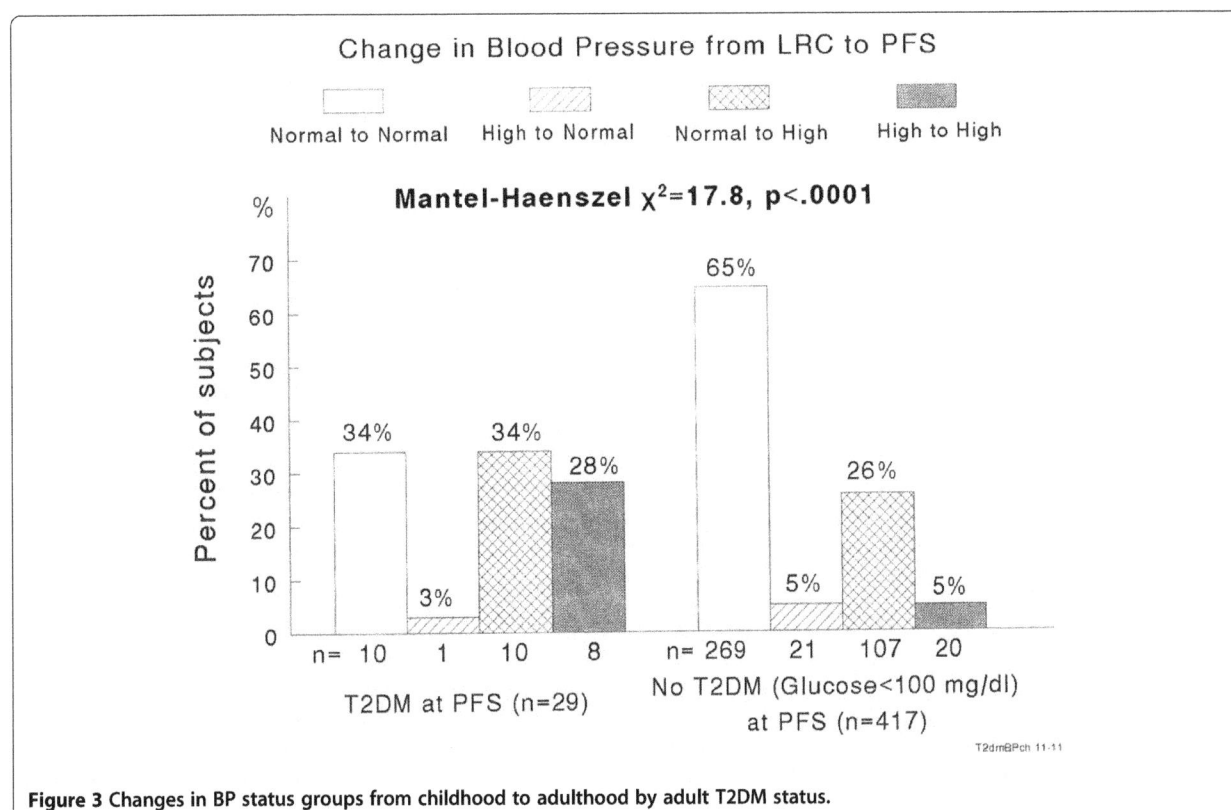

Figure 3 Changes in BP status groups from childhood to adulthood by adult T2DM status.

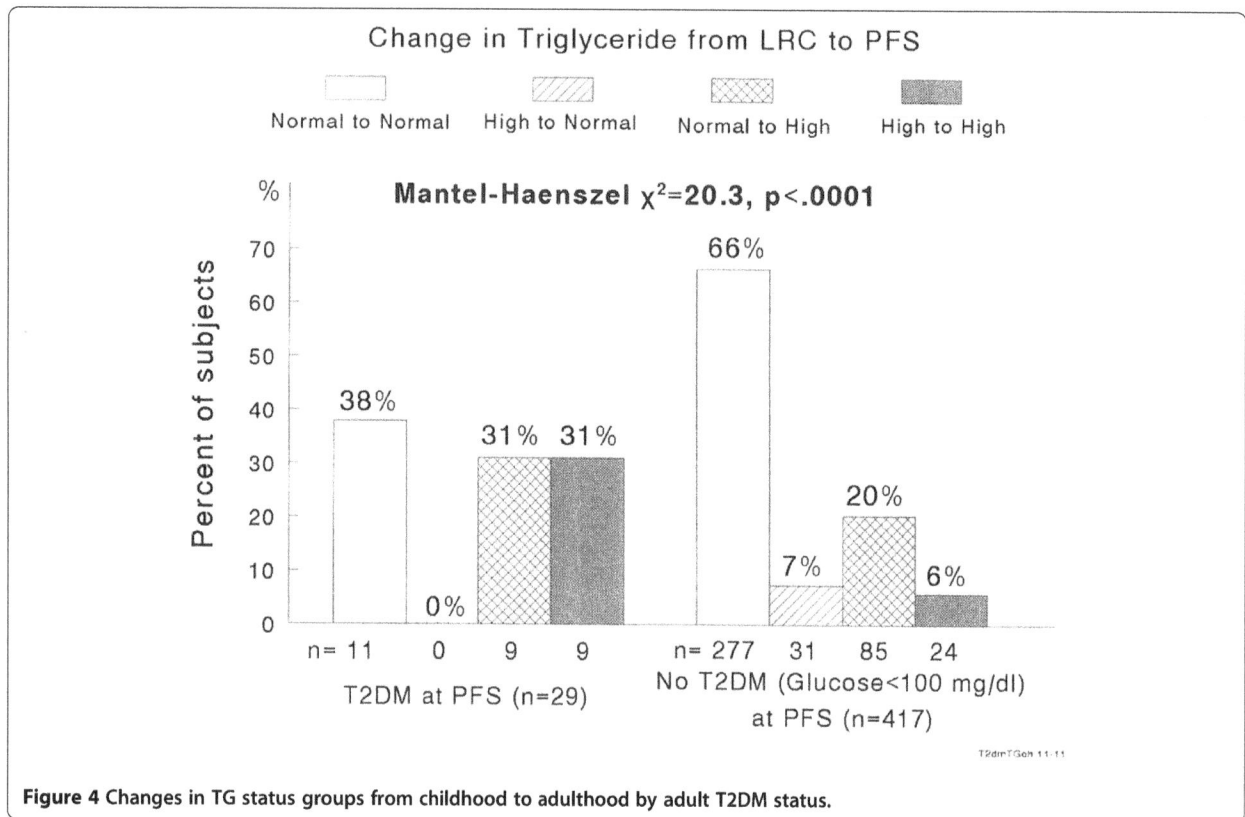

Figure 4 Changes in TG status groups from childhood to adulthood by adult T2DM status.

Adult IFG (88 yes, 617 no) was positively associated with adult BP and TG (high vs not high), $p < .0001$, $p = .0009$, respectively, and with cigarette smoking, $p = .018$, Table 3.

Neither pediatric nor young adult LDLC was associated with young adult CVD, $p > .05$.

Discussion

In the current study, risk factors for CVD retained from childhood to adulthood predicted CVD in young adulthood. Risk for CVD was attenuated when childhood risk factors were not maintained into adulthood, congruent with the report by Juonala et al. [12]. Children who had high TG and retained high TG as adults had increased CVD events. Children who had normal BMI and retained normal BMI as adults had reduced CVD events. Children who had high childhood BP and TG and retained these into adulthood were more likely to have adult T2DM, children with childhood risk factors not retained were not associated with increased adult T2DM, congruent with the report by Juonala et al. [12].

In contrast to CVD and T2DM, adult IFG was associated with adult high BP, TG, and cigarette smoking, and was not associated with retention of risk factors from childhood to adulthood.

Our finding of a significant association of high TG retained from childhood to adulthood with young adult CVD is consistent with pediatric [8] and adult studies

where non-fasting [23-25] and fasting TG [26-29] are independent risk factors for CVD and for ischemic stroke [30]. The association of TG high from childhood through young adulthood with adult CVD may, speculatively, reflect the presence of pediatric metabolic syndrome, a known predictor of adult CVD [18]. Moreover, TG levels in adolescent males have been related to coronary artery calcification 15 to 20 years later in young adults [31]. Coronary artery streaks in 6 to 30 year olds are significantly correlated with antecedent TG and very low density lipoprotein cholesterol [32,33]. In a postmortem study of 15 to 34 year old men, the percentage of the right coronary arterial intima involved with atherosclerosis correlated with a combination of LDL and VLDL cholesterol levels, and was inversely associated with HDL cholesterol [34].

Normal childhood BMI retained to adulthood was a significant negative risk factor for adult CVD. The association of normal BMI retained from childhood to adulthood with low young adult CVD events is consistent with the report by Chen et al. [35] where clustering of bottom quartile BMI, HOMA IR, SBP, and the ratio of total/HDL cholesterol was associated with decreasing mean values of carotid intima-media thickness in adulthood.

High childhood BP and TG, two components of the metabolic syndrome complex, retained into adulthood were associated with adult T2DM, findings broadly in agreement

Table 3 Childhood (LRC) and adulthood (PFS) predictors for cardiovascular disease (CVD), type 2 diabetes (T2DM) and impaired fasting glucose (IFG) at PFS

Young adult outcome	Childhood Predictors	p	Odds Ratio, 95% Confidence Intervals
CVD (19 Yes, 751 no) [a] **770 observations used AUC = 0.843**	TG at LRC and PFS (high to high vs others)	.0005	6.06, 2.20–16.7
	Age at PFS (year)	.0009	1.30, 1.11–1.53
	BMI at LRC and PFS (low to low vs others)	.019	0.25, 0.077–0.79
T2DM (29 Yes, 417 normal) [b] **446 observations used AUC = 0.842**	BP at LRC and PFS (high to high vs others)	.0006	6.74, 2.26–20.07
	TG at LRC and PFS (high to high vs others)	.0026	4.95, 1.75–14.06
	BMI at PFS (high vs not high)	.0010	4.56, 1.85–11.23
	Glucose at LRC (high vs not high)	.0057	5.93, 1.68–20.95
	Age at PFS	.0016	1.26, 1.09–1.45
	Black race	.043	2.53, 1.03–6.24
IFG (88 Yes, 617 normal) [b] **705 observations used AUC = 0.699**	BP at PFS (high vs not high)	<.0001	2.63, 1.64–4.23
	TG at PFS (high vs not high)	.0009	2.24, 1.39–3.60
	Cigarette smoking (yes vs no)	.018	1.78, 1.10–2.89

[a] Logistic regression model fit after stepwise selection (SLE = .15, SLS = .05) from categorical explanatory variables: race, risk factors at LRC and at PFS (TG, HDLC, LDLC, BMI, BP and glucose), changes of risk factors from LRC to PFS (TG, HDLC, LDLC, BMI, BP and glucose), cigarette smoking (yes/no), parents had CVD (yes/no), parents had CVD before age 50 (yes/no), and parents had CVD before age 60 (yes/no), and age at PFS.

[b] Logistic regression model fit after stepwise selection (SLE = .15, SLS = .05) from categorical explanatory variables: race, risk factors at LRC (TG, HDLC, LDLC, BMI, BP and glucose), risk factors at PFS (TG, HDLC, LDLC and BMI), changes of risk factors from LRC to PFS (TG, HDLC, LDLC, BMI and BP), cigarette smoking (yes/no), parents had T2DM (yes/no), and age at PFS.

with those of Everhart et al. [15] and Lee et al. [16], which suggested that the duration of the risk factor presence from childhood to young adulthood and the cumulative exposure to risk factors predict adult outcomes.

Our finding of an association of glucose levels in childhood with the development of T2DM in adulthood is consistent with a recent report from the Bogalusa Heart Study that fasting plasma glucose in childhood is a predictor of T2DM in young adulthood even when the pediatric glucose is within the normal range [36]. Moreover, childhood insulin response during an oral glucose challenge predicts adult acute insulin response [37].

Given the significant tracking of risk factors for CVD and T2DM as observed in the current and previous studies [11,38-40], failure to act on such childhood risk factors high TG, high BP, and obesity [12,16] means the underlying pathology may continue into young adulthood, increasing the likelihood of an adverse outcome [10,41]. These findings emphasize the importance of risk factor screening in childhood [1]. Lifestyle [1] and pharmacologic intervention [1,42,43] in childhood-adolescence might prevent development of CVD or T2DM in young adulthood.

A weakness in the current study is the absence of knowledge concerning when (at what age) participants with normal factors in childhood developed abnormal risk factors and when participants with abnormal factors in childhood developed normal risk factors. Thus, it was not possible to evaluate more precisely the length of time the at-risk state existed.

In the current study, neither pediatric nor young adult LDLC was associated with young adult CVD, perhaps attributable to treatment of high LDLC in 26 of 770 (3. 4%) young adults at PFS, or to the fact that with only 19 CVD endpoints by mean age 38, the study may not have had adequate power to declare an LDLC effect significant. Treatment to lower LDLC might, speculatively, also have reduced the power of LDLC to predict CVD.

Conventionally, parental history of CVD serves as an indication for screening for lipid abnormalities in children [44,45]. After detailed review of basing childhood screening on parental history, the recent Expert Panel statement [1] called for universal risk factor screening in children [1]. Identification of CVD risk factors in a child can directly facilitate primary prevention [1] in the child through young adulthood, and also focus diagnostic attention on the potentially high-risk parent.

Conclusions

Risk factors for CVD and T2DM retained from childhood to adulthood predict CVD and T2DM in young adulthood and support universal childhood screening.

Abbreviations

LRC: Lipid Research Clinics; PFS: Princeton School Follow-up Study; CVD: cardiovascular disease; CHD: coronary heart disease; CIMT: carotid intima-media thickening; IFG: impaired fasting glucose; T2DM: type 2 diabetes mellitus; HBP: high blood pressure; DBP: diastolic blood pressure; SBP: systolic blood pressure; TG: triglyceride; MetS: metabolic syndrome; HDLC: high density lipoprotein cholesterol; LDLC: low density lipoprotein cholesterol; BMI: body mass index; NCEP: National Cholesterol Education Program; NHLBI: National Heart, Lung, and Blood Institute; AHA: American Heart Association.

Competing interests
The authors declare that they have no competing interests.

Authors' contributions
JAM and CJG designed the study. JAM supervised the initial study in children and the prospective follow-up study in young adulthood. CJG, JAM, and PW edited, analyzed, and assessed the data. PW provided the major biostatistical expertise, JAM, the major epidemiologic expertise. All authors read and approved the final manuscript.

Acknowledgements
Supported by American Heart Association (National) 9750129 N and NIH-HL62394 (Dr Morrison), Lipoprotein Research Fund of the Jewish Hospital of Cincinnati (Dr Glueck).

Author details
[1]From the Division of Cardiology, Children's Hospital of Cincinnati, 3333 Burnet Avenue, 45229, Cincinnati, USA. [2]From the Cholesterol and Metabolism Center, Jewish Hospital of Cincinnati, Cincinnati, USA. [3]Cholesterol Center, UC Health Business Center, 3200 Burnet Avenue, Cincinnati, OH 45229, USA.

References
1. Expert panel on integrated guidelines for cardiovascular health and risk reduction in children and adolescents: Summary Report. Pediatrics. 2011;128, Supplement 5:S1-S45.
2. McMahan CA, Gidding SS, Malcom GT, Tracy RE, Strong JP, McGill HC Jr: Pathobiological determinants of atherosclerosis in youth risk scores are associated with early and advanced atherosclerosis. Pediatrics 2006, 118:1447-1455.
3. Juonala M, Magnussen CG, Venn A, Dwyer T, Burns TL, Davis PH, Chen W, Srinivasan SR, Daniels SR, Kahonen M, Laitinen T, Taittonen L, Berenson GS, Viikari JS, Raitakari OT: Influence of age on associations between childhood risk factors and carotid intima-media thickness in adulthood: the Cardiovascular Risk in Young Finns Study, the Childhood Determinants of Adult Health Study, the Bogalusa Heart Study, and the Muscatine Study for the International Childhood Cardiovascular Cohort (i3C) Consortium. Circulation 2010, 122:2514-2520.
4. Juonala M, Viikari JS, Kahonen M, Taittonen L, Laitinen T, Hutri-Kahonen N, Lehtimaki T, Jula A, Pietikainen M, Jokinen E, Telama R, Rasanen L, Mikkila V, Helenius H, Kivimaki M, Raitakari OT: Life-time risk factors and progression of carotid atherosclerosis in young adults: the Cardiovascular Risk in Young Finns study. Eur Heart J 2010, 31:1745-1751.
5. Magnussen CG, Venn A, Thomson R, Juonala M, Srinivasan SR, Viikari JS, Berenson GS, Dwyer T, Raitakari OT: The association of pediatric low- and high-density lipoprotein cholesterol dyslipidemia classifications and change in dyslipidemia status with carotid intima-media thickness in adulthood evidence from the cardiovascular risk in Young Finns study, the Bogalusa Heart study, and the CDAH (Childhood Determinants of Adult Health) study. J Am Coll Cardiol 2009, 53:860-869.
6. Freedman DS, Dietz WH, Tang R, Mensah GA, Bond MG, Urbina EM, Srinivasan S, Berenson GS: The relation of obesity throughout life to carotid intima-media thickness in adulthood: the Bogalusa Heart Study. Int J Obes Relat Metab Disord 2004, 28:159-166.
7. Davis PH, Dawson JD, Riley WA, Lauer RM: Carotid intimal-medial thickness is related to cardiovascular risk factors measured from childhood through middle age: the Muscatine Study. Circulation 2001, 104:2815-2819.
8. Morrison JA, Glueck CJ, Horn PS, Yeramaneni S, Wang P: Pediatric triglycerides predict cardiovascular disease events in the fourth to fifth decade of life. Metabolism 2009, 58:1277-1284.
9. Raitakari OT, Juonala M, Kahonen M, Taittonen L, Laitinen T, Maki-Torkko N, Jarvisalo MJ, Uhari M, Jokinen E, Ronnemaa T, Akerblom HK, Viikari JS: Cardiovascular risk factors in childhood and carotid artery intima-media thickness in adulthood: the Cardiovascular Risk in Young Finns Study. JAMA 2003, 290:2277-2283.
10. Daniels SR: Can lipid and lipoprotein concentrations in childhood predict adult atherosclerosis? J Am Coll Cardiol 2009, 53:870-871.
11. Magnussen CG, Koskinen J, Chen W, Thomson R, Schmidt MD, Srinivasan SR, Kivimaki M, Mattsson N, Kahonen M, Laitinen T, Taittonen L, Ronnemaa T, Viikari JS, Berenson GS, Juonala M, Raitakari OT: Pediatric metabolic syndrome predicts adulthood metabolic syndrome, subclinical atherosclerosis, and type 2 diabetes mellitus but is no better than body mass index alone: the Bogalusa Heart Study and the Cardiovascular Risk in Young Finns Study. Circulation 2010, 122:1604-1611.
12. Juonala M, Magnussen CG, Berenson GS, Venn A, Burns TL, Sabin MA, Srinivasan SR, Daniels SR, Davis PH, Chen W, Sun C, Cheung M, Viikari JS, Dwyer T, Raitakari OT: Childhood adiposity, adult adiposity, and cardiovascular risk factors. N Engl J Med 2011, 365:1876-1885.
13. Lauer RM, Clarke WR: Childhood risk factors for high adult blood pressure: the Muscatine Study. Pediatrics 1989, 84:633-641.
14. Lloyd LJ, Langley-Evans SC, McMullen S: Childhood obesity and adult cardiovascular disease risk: a systematic review. Int J Obes (Lond) 2010, 34:18-28.
15. Everhart JE, Pettitt DJ, Bennett PH, Knowler WC: Duration of obesity increases the incidence of NIDDM. Diabetes 1992, 41:235-240.
16. Lee J, Gebremariam A, Vijan S, Gurney JG. Excess body mass index-years, a measure of degree and duration of excess weight and risk for incident diabetes. Archives of Pediatrics and Adolescent Medicine. 2011, 166(1):42-48.
17. Morrison JA, Friedman LA, Wang P, Glueck CJ: Metabolic syndrome in childhood predicts adult metabolic syndrome and type 2 diabetes mellitus 25 to 30 years later. J Pediatr 2008, 152:201-206.
18. Morrison JA, Friedman LA, Gray-McGuire C: Metabolic syndrome in childhood predicts adult cardiovascular disease 25 years later: the Princeton Lipid Research Clinics Follow-up Study. Pediatrics 2007, 120:340-345.
19. Dabelea D, Bell RA, D'Agostino RB Jr, Imperatore G, Johansen JM, Linder B, Liu LL, Loots B, Marcovina S, Mayer-Davis EJ, Pettitt DJ, Waitzfelder B: Incidence of diabetes in youth in the United States. JAMA 2007, 297:2716-2724.
20. Magnussen CG, Raitakari OT, Thomson R, Juonala M, Patel DA, Viikari JS, Marniemi J, Srinivasan SR, Berenson GS, Dwyer T, Venn A: Utility of currently recommended pediatric dyslipidemia classifications in predicting dyslipidemia in adulthood: evidence from the Childhood Determinants of Adult Health (CDAH) study, Cardiovascular Risk in Young Finns Study, and Bogalusa Heart Study. Circulation 2008, 117:32-42.
21. Cook S, Weitzman M, Auinger P, Nguyen M, Dietz WH: Prevalence of a metabolic syndrome phenotype in adolescents: findings from the third National Health and Nutrition Examination Survey, 1988-1994. Arch Pediatr Adolesc Med 2003, 157:821-827.
22. Grundy SM, Cleeman JI, Daniels SR, Donato KA, Eckel RH, Franklin BA, Gordon DJ, Krauss RM, Savage PJ, Smith SC Jr, Spertus JA, Costa F: Diagnosis and management of the metabolic syndrome: an American Heart Association/National Heart, Lung, and Blood Institute scientific statement. Curr Opin Cardiol 2006, 21:1-6.
23. Bansal S, Buring JE, Rifai N, Mora S, Sacks FM, Ridker PM: Fasting compared with nonfasting triglycerides and risk of cardiovascular events in women. JAMA 2007, 298:309-316.
24. McBride PE: Triglycerides and risk for coronary heart disease. JAMA 2007, 298:336-338.
25. Nordestgaard BG, Benn M, Schnohr P, Tybjaerg-Hansen A: Nonfasting triglycerides and risk of myocardial infarction, ischemic heart disease, and death in men and women. JAMA 2007, 298:299-308.
26. Sarwar N, Danesh J, Eiriksdottir G, Sigurdsson G, Wareham N, Bingham S, Boekholdt SM, Khaw KT, Gudnason V: Triglycerides and the risk of coronary heart disease: 10,158 incident cases among 262,525 participants in 29 Western prospective studies. Circulation 2007, 115:450-458.
27. Austin MA, McKnight B, Edwards KL, Bradley CM, McNeely MJ, Psaty BM, Brunzell JD, Motulsky AG: Cardiovascular disease mortality in familial forms of hypertriglyceridemia: a 20-year prospective study. Circulation 2000, 101:2777-2782.
28. Kannel WB, Vasan RS: Triglycerides as vascular risk factors: new epidemiologic insights. Curr Opin Cardiol 2009, 24:345-350.
29. Onat A, Sari I, Yazici M, Can G, Hergenc G, Avci GS: Plasma triglycerides, an independent predictor of cardiovascular disease in men: a prospective

study based on a population with prevalent metabolic syndrome. *Int J Cardiol* 2006, **108**:89–95.

30. Varbo A, Nordestgaard BG, Tybjaerg-Hansen A, Schnohr P, Jensen GB, Benn M: Nonfasting triglycerides, cholesterol, and ischemic stroke in the general population. Ann Neurol. 2011, **69**:628–634.

31. Mahoney LT, Burns TL, Stanford W, Thompson BH, Witt JD, Rost CA, Lauer RM: Coronary risk factors measured in childhood and young adult life are associated with coronary artery calcification in young adults: the Muscatine Study. *J Am Coll Cardiol* 1996, **27**:277–284.

32. Berenson GS, Wattigney WA, Tracy RE, Newman WP 3rd, Srinivasan SR, Webber LS, Dalferes ER Jr, Strong JP: Atherosclerosis of the aorta and coronary arteries and cardiovascular risk factors in persons aged 6 to 30 years and studied at necropsy (The Bogalusa Heart Study). *Am J Cardiol* 1992, **70**:851–858.

33. Newman WP 3rd, Freedman DS, Voors AW, Gard PD, Srinivasan SR, Cresanta JL, Williamson GD, Webber LS, Berenson GS: Relation of serum lipoprotein levels and systolic blood pressure to early atherosclerosis. The Bogalusa Heart Study. *N Engl J Med* 1986, **314**:138–144.

34. Relationship of atherosclerosis in young men to serum lipoprotein cholesterol concentrations and smoking. A preliminary report from the Pathobiological Determinants of Atherosclerosis in Youth (PDAY) Research Group. JAMA. 1990;264:3018–24.

35. Chen W, Srinivasan SR, Li S, Xu J, Berenson GS: Metabolic syndrome variables at low levels in childhood are beneficially associated with adulthood cardiovascular risk: the Bogalusa Heart Study. *Diabetes Care* 2005, **28**:126–131.

36. Nguyen QM, Srinivasan SR, Xu JH, Chen W, Berenson GS: Fasting plasma glucose levels within the normoglycemic range in childhood as a predictor of prediabetes and type 2 diabetes in adulthood: the Bogalusa Heart Study. *Arch Pediatr Adolesc Med* 2010, **164**:124–128.

37. Thearle MS, Bunt JC, Knowler WC, Krakoff J. Childhood Predictors of Adult Acute Insulin Response and Insulin Action. Diabetes Care. 2009, **32**:938–943.

38. Nicklas TA, von Duvillard SP, Berenson GS: Tracking of serum lipids and lipoproteins from childhood to dyslipidemia in adults: the Bogalusa Heart Study. *Int J Sports Med* 2002, **23**(Suppl 1):S39–S43.

39. Eisenmann JC, Welk GJ, Wickel EE, Blair SN: Stability of variables associated with the metabolic syndrome from adolescence to adulthood: the Aerobics Center Longitudinal Study. *Am J Hum Biol* 2004, **16**:690–696.

40. Webber LS, Srinivasan SR, Wattigney WA, Berenson GS: Tracking of serum lipids and lipoproteins from childhood to adulthood. The Bogalusa Heart Study. *Am J Epidemiol* 1991, **133**:884–899.

41. Nadeau KJ, Maahs DM, Daniels SR, Eckel RH: Childhood obesity and cardiovascular disease: links and prevention strategies. *Nat Rev Cardiol* 2011, **8**:513–525.

42. Manlhiot C, Larsson P, Gurofsky RC, Smith RW, Fillingham C, Clarizia NA, Chahal N, Clarke JT, McCrindle BW: Spectrum and management of hypertriglyceridemia among children in clinical practice. *Pediatrics* 2009, **123**:458–465.

43. McCrindle BW, Urbina EM, Dennison BA, Jacobson MS, Steinberger J, Rocchini AP, Hayman LL, Daniels SR: Drug therapy of high-risk lipid abnormalities in children and adolescents: a scientific statement from the American Heart Association Atherosclerosis, Hypertension, and Obesity in Youth Committee, Council of Cardiovascular Disease in the Young, with the Council on Cardiovascular Nursing. *Circulation* 2007, **115**:1948–1967.

44. Schwandt P, Haas GM, Liepold E: Lifestyle and cardiovascular risk factors in 2001 child–parent pairs: the PEP Family Heart Study. *Atherosclerosis* 2010, **213**:642–648.

45. Dennison BA, Kikuchi DA, Srinivasan SR, Webber LS, Berenson GS: Parental history of cardiovascular disease as an indication for screening for lipoprotein abnormalities in children. *J Pediatr* 1989, **115**:186–194.

4

Testicular volumes revisited: A proposal for a simple clinical method that can closely match the volumes obtained by ultrasound and its clinical application

Juan F Sotos[1]* and Naomi J Tokar[2]*

Abstract

Background: The testicular volumes obtained with the clinical methods, calculated using the ellipsoid equation $W^2 \times L \times \pi/6$, correlate with those obtained by ultrasound (US) and are useful clinically, but overestimate ultrasound values, mainly because of the inclusion of the scrotal skin and epididymis, have much variability, and may not be accurate or reproducible.

The US measurement is somewhat inconvenient, because it requires another procedure and, mainly, is costly.

It would be helpful to have a simple, low cost clinical method that approximates or closely matches the results obtained by ultrasound.

Formulas, equivalent to the ellipsoid equations, were developed to calculate testicular volumes with corrections of the width (W), length (L), and height (H) of the testis obtained in the scrotum to avoid the inclusion of the scrotal skin and epididymis.

Subjects & methods: The US observations in our hospital of the width, height, length, height/width, and length/width ratios and volumes of 110 testes from 55 children from 1 month to 17 ½ years of age were reviewed. Based on these observations and those reported by others, formulas to apply to the clinical measurements were developed to approximate the volumes obtained by ultrasound. The validity and accuracy of the formulas were determined. For the clinical application of the formulas, measurements of the width of the testis in the scrotum, with a centimeter ruler, were obtained in 187 study subjects in different stages of puberty and adults, for a total of 374 testicular determinations.

Results: The widths obtained in the scrotum were corrected by subtracting the values of the double scrotal skin. The formulas were then applied and the testicular volumes determined. The testicular volumes were then compared to the ultrasound values reported in hundreds of subjects by four different groups and statistically analyzed. The volumes obtained by the formulas (means ± SD) closely matched the volumes obtained by ultrasound.

Conclusion: A simple clinical method, based on the width of the testis obtained in the scrotum with a centimeter ruler, which can determine testicular volumes closely matching those reported by ultrasound, is proposed.

Keywords: Testicular volume, Gonadal development, Pubertal changes

* Correspondence: Juan.Sotos@NationwideChildrens.org; Naomi.Tokar@NationwideChildrens.org
[1]Department of Pediatric, College of Medicine, The Ohio State University, Nationwide Children's Hospital, Section of Pediatric Endocrinology, Metabolism & Diabetes, 700 Children's Drive, Columbus, OH 43205, USA
[2]Nationwide Children's Hospital, Section of Pediatric Endocrinology, Metabolism & Diabetes, 700 Children's Drive, Columbus, OH 43205, USA

Background

For more than 50 years there has been [1-4] and continues to be [5-7] an interest in the subject. The determination of the testicular volume is of considerable importance to assess for a number of conditions: the onset, progression and disorders of puberty, the effect of cryptorchidism and orchiopexy, hypogonadism with respect to tubular function, the effect of a varicocele, abnormal testicular development, damage to the testis by torsion or inflammation, compensatory hypertrophy, detection of Klinefelter syndrome, effect of the administration of sexual steroids or drugs, and, in adults, assessment of fertility. Testicular size correlates with tubular size, function and spermatogenesis [8].

In addition, the testicular volume is of interest to assess macroorchidism, such as in Fragile X syndrome, FSH secreting pituitary macroadenomas, long-standing hypothyroidism, adrenal rest cell tumors in congenital adrenal hyperplasia, lymphomas and so on.

A number of clinical methods have been used for the measurement of testicular volumes in the scrotum. Some use the length and width or the testis obtained with an ordinary ruler or with sliding calipers [2,3]. Others use orchidometers by comparative palpation with ellipsoid models of known volume [1,9,10] or by a series of punch out elliptical rings of varying sizes that fit over the testis [11,12]. All the clinical methods calculate the volumes following the ellipsoid equation $W^2 \times L \times 0.52$.

Ultrasound measurements of testicular volume have a high degree of accuracy and reproducibility and are the standard for quantitation of testicular volume [13-15]. The volumes obtained with the clinical methods correlate with those obtained by ultrasound and are useful clinically, but overestimate ultrasound values [14-17], by two to three folds [7,16], mainly because the inclusion of the scrotal skin and epididymis, have much intraobserver and interobserver variability and may not be accurate or reproducible [13]. The ultrasound measurement, however, is somewhat inconvenient, because it requires another procedure, and, mainly, is costly. It does not appear practical or reasonable to use ultrasound to assess the onset and progression of puberty or to assess some of the other conditions that have been mentioned.

It would be helpful to have a clinical method that is simple, low cost, and that approximates or closely matches the results obtained by ultrasound.

The volumes obtained by ultrasound have been calculated by different ellipsoid equations. Some have used only the width (W) and length (L) of the testes, $W^2 \times L \times \pi/6$ that when resolved is $W^2 \times L \times 0.52 =$ Volume. More frequently they have included the height (H), $W \times H \times L \times 0.52$ and others, recently, have used the constant 0.71 to closely match the "true" testicular volumes obtained by water displacement, $W \times H \times L \times 0.71 =$ Volume.

Three formulas, equivalent to the 3 ellipsoid equations used in ultrasound measurements, were developed with corrections of the width, length, and height of the testis obtained in the scrotum, to avoid the inclusion of the scrotal skin and epididymis and to approximate testicular volumes obtained by ultrasound.

The aim of this report is to describe a simple clinical method based on the width of the testis obtained in the scrotum with a centimeter ruler that can determine testicular volumes closely matching those reported by ultrasound. 1) The basis for the development of the formulas to do so, 2) their validity and accuracy, and 3) the volumes obtained with the formulas in our children, adolescents and adults will be presented.

Subjects and methods

The ultrasound observations in our hospital, of the width, height, length, height/width and length/width ratios, and volumes of 110 testes from 55 children, from 1 month to 17 ½ years of age (using Phillips, Model iu22 and Siemens S2000 with linear array transducers and imaging frequencies of 17-5 MHz and 18-16 MHz respectively) were reviewed.

Based on these observations and those reported by others, formulas were developed to approximate the volumes obtained by ultrasound, by expressing the width (W), without the scrotal skin (W-ss) and the height (H) (anterior-posterior diameter or depth) and length (L) in the ellipsoid equation $W \times H \times L \times 0.52$ with values based on the ratios of the Width-ss; the height as a ratio of the width (H/(W-ss)), to avoid the inclusion of the scrotal skin and body of the epididymis, and the length as a ratio of the width (L/(W-ss)) to avoid the inclusion of the head of the epididymis and scrotal skin. Three formulas were developed to be equivalent to the ellipsoid equations used in US measurements: to the equation $W^2 \times L \times 0.52$ (Formula 1); to the equation $W \times H \times L \times 0.52$ (Formula 2); and to the equation $W \times H \times L \times 0.71$ (Formula 3).

The validity and accuracy of the formulas were determined by the significance of Pearson's linear correlations coefficient (r) and by the comparison of the volumes obtained by ultrasound and by the formulas.

For the clinical application of the formulas, 163 measurements of the double scrotal skin (ss) were obtained with a Harpenden Skinfold caliper in boys in different stages of puberty and in adults. Measurements of the width and length of the testis in the scrotum, with a centimeter ruler, were obtained in 187 study subjects in different stages of puberty and in adults, for a total of 374 testicular determinations. The 187 subjects consisted of 42 normal and 145 patients attending the endocrine clinic who had normal growth and gonadal development. The widths obtained in the scrotum were corrected by subtracting the values for the double scrotal skin, in accordance with their gonadal stage, to approximate or match the width of the testis. The formulas were then applied and the testicular volumes determined. The testicular volumes obtained were then compared to the ultrasound volumes reported by four different groups.

To avoid confusion, the term "equation" has been used for the determination of testicular volumes by ultrasound and "formula" for the calculation of volumes in study subjects.

Basis for the development of the formulas

The testis is assumed and generally accepted to be an ellipsoid. When the width and the height are the same (a prolate spheroid, like a rugby ball), the equation for the volume would be: W^2 x L x $\pi/6$ = volume or W^2 x L x 0.52 = volume – that comes for the resolution of the equation: $(W/2)^2$ x π x $4/3$ x $L/2$ = volume. If the width and the height are different, as in a rotational ellipsoid, then the equation would be W x H x L x 0.52.

As previously mentioned, all the clinical measurements of the testes overestimate the US volumes, mainly because of the inclusion of the scrotal skin and the epididymis.

Formulas, to apply to the clinical measurements obtained in the scrotum of the study subjects, were developed to approximate the volumes obtained by US, by expressing the width (W) without the scrotal skin (W-ss), the height (H) as a ratio of the width (H/(W-ss)) and the length and a ratio of the width (L/(W-ss)). The numbers for the last two ratios can be obtained by the measurements usually observed in ultrasound determinations.

A. *Length/width ratio*

With the development and growth of the testes, the dimensions of the testes width and length remain proportional with the width being approximately 2/3 of the length [9,11]. The width/length ratio in a number of testes (number 110) in our hospital by US was 0.64 ± 0.09 (length/width ratio = 1.55 ± 0.21). The width/length ratio determined by ultrasound in a number of children by others was 0.67 ± 0.12 (length/width ratio = 1.5) [13]. Of note is that the width/length ratio of all the ellipsoid models from 1 ml to 25 ml in the Prader orchidometer is the same, 0.638 (length/width = 1.57), and of all the punch out elliptical rings in the Takihara (also known as the Rochester Orchidometer) is 0.666 (length/width = 1.50) [12]. Thus, knowing the width, the length of the testis can be calculated (L = (W-ss) x 1.55 or 1.50) and the length would not include the epididymis and the scrotal skin. So the length in the formula can be expressed as 1.55 x (W-ss) = L.

B. *Height/width ratio*

The testis is not a perfect prolate spheroid, but an ellipsoid. The height or depth is usually less than the width by ultrasound measurements. As a consequence the US volumes obtained by the equations W^2 x L x 0.52 or W x H x L x 0.52 are different. The volumes are lower with the equation that includes the height.

By report of US measurements, it seems that the height is variable. In our hospital the H/W ratio in 110 testes was 0.76 ± 0.12 (minimum 0.5 to maximum 1.0). The H/W ratio of 0.69 ± 0.04 (minimum 0.69 to maximum 0.8) was reported by Osemlak [6]. Thus, the H/W ratio to be included in the formula may need to be adjusted in different institutions. With our data the best correlation was obtained with an H/W ratio of 0.8.

Thus, the H in the formula could be expressed as 0.8 x (W-ss) = H. Because of the variability of the shape in the testes (or in the US measurements), there would be a variability of the results. Higher values of the H/W ratio of the testes by US than in the formula will yield higher values by US than the formula and vice versa.

C. *Formulas*

Thus, Formula 1, equivalent to the ellipsoid equation W^2 x L x 0.52, would be $(W-ss)^2$ x ((W-ss) x 1.55) x 0.52 = volume or $(W-ss)^3$ x 0.80.

Formula 2, equivalent to the ellipsoid equation W x H x L x 0.52, would be (W-ss) x (0.8 x (W-ss)) x (1.55 x (W-ss)) x 0.52 = volume or $(W-ss)^3$ x 0.64.

Formula 3, equivalent to the ellipsoid equation W x H x L x 0.71 would be the same as formula 2, except for the constant of 0.71 instead of 0.52, (W-ss) x (0.8 x (W-ss)) x (1.55 x (W-ss)) x 0.71 = volume or $(W-ss)^3$ x 0.88.

The equation W x H x L x 0.71 = volume comes from the observations of Lambert [18]. In postmortem dissections, Lambert found that the constant of 0.52 results in too small of a value for testicular size and concluded that the constant to be used in practice should be 0.71. The values of the constant, however, varied from 0.37 to 1.08, depending on the shape and size of the testis. Consequently, he recognized that the error (or variability) of the method was quite large. This variability relates to the different shape of the testis, and would be difficult to resolve.

Ultrasound measurement of the testicular volume is acknowledged to be the best method to quantitate the size of the testis. There is some question regarding the equation that should be used to obtain the volume of the testis.

The equation W x H x L x 0.52 = volume, is probably the most frequently used for ultrasound measurements. According to some authors that equation underestimates the "true" volumes determined by water displacement and the equation W x H x L x 0.71 is the best and should be used [19,20].

Thus, with the measurement of the width of the testis in the scrotum, and subtraction of the double scrotal skin one could determine the volume.

Some variability related to the variability of the shape of the testis itself and intra and interobserver variability would be expected.

The formula or ellipsoid equation used should be the same for clinical and for US methods.

If no height is included: W^2 x L x 0.52 = volume – for the ultrasound,

$$(W-ss)^3 \times 0.80 = \text{volume } for \text{ } the \text{ } clinical \text{ } method.$$

If height is included: W x H x L x 0.52 = volume for the ultrasound,

$$(W-ss)^3 \times 0.64 = \text{volume } for \text{ } the \text{ } clinical \text{ } method.$$

If the constant of 0.71 instead of 0.52 is used: W x H x L x 0.71 = volume for the ultrasound,

$$(W-ss)^3 \times 0.88 = \text{volume } for \text{ } the \text{ } clinical \text{ } method.$$

The constant will change, depending on the H/W ratio included in the formula, which should be based on the H/W ratio in the institution.

Statistics

The correlations between the volumes obtained by ultrasound and by the formulas were measured using the Pearson's correlation coefficients (r). The significance of the difference between the means of the samples was calculated by paired *t*-test. All tests were two-tailed and significance was set at $p < 0.05$.

Results

Validity and accuracy of the formulas

The validity and accuracy of the formulas were determined by the significance of the linear correlations and by the comparison of the volumes obtained by ultrasound and by the formulas.

The ultrasound results of 110 testicular measurements (width, height, length) and volumes obtained in our hospital were used.

To assess the validity of the formulas, the same widths were used for the ultrasound and for the formulas.

Formula 1

The correlation of the testicular volumes obtained by ultrasound, without the inclusion of height (W^2 x L x 0.52 = volume) and the formula (W^2 x (1.55 x W) x 0.52) W^3 x 0.8 = volume is illustrated in Figure 1a. In 110 determinations, the correlation coefficient was r = 0.9945, highly significant (p <0.001) and the regression equation y = 0.9991x – 0.0232. The mean of the volumes of 5.27 ± 6.90 ml by US and 5.24 ± 6.93 ml by formula were not different (p = >0.5)(not shown). Because when one has large numbers and differences in

gonadal development the means may not reflect the large variation, the volumes by age groups were compared (Table 1). Again, the volumes were not different (p >0.5).

Formula 2

The correlation of the testicular volumes obtained by ultrasound in 110 testes, when the height was included (W x H x L x 0.52), and by the formula (W x (0.8 x W) x (1.55 x W) x 0.52) W^3 x 0.64 = volume, is shown in Figure 1b.

The correlation coefficient was r = 0.97545, highly significant (p <0.001), and the regression equation Y = 0.9599x +0.1679.

The mean of the volumes by US and the formula were not different (p >0.5), 4.19 ± 5.63 ml and 4.19 ± 5.54 ml (not shown). Again the volumes were compared by age groups. The volumes were not different (p >0.1 or >0.5) (Table 1).

Formula 3

Because of reports [19,20] that using the constant 0.71, instead of 0.52, is the best to determine the true volume of the testis, obtained by water displacement, calculations and comparisons were made using the 0.71 constant.

The correlation of the testicular volumes obtained by US (W x H x L x 0.71 = volume) and by the formula (W x (0.8 x W) x (1.55 x W) x 0.71) W^3 x 0.88 is shown in Figure 1c.

The correlation coefficient was r = 0.9754, highly significant (p <0.001), and the regression equation y = 0.9667x + 0.2308.

The means of the volumes by US and by the formula were 5.73 ± 7.69 ml and 5.77 ± 7.62 ml, respectively, not different (not shown). Again the volumes were compared by age groups. The volumes were not different (p >0.1 or >0.5) (Table 1).

By the aforementioned, the formulas seem valid and accurate. The variability of results is owing to the variability of the shape of the testis, variability on the length/width ratio or height/width ratio. This variability is difficult to resolve, because the US measurements are individual and the method applies the same formula for all.

Clinical application of the formulas to our study subjects

Measurements of the double scrotal skin were obtained (Table 2), so that the width of the testis obtained in the scrotum could be corrected to approximate or equal the width of the testis.

The double scrotal skin measured 0.17 cm for G-1, 0.15 for G-2, 0.15 for G-3, 0.19 for G-4, 0.2 for G-5 and 0.21 for adults.

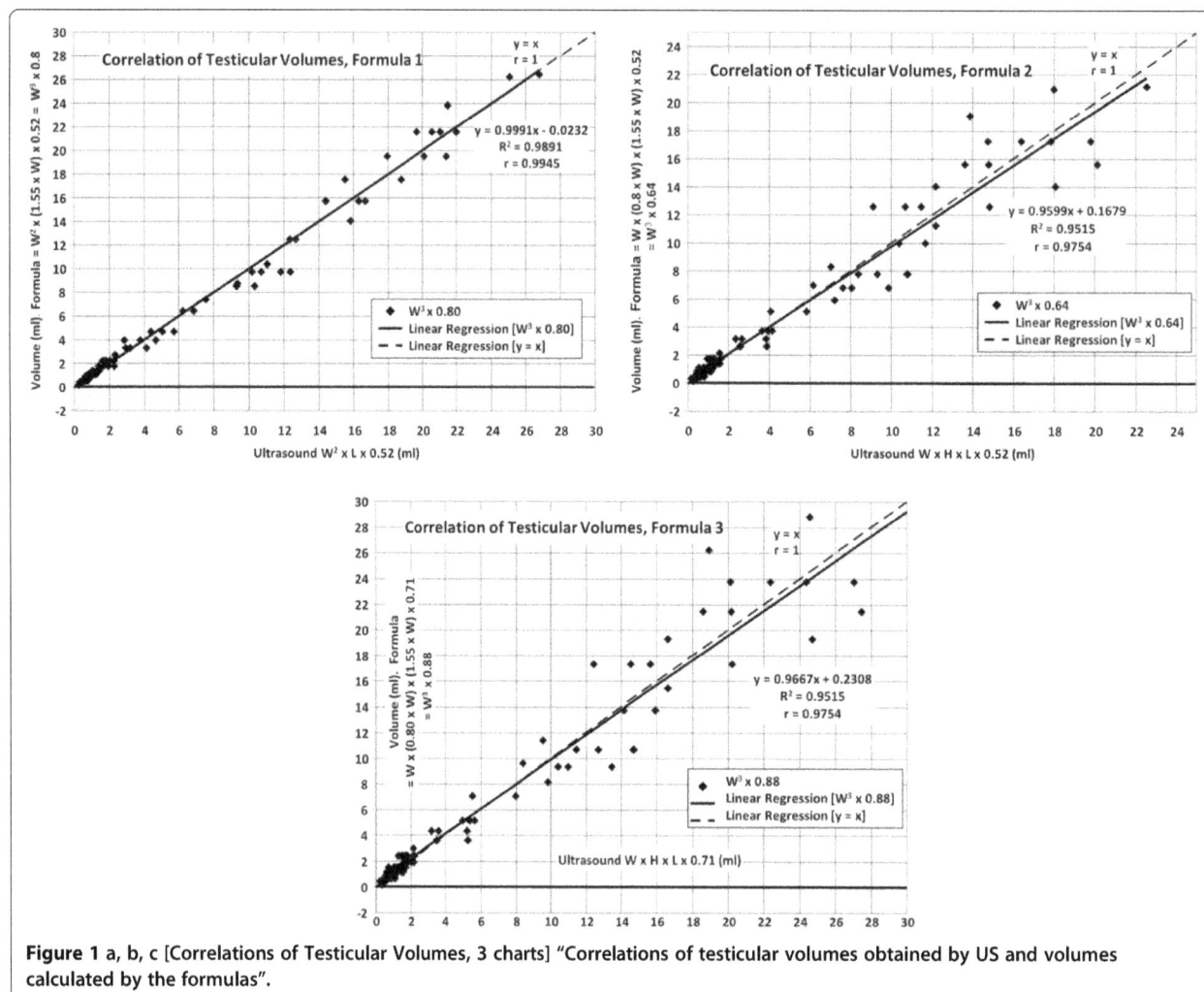

Figure 1 a, b, c [Correlations of Testicular Volumes, 3 charts] "Correlations of testicular volumes obtained by US and volumes calculated by the formulas".

The width and length of the testis in the scrotum were measured, with a centimeter ruler, in 187 boys in different stages of puberty and in adults, for a total of 374 testes. Our study subjects were divided in groups by age (to permit comparison with other published reports) or by Tanner stages of pubertal development.

With the widths obtained after subtracting the double scrotal skin, the formulas were applied to our study subjects and the volumes were compared to the testicular volumes obtained by ultrasound by others: to P Osemlak [6] who reported volumes in 309 boys from 1 day to 17 years of age (linear array transducer 12 MHz LA523); to J Goede et al. [7] who obtained volumes in 769 boys 6 months to 19 years of age (using a 12 MHz linear array transducer – Falco AutoImage, Falco Software, Tomsk, Russia); to Kuijper et al. [21] who reported volumes in the first 6 years of life in 344 boys obtained with a linear array transducer 7.5 MHz (Aloka SSD-900); and to JY Bahk et al. [22] who determined volumes in 1,139 normal young men, 19 -27 year old by ultrasound (model SSD, 1700 Aloka, Japan) (Table 3).

For the first nine years, all the volumes, on the average, are less than 1 ml and the means of our children are on the range reported by others.

Our values seem lower than those reported by Osemlak and Goede et al. by 0.1 to 0.2 ml for the first 9 years of age. Although this difference is statistically significant ($p < 0.05$), it does not appear of clinical importance. This difference could result from a 0.5 to 1 mm difference in the measurement of the width, by manual compression. Kuijper et al. reported an increase of the volumes from 0.27 ml at 1 month to 0.44 at five months (minipuberty), and a decrease to 0.31 ml at 9 months. The volumes remain stable after that. They did not report the number of observations or standard deviations of the 97 children 1 to 6 years of age, so no comparison could be analyzed.

The volumes after 10 years seem similar, even though the age of some groups was not the same. Statistical comparisons showed no differences ($p > 0.1$ or > 0.5) (Table 4). Figure 2 showing the means and standard deviations of the different groups is rather convincing that the

Table 1 Comparison of Testicular Volumes Obtained by Ultrasound (US) in our Hospital with those obtained by Formulas (means ± SD) All using the US Width

Age range years	Number	US (ml) equation W^2 x L x 0.52	Formula (ml)W^3 X 0.8	p value
1 to 2	19	0.64 ± 0.25	0.64 ± 0.24	>0.5
3 to 6	26	1.05 ± 0.44	1.08 ± 0.50	>0.5
7 to 9	15	1.37 ± 0.56	1.46 ± 0.63	>0.5
10 to 11	9	1.40 ± 0.60	1.57 ± 0.77	>0.5
12 to 13	18	7.79 ± 4.40	7.83 ± 4.81	>0.5
14 to 15	10	12.87 ± 7.12	12.50 ± 7.43	>0.5
16 to 17	13	18.31 ± 4.63	18.02 ± 5.54	>0.5

Age range years	Number	US (ml) equation W x H x L x 0.52	Formula (ml)W^3 x 0.64	p value
1 to 2	19	0.48 ± 0.17	0.51 ± 0.20	>0.5
3 to 6	26	0.78 ± 0.34	0.87 ± 0.40	>0.1
7 to 9	15	0.95 ± 0.42	1.17 ± 0.51	>0.1
10 to 11	9	1.06 ± 0.35	1.26 ± 0.61	>0.1
12 to 13	18	5.94 ± 3.31	6.26 ± 3.85	>0.5
14 to 15	10	10.02 ± 4.76	9.99 ± 5.95	>0.5
16 to 17	13	15.49 ± 4.06	14.42 ± 4.44	>0.5

Age range years	Number	US (ml) equation W x H x L x 0.71	Formula (ml)W^3 x 0.88	p value
1 to 2	19	0.65 ± 0.24	0.70 ± 0.27	>0.5
3 to 6	26	1.06 ± 0.46	1.19 ± 0.55	>0.1
7 to 9	15	1.30 ± 0.58	1.61 ± 0.70	>0.1
10 to 11	9	1.45 ± 0.48	1.73 ± 0.84	>0.1
12 to 13	18	8.10 ± 4.52	8.61 ± 5.21	>0.5
14 to 15	10	13.68 ± 6.50	13.75 ± 8.18	>0.5
16 to 17	13	21.15 ± 5.54	19.83 ± 6.10	>0.5

volumes of our study subjects, based on the formula, closely match the volumes obtained by ultrasound in different institutions. This, in itself, is additional evidence in support of the validity and accuracy of the formulas.

Because of the wide range of ages for the development of gonadal stages and the overlapping of ages for different stages (i.e. G-1 up to 13 9/12 years; G-2, 9 to 13; G-3, 12 to 16), it seems preferable to report the volumes obtained in study subjects with the formulas by the gonadal stage (Table 5 and Figure 3). Pubertal stages were determined by the method of Tanner.

One can convert the volumes and standard deviations from one formula to another by multiplying or dividing

$$\text{From}(W - ss)^3 \times 0.8 \text{ to}(W - ss)^3 \times 0.88,$$
$$\text{multiply by } 1.1$$
$$(\text{since } 0.88/0.8 = 1.1)$$
$$\text{From}(W - ss)^3 \times 0.8 \text{ to } (W - ss)^3$$
$$\times 0.64 (0.8/0.64 = 1.25)$$
$$\text{divide by } 1.25 \text{ or vice versa.}$$

If one prefers the formula with the constant 0.71 to obtain the volumes that approximate "true" testicular volumes, then multiply $(W\text{-ss})^3$ x 0.64 by 1.365, since 0.88/0.6448 = 1.365].

Discussion

The measurement of the testicular volume is not an exact science. After the advent in 1970, ultrasound has been recognized as the most accurate and reproducible method, even though variability related to the transducer used, possibility of compression of the testis, and intra and interobserver variation in the measurements (width, height, length, and volumes), among other factors exists [13,19,21].

Different methods have been used for the clinical measurement of testicular volumes: measurements of the testis in the scrotum by a ruler or by a caliper or by orchidometers. A number of orchidometers have been described: the Prader orchidometer, described in 1966 [9], and the Takihara (also known as the Rochester orchidometer), described in 1983 [12], are probably the most frequently used.

There have been multiple publications comparing the volumes obtained by the orchidometers and by ultrasound. The volumes obtained with the clinical methods correlate with those obtained by ultrasound and are useful clinically, but all overestimate the volumes obtained by ultrasound, have much variability and may not be accurate or reproducible.

A simple clinical method that would approximate or closely match the ultrasound values would be quite helpful.

In 1966, Prader stated [9] that "knowing the width of the testis in the scrotum (obtained by a caliper), one can calculate the volume, being assumed that the testicle is an ellipsoid of revolution, corresponding to the equation 0.52 x W^2 x L or 0.71 x W^2 x L". In the ellipsoid the width is about 2/3 of the length. Since he felt that the use of the caliper was laborious and required considerable manipulation, he developed ellipsoid models of known volumes for comparison, all of them with an L/W ratio of 1.57 (W/L = 0.638), and volumes calculated using the equation 0.52 x W^2 x L.

The ultrasound method was not available then. The volumes obtained with the Prader orchidometer overestimate those obtained by ultrasound [7,13,14,16,19,20] usually by 2 to 3 folds, because of the inclusion of the scrotal skin and epididymis, the lack of including the height of the testis, and the intraobserver and, particularly, the interobserver variability.

The method presented here, more or less, states the same as was stated in 1966. Knowing the width of the testis in the scrotum (with a centimeter ruler), one can calculate the volume, but this time closely matching the

Table 2 Double Scrotal Skin (cm)

Gonadal stage	Number of measurements	Mean ± SD
G-1	36	0.17 ± 0.02
G-2	28	0.15 ± 0.02
G-3	18	0.16 ± 0.01
G-4	31	0.19 ± 0.02
G-5	22	0.20 ± 0.03
Adults	28	0.21 ± 0.03

Legend: Measurement obtained within 1 to 2 seconds after releasing the grip using a Harpenden Skinfold Caliper HSK-BI.

ultrasound values. To do that, the width was subtracted by the double scrotal skin to approximate the width obtained by US, the length was expressed as a ratio of the width to avoid the inclusion of the epididymis and scrotal skin, and the height was expressed as a ratio of the width, to take into consideration the inclusion of the height in the ultrasound measurements and to avoid the inclusion of the scrotal skin and the body of the epididymis.

Thus, formulas were developed to be equivalent to ultrasound equations (W^2 x L x 0.52, W x H x L x 0.52, or W x H x L x 0.71).

The validity and accuracy of the formulas were determined by the significance of the linear correlations and by the comparison of the volumes obtained by ultrasound and by the formulas.

The formulas were applied to the clinical measurements obtained in 374 testes in our study subjects and the volumes compared to the volumes obtained by ultrasound by 4 different groups.

The results seem rather convincing that the testicular volumes of our study subjects, based on the formulas,

Table 3 Testicular Volumes (ml) Obtained by Ultrasound in Normal Children and Adults Reported by 4 Groups Compared with Volumes in Our Study Subjects Obtained Clinically by Formula

Age group	Osemlak [6] Mean ± SD	Goede et al. [7] Mean ± SD	Kuijper et al. [21] Mean ± SD	Our study subjects $(W-ss)^3$ x 0.64 Mean ± SD
1 month	(17) 0.35 ± 0.12		(31) 0.27 ± 0.02	
2 to 12 months	(17) 0.5 ± 0.24	(40) 0.48 ± 0.13	(216) 0.44 ± 0.03 0.31 ± 0.02	
2 years	(17) 0.55 ± 0.22	(38) 0.46 ± 0.09	0.31	
3 years	(17) 0.64 ± 0.19	(36) 0.51 ± 0.15	0.31	(24) 0.46 ± 0.07
4 years	(17) 0.78 ± 0.21	(38) 0.51 ± 0.16	0.31	
5 years	(17) 0.67 ± 0.19	(48) 0.58 ± 0.15	0.31	
6 years	(17) 0.78 ± 0.24	(42) 0.63 ± 0.26	0.31	
7 years	(17) 0.68 ± 0.21	(62) 0.65 ± 0.17		(22) 0.56 ± 0.09
8 years	(17) 0.81 ± 0.23	(59) 0.66 ± 0.22		
9 years	(17) 0.85 ± 0.31	(53) 0.79 ± 0.46		(36) 0.65 ± 0.19
10 years	(18) 1.36 ± 0.61	(49) 0.97 ± 0.51		
11 years	(18) 1.94 ± 1.41	(60) 1.33 ± 1.03		(50) 2.56 ± 1.24
12 years	(17) 3.29 ± 2.99	(55) 2.33 ± 1.77		
13 years	(18) 5.37 ± 2.92	(47) 4.42 ± 2.66		(18) 4.28 ± 0.96
14 years	(17) 4.98 ± 2.68	(35) 7.31 ± 4.11		(58) 8.01 ± 2.58
15 years	(17) 8.71 ± 2.52	(26) 8.69 ± 2.91		
16 years	(17) 11.8 ± 4.91	(31) 11.51 ± 3.03		(36) 12.45 ± 1.99
17 years	(17) 12.83 ± 3.94	(27) 12.12 ± 2.8		
18 years		(23) 13.73 ± 3.51		(56) 13.16 ± 2.67
Adults		**Bahk et al.** [22] W x H x L x 0.52		$(W-ss)^3$ x 0.64
	(1139)	*Lt. 13.46 ± 2.65 Rt. 13.29 ± 2.82		(102) 13.12 ± 3.17
		W x H x L x 0.71		$(W-ss)^3$ x 0.88
	(1139)	Lt. 18.37 ± 3.62 Rt. 18.13 ± 3.85		(102) 18.05 ± 4.36

Legend: (#) Number of observations. The US equation used by Osemlak and Goede et al. and Kuijper et al. was W x H x L x 0.52.
* The equation used by Bahk et al. was W x H x L x 0.71. The volumes were divided by 1.365 to obtain volumes determined with the constant 0.52 (0.71/0.52 = 1.365).

Table 4 Comparison of Testicular Volumes (ml) Obtained by Ultrasound in Normal Children and Adults at different ages Reported by 3 Groups with Volumes in Our Study Subjects Obtained Clinically (means ± SD)

Age group	Osemlak [6]	Goede et al. [7]	Bahk et al. [22] (W x H x L x 0.52)	Our study subjects (W-ss)³ x 0.64	p value Osemlak to Our	p value Goede et al. To Our	p value Bahk et al. To Our
5 years	(17) 0.67 ± 0.19	(48) 0.58 ± 0.15		(24) 0.46 ± 0.07	<0.001	<0.001	
7 years	(17) 0.68 ± 0.21	(62) 0.65 ± 0.17		(22) 0.56 ± 0.09	<0.05	<0.01	
9 years	(17) 0.85 ± 0.31	(53) 0.79 ± 0.46		(36) 0.65 ± 0.19	<0.02	>0.05	
12 years	(17) 3.29 ± 2.99	(55) 2.33 ± 1.77		(50) 2.56 ± 1.24	>0.1	>0.05	
13 years	(18) 5.37 ± 2.92	(47) 4.42 ± 2.66		(18) 4.28 ± 0.96	>0.1	>0.05	
15 years	(17) 8.71 ± 2.52	(26) 8.69 ± 2.91		(58) 8.01 ± 2.58	>0.1	>0.1	
17 years	(17) 12.83 ± 3.94	(27) 12.12 ± 2.8		(36) 12.45 ± 1.99	>0.5	>0.5	
18 years		(23) 13.73 ± 3.51		(56) 13.16 ± 2.67		>0.1	
Adults			(1139)*13.29 ± 2.82	(102) 13.12 ± 3.17			>0.1
			(W x H x L x 0.71) 18.37 ± 3.62	((W-ss)³ x 0.88) (102) 18.05 ± 4.36			>0.1

Legend: (#) Number of observations.
The equation used by Osemlak and Goede et al. was W x H x L x 0.52 and our formula (W-ss)³ x 0.64.
* Calculated from the values using 0.71 as a constant.

closely match the volumes obtained by ultrasound in different institutions.

The proposed method should be helpful to assess the onset and progression and disorders of puberty and the disorders previously mentioned.

The US remains the method of choice for the evaluation of extratesticular (i.e. hydrocele, spermatocele, epididymal cyst, varicocele) or intratesticular (i.e. tumors) abnormalities.

As always, there may be limitations. The clinical measurements were obtained by one observer. The interobserver variability remains to be determined.

Ultrasound determinations could be obtained in the same subjects whom the clinical measurements are made and then compare US volumes with those obtained by formulas. Comparison with US volumes reported by others, as done, would seem to be a more difficult test, so different results may not be likely.

In summary: A simple clinical method, based on the width of the testis obtained in the scrotum with a centimeter ruler that can determine testicular volumes closely matching those reported by ultrasound is proposed. This

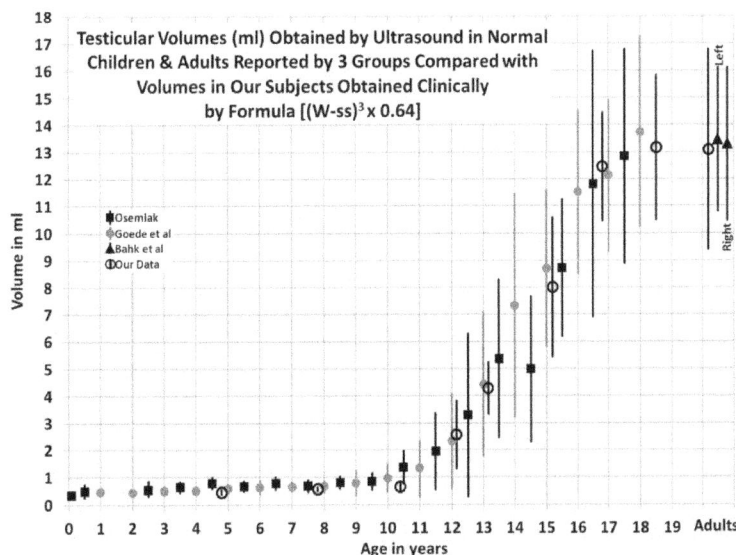

Figure 2 [Comparison of Testicular Volumes obtained by the formula & those published by 3 groups, chart] "Illustration of the means ± SD of volumes obtained by US by Osemlak [6], Goede et al. [7], Bahk et al. [22], and our formula. The formula (W-ss)³ x 0.64 is equivalent to the US equation W x H x L x 0.52".

Table 5 Testicular Volumes (ml) of Study Subjects Obtained Clinically by Described Formulas

	Formulas equivalent to the following US Equations		
Gonadal Stage (number in group)	W^2 x L x 0.52 $(W-ss)^3$ x 0.8 (mean ± SD)	W x H x L x 0.52 $(W-ss)^3$ x 0.64 (mean ± SD)	W x H x L x 0.71 $(W-ss)^3$ x 0.88 (mean ± SD)
G-1 3 to 7 yr (24)	0.57 ± 0.09	0.46 ± 0.07	0.63 ± 0.10
7 to 9 yr (22)	0.70 ± 0.11	0.56 ± 0.09	0.77 ± 0.12
9 to 11 yr (36)	0.81 ± 0.24	0.65 ± 0.19	0.90 ± 0.26
G-2 (50)	3.20 ± 1.56	2.56 ± 1.24	3.52 ± 1.71
G-3 (18)	5.36 ± 1.20	4.28 ± 0.96	5.89 ± 1.32
G-4 (58)	10.01 ± 3.22	8.01 ± 2.58	11.01 ± 3.55
G-5 (36)	15.57 ± 2.49	12.45 ± 1.99	17.12 ± 2.74
Adults (102)	16.41 ± 3.96	13.12 ± 3.17	18.05 ± 4.36

method should be helpful for the assessment of the onset and progression of puberty, of disorders of puberty and of conditions associated with differential testicular volumes. (Appendix)

A centimeter ruler is usually available to any provider and should be less intrusive than the use of a caliper or orchidometer.

The process for the determination of the testicular volume seems simple:

1. Measurement of the width of testis in the scrotum can be obtained by smoothing the scrotal skin around the testis with the thumb and index finger of one hand, avoiding compression of the testis and using the ruler with the other hand.

2. The Tanner Stage of pubertal (gonadal) development is determined.

3. The width is subtracted by the double scrotal skin, for the gonadal stage – shown in Table 2. One could make it simpler by subtracting 1.5 mm for Tanner stages 1, 2, and 3 and 2 mm for Tanner 4, 5, and adult. The error or variation would be minor.

4. The volume, then, is calculated by the formula: $(W-ss)^3$ x 0.88, if one would like to obtain the "true" volume of the testis matching volumes determine by water displacement, or by $(W-ss)^3$ x 0.64 or $(W-ss)^3$ x 0.8 and compared with the normal values for the Tanner (gonadal) stage and adults shown in Tables 5 and Figure 3.

5. If one would like to compare the values obtained by the formula with those obtained by ultrasound in the institution, one should use the formula equivalent to the ellipsoid equation that they use for the calculation of US volumes: for US equation W^2 x L x 0.52 use formula $(W-ss)^3$ x 0.8; for US equation W x H x L x 0.52 use formula $(W-ss)^3$ x 0.64; and for US equation W x H x L x 0.71 use formula $(W-ss)^3$ x 0.88.

Appendix
Assessment of differential testicular volumes

The formulas can also provide information on the testicular volumes expected from the changes in millimeters of the width (Table 6) and be helpful for evaluation of disorders associated with discrepancies in testicular volumes.

Of particular interest is the effect of a varicocele, occurring in approximately 10 to 25% of adolescents and

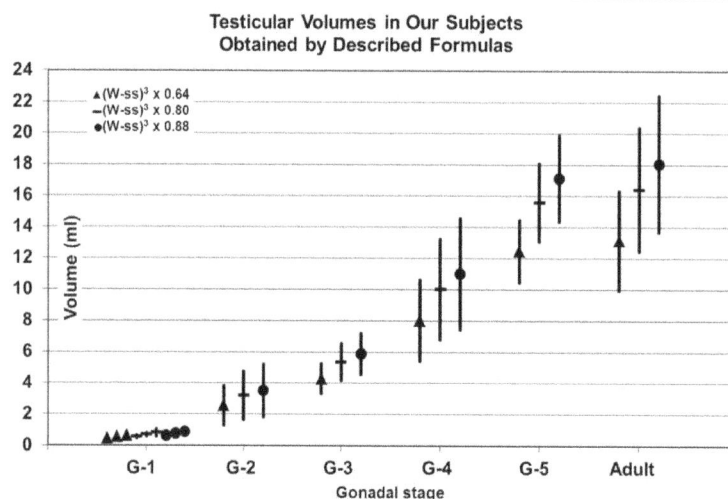

Figure 3 [Testicular Volumes at gonadal stages with 3 formulas, chart] "Illustration of the means ± SD of volumes at different stages of gonadal (G) development. The formula with the constant 0.64 is equivalent to the equation W x H x L x 0.52; the one with the constant 0.80 is equivalent to W^2 x L x 0.52; the one with the constant 0.88 is equivalent to W x H x L x 0.71".

Table 6 Testicular Volumes (ml)

Width of testis (cm) (ss subtracted)	Formulas equivalent to the following US Equations		
	$W^2 \times L \times 0.52$ $(W-ss)^3 \times 0.8$	$W \times H \times L \times 0.52$ $(W-ss)^3 \times 0.64$	$W \times H \times L \times 0.71$ $(W-ss)^3 \times 0.88$
1.0	0.80	0.64	0.88
1.1	1.06	0.85	1.17
1.2	1.38	1.11	1.52
1.3	1.76	1.41	1.93
1.4	2.20	1.76	2.41
1.5	2.70	2.16	2.97
1.6	3.28	2.62	3.60
1.7	3.93	3.14	4.32
1.8	4.67	3.73	5.13
1.9	5.49	4.39	6.04
2.0	6.40	5.12	7.04
2.1	7.41	5.93	8.15
2.2	8.52	6.81	9.37
2.3	9.73	7.79	10.71
2.4	11.06	8.85	12.17
2.5	12.50	10.00	13.75
2.6	14.06	11.25	15.47
2.7	15.75	12.60	17.32
2.8	17.56	14.05	19.32
2.9	19.51	15.61	21.46
3.0	21.60	17.28	23.76
3.1	23.83	19.07	26.22
3.2	26.21	20.97	28.84
3.3	28.75	23.00	31.62

Legend: Volumes expected from different widths of the testis depending on the formulas used, which could be helpful to assess differential volumes.

adults, more commonly (85 to 95%) in the left scrotum. The varicocele may lead to testicular asymmetry from an arrest of growth of the testis in adolescents and to testicular atrophy in adults, thought to result from apoptosis of Sertoli cells owing to increased temperature from blood. Small size discrepancy may occur normally without varicocele.

There are no clear guidelines established for treatment of a varicocele. Most varicoceles in adolescents are managed conservatively with observation. Surgical ligation of the spermatic vein, however, is usually indicated for adolescents who demonstrate retarded growth of the left testis and in young men who develop testicular atrophy [1-3]. The discrepancy of testicular volumes is the main criterion for performing surgery and may be assessed by ultrasound [4]. At times there is no asymmetry and the levels of FSH and LH may be helpful to identify patients who need surgical treatment [5]. One can easily see,

looking at the table, the volume change expected from the difference of 1, 2, or 3, mm in the width. A difference of 3 mm in the width should easily be detected by the same observer (i.e. 2.0 cm to 2.3 or 2.3 to 2.6).

Appendix B. References

1. Costabile RA, Skoog S, Radowich M. Testicular volume assessment in the adolescent with a varicocele. *J Urol.* 1992, 147(5):1348-50.
2. Paduch DA, Niedzielski J. Repair versus observation in adolescent varicocele: a prospective study. *J Urol.* 1997, 158(3 Pt 2):1128-32.
3. Sayfan J, Siplovich L, Koltun L, Benyamin N. Varicocele treatment in pubertal boys prevents testicular growth arrest. *J Urol.* 1997, 157(4):1456-7.
4. Diamond DA, Paltiel HJ, DiCanzio J, Zurakowski D, Bauer SB, Atala A, Ephraim PL, Grant R, Retik AB. Comparative assessment of pediatric testicular volume: orchidometer versus ultrasound. *J Urol.* 2000, 164(3 Pt 2):1111-4.
5. Guarino N, Tadini B, Bianchi M. The adolescent varicocele: the crucial role of hormonal tests in selecting patients with testicular dysfunction. *J Pediatr Surg.* 2003, 38(1):120-3.

Competing interests
The authors declare that they have no competing interests.

Authors' contributions
JFS contributed to conception and design, acquisition of data, analysis and interpretation of data. NJT contributed to collection, analysis and presentation of data. Both contributed to the drafting of the manuscript and the final version.

Acknowledgements
Our appreciation to Dr. Robert Hoffman for the review of the article and helpful suggestions and to Dr. Jennifer Klima, PhD, for the review of the statistical analysis and helpful recommendations.

References
1. Schonfeld WA, Beebe GW: **Normal growth and variation in the male genitalia from birth to maturity.** *J Urol* 1942, **48:**759–777.
2. Hansen PF, With TK: **Clinical measurements of the testes in boys and men.** *Acta Med Scand Suppl* 1952, **266:**457–65.
3. Rundle AT, Sylvester PE: **Measurement of testicular volume. Its application to assessment of maturation, and its use in diagnosis of hypogonadism.** *Arch Dis Child* 1962, **37:**514–7.
4. Behre HM, Nashan D, Nieschlag E: **Objective measurement of testicular volume by ultrasonography: evaluation of the technique and comparison with orchidometer estimates.** *Int J Androl* 1989, **12**(6):395–403.
5. Tomova A, Deepinder F, Robeva R, Lalabonova H, Kumanov P, Agarwal A: **Growth and development of male external genitalia: a cross-sectional study of 6200 males aged 0 to 19 years.** *Arch Pediatr Adolesc Med* 2010, **164**(12):1152–7.
6. Osemlak P: **Size of testes and epididymes in boys up to 17 years of life assessed by ultrasound method and method of external linear measurements.** *Med Wieku Rozwoj* 2011, **15**(1):39–55.
7. Goede J, Hack WW, Sijstermans K, van der Voort-Doedens LM, Van der Ploeg T, Meij-de Vries A, de Waal HA Delemarre-van: **Normative values for**

testicular volume measured by ultrasonography in a normal population from infancy to adolescence. *Horm Res Paediatr* 2011, **76**(1):56–64.

8. Sakamoto H, Yajima T, Nagata M, Okumura T, Suzuki K, Ogawa Y: **Relationship between testicular size by ultrasonography and testicular function: measurement of testicular length, width, and depth in patients with infertility.** *Int J Urol* 2008, **15**(6):529–33.

9. Prader A: **Testicular size: assessment and clinical importance.** *Triangle* 1966, **7**(6):240–3.

10. Zachmann M, Prader A, Kind HP, Häfliger H, Budliger H: **Testicular volume during adolescence. Cross-sectional and longitudinal studies.** *Helv Paediatr Acta* 1974, **29**(1):61–72.

11. Nahoum CR: **A new orchidometer.** *Arch Androl* 1978, **1**(4):355–9.

12. Takihara H, Sakatoku J, Fujii M, Nasu T, Cosentino MJ, Cockett AT: **Significance of testicular size measurement in andrology. I. A new orchiometer and its clinical application.** *Fertil Steril* 1983, **39**(6):836–40.

13. Rivkees SA, Hall DA, Boepple PA, Crawford JD: **Accuracy and reproducibility of clinical measures of testicular volume.** *J Pediatr* 1987, **110**(6):914–7.

14. Diamond DA, Paltiel HJ, DiCanzio J, Zurakowski D, Bauer SB, Atala A, Ephraim PL, Grant R, Retik AB: **Comparative assessment of pediatric testicular volume: orchidometer versus ultrasound.** *J Urol* 2000, **164**(3 Pt 2):1111–4.

15. Fuse H, Takahara M, Ishii H, Sumiya H, Shimazaki J: **Measurement of testicular volume by ultrasonography.** *Int J Androl* 1990, **13**(4):267–72.

16. al Salim A, Murchison PJ, Rana A, Elton RA, Hargreave TB: **Evaluation of testicular volume by three orchidometers compared with ultrasonographic measurements.** *Br J Urol* 1995, **76**(5):632–5.

17. Sakamoto H, Saito K, Ogawa Y, Yoshida H: **Testicular volume measurements using Prader orchidometer versus ultrasonography in patients with infertility.** *Urology* 2007, **69**(1):158–62.

18. Lambert B: **The frequency of mumps and of mumps orchitis and the consequences for sexuality and fertility.** *Acta Genet Stat Med* 1951, **2**(Suppl. 1):1–166.

19. Paltiel HJ, Diamond DA, Di Canzio J, Zurakowski D, Borer JG, Atala A: **Testicular volume: comparison of orchidometer and US measurements in dogs.** *Radiology* 2002, **222**(1):114–9.

20. Sakamoto H, Saito K, Oohta M, Inoue K, Ogawa Y, Yoshida H: **Testicular volume measurement: comparison of ultrasonography, orchidometry, and water displacement.** *Urology* 2007, **69**(1):152–7.

21. Kuijper EA, van Kooten J, Verbeke JI, van Rooijen M, Lambalk CB: **Ultrasonographically measured testicular volumes in 0- to 6-year-old boys.** *Hum Reprod* 2008, **23**(4):792–6. Epub 2008 Feb 15.

22. Bahk JY, Jung JH, Jin LM, Min SK: **Cut-off value of testes volume in young adults and correlation among testes volume, body mass index, hormonal level, and seminal profiles.** *Urology* 2010, **75**(6):1318–23.

5

Fulvestrant treatment of precocious puberty in girls with McCune-Albright syndrome

Emily K Sims[1*], Sally Garnett[2], Franco Guzman[3], Françoise Paris[4], Charles Sultan[4] and Erica A Eugster[1]
On behalf of the fulvestrant McCune-Albright study group

Abstract

Background: McCune-Albright Syndrome (MAS) is usually characterized by the triad of precocious puberty (PP), fibrous dysplasia, and café au lait spots. Previous treatments investigated for PP have included aromatase inhibitors and the estrogen receptor modulator, tamoxifen. Although some agents have been partially effective, the optimal pharmacologic treatment of PP in girls with MAS has not been identified. The objective of this study was to evaluate the safety and efficacy of fulvestrant (Faslodex™), a pure estrogen receptor antagonist, in girls with progressive precocious puberty (PP) associated with McCune-Albright Syndrome (MAS).

Methods: In this prospective international multicenter trial, thirty girls ≤ 10 years old with MAS and progressive PP received fulvestrant 4 mg/kg via monthly intramuscular injections for 12 months. Changes in vaginal bleeding, rates of bone age advancement, growth velocity, Tanner staging, predicted adult heights, and uterine and ovarian volumes were measured.

Results: Median vaginal bleeding days decreased from 12.0 days per year to 1.0 day per year, with a median change in frequency of -3.6 days, (95% confidence interval (CI) -10.10, 0.00; p = 0.0146). Of patients with baseline bleeding, 74% experienced a ≥50% reduction in bleeding, and 35% experienced complete cessation during the study period (95% CI 51.6%, 89.8%; 16.4%, 57.3%, respectively). Average rates of bone age advancement (ΔBA/ΔCA) decreased from 1.99 pre-treatment to 1.06 on treatment (mean change -0.93, 95% CI -1.43, -0.43; p = 0.0007). No significant changes in uterine volumes or other endpoints or serious adverse events occurred.

Conclusions: Fulvestrant was well tolerated and moderately effective in decreasing vaginal bleeding and rates of skeletal maturation in girls with MAS. Longer-term studies aimed at further defining potential benefits and risks of this novel therapeutic approach in girls with MAS are needed.

Keywords: McCune Albright syndrome, Peripheral precocious puberty, Estrogen receptor antagonist

Background

McCune-Albright syndrome (MAS) is characterized by the triad of peripheral precocious puberty (PP), fibrous dysplasia of bone, and café au lait spots [1,2]. This disorder develops secondary to a post-zygotic gain of function mutation in the gene encoding the alpha subunit of the heterotrimeric G-protein (Gsα) on chromosome 20, resulting in constitutive activation in affected cells [3,4].

PP, the most common manifestation of MAS, is diagnosed more frequently in girls than boys [5]. Autonomous activation of ovarian tissue leads to intermittent development of ovarian cysts, resulting in vaginal bleeding upon resolution and subsequent estrogen withdrawal [5,6]. A subset of girls develop progressive PP marked by recurrent vaginal bleeding, increased breast development, accelerated growth velocity, and bone age (BA) advancement with the potential for significant compromise in adult height [5]. Although the PP in MAS is gonadotropin independent, secondary activation of the hypothalamic-pituitary-gonadal axis may occur, resulting in concurrent central precocious puberty (CPP) [7].

* Correspondence: eksims@iupui.edu
[1]Section of Pediatric Endocrinology/Diabetology, Riley Hospital for Children, Indiana University School of Medicine, 705 Riley Hospital Drive, Room 5960, Indianapolis, IN 46202, USA
Full list of author information is available at the end of the article

Thus far, treatment options for PP in girls with MAS have met with mixed success. Fulvestrant (Faslodex[TM]) is a pure antiestrogen that binds to the estrogen receptor, triggering rapid degradation [8]. The objective of our study was to evaluate the safety and efficacy of fulvestrant in girls with progressive PP associated with MAS.

Methods

This international prospective open-label trial recruited girls from 15 centers and was approved by an Institutional Review Board at each site. Because of the rarity of MAS, a study based on formal power calculations was not feasible. However, based on a similar AstraZeneca study evaluating tamoxifen in this population, an assumed proportion of 0.67 patients with a ≥ 50% reduction in vaginal episodes was used to determine that a group of 20 patients would generate a 95% confidence interval (CI) of 0.46-0.87 [9]. Thus, 30 patients were recruited with the goal of having 20 patients complete 12 months of treatment. Inclusion criteria included age ≤ 10 years at the start of therapy, and a diagnosis of MAS and progressive PP (onset before 8 years of age) made by a pediatric endocrinologist. MAS was diagnosed based on the presence of PP combined with café au lait spots, fibrous dysplasia, or a documented Gsα mutation. Subjects had clinical evidence of pubertal progression along with BA advancement (BA ≥ 12 months above chronologic age) or growth velocity > 2 standard deviations (SD) above the mean for age. Previously treated patients must have had documented progression on treatment with a 1 month washout period, or have stopped treatment for 6 months with subsequent progression of disease. Patients with CPP must have received at least 6 months of treatment with a gonadotropin-releasing hormone analog (GnRHa). Written informed consent of all parents/legal guardians and patient assent as locally required was obtained.

Patients were excluded if they had previously received fulvestrant, were currently receiving treatment for peripheral PP, had liver function tests ≥ 3 times the upper limit of normal, an International Normalized Ratio (INR) > 1.6, a history of bleeding diathesis or long-term anticoagulation, any severe comorbidities, or known hypersensitivity to any component of the study drug product.

Initial assessment occurred at a screening visit, followed by 13 monthly visits. Six months of pre-treatment data, including height, weight, Tanner stage, BA, and parental recall of vaginal bleeding history, were retrospectively reviewed. Physical exam including Tanner staging for breasts and pubic hair was performed at screening and at the 0, 3, 6, and 12 month visits.

BA radiographs were obtained at baseline, 6 and 12 months. Rate of skeletal maturation was defined as the change in BA divided by the change in chronological age. Pre-treatment BAs obtained at a minimum of 6 and maximum of 15 months apart were used to determine pre-treatment rates of skeletal maturation. Predicted adult heights (PAHs) were calculated based on the method of Bayley and Pinneau for patients 6 years or older. Vaginal bleeding data were obtained from patient diaries and reviewed monthly. Any missing days on diary cards were reported as bleeding days. Pelvic ultrasounds were obtained at the screening, 6 month, and 12 month visits. All radiographs were centrally read at Lifespan Health Research Center, at Wright State University, in Kettering, Ohio and all ultrasounds were read at Bio Clinica Inc., in Newton, Pennsylvania. Radiologists were blinded to patient diagnosis.

Chemiluminescent serum estradiol, testosterone, luteinizing hormone (LH), and follicle stimulating hormone (FSH) assays were obtained at screening and at 3, 6, and 12 months. Thyroxine and thyrotropin levels were drawn at baseline. Complete blood count, INR, alanine aminotransferase, and aspartate transaminase levels were obtained during screening. Liver function tests were repeated at the last visit. Laboratory assays were performed by Quintiles Laboratories North America (Marietta, GA).

The dose of fulvestrant was derived from studies in breast cancer patients, and was initiated at 2 mg/kg via monthly intramuscular injections in the first 10 patients [10]. Based on pharmacokinetics from the first 6 patients, the dose was increased to 4 mg/kg injections monthly, which corresponds to a dose of 250 mg/month in adult patients. All remaining patients received this dose for the entire study period. At 2 different time points between the 6 and 12 month visits, serum trough levels of medication were obtained to ensure that steady state drug concentrations were similar to those of patients in the breast cancer studies. Participants who completed the study were offered the option of continuing on treatment for an extension period with yearly data collection.

Intention-to-treat as well as per-protocol statistical analyses were performed. Results from both evaluations were consistent and so outcomes of the intention-to-treat analysis are reported. Analysis of hormone changes was performed retrospectively. For continuous efficacy endpoints with normal distributions, the mean changes from baseline to the treatment period were analyzed using the 2-sided paired t-test at the 5% level of significance, with a 95% CI using SAS PROC MEANS. A Signed rank test or a Sign test was used to analyze median changes (with SAS PROC UNIVARIATE) for endpoints with non-normal distributions. A distribution-free 95% CI of the median was obtained using SAS PROC UNIVARIATE with CIPCTLDF option. To evaluate the impact of outliers on BA advancement data, post-hoc analysis replacing the most extreme negative value with the second most extreme value was undertaken. No adjustments were made for multiple comparisons.

Results

A total of 30 girls aged 5.86 ± 1.8 years were enrolled, of whom 29 completed 12 months of treatment. All patients had at least 2 of the classic components of MAS, and all had evidence of progressive PP. Three girls were receiving a GnRHa at baseline. Four girls had received aromatase inhibitors in the past, and none had been treated with tamoxifen. Twenty-three (77%) had vaginal bleeding during the pre-study interval. Baseline as well as pretreatment participant characteristics are provided in Table 1.

Pharmacokinetic data revealed that patients on the 4 mg/kg dose reached steady-state serum concentrations consistent with patients effectively treated with fulvestrant for breast cancer. The mean serum half-life of the drug was 70.4 ± 8.1 days.

Median vaginal bleeding days on treatment decreased from 12.0 days per year to 1.0 day per year, with a median change in frequency of -3.6 days (p = 0.0146). Of the patients with baseline bleeding, 17 (74%) experienced a ≥50% reduction in bleeding, and 8 (35%) experienced complete cessation during the year of study (CI 51.6%, 89.8%; 16.4%, 57.3%, respectively). One patient was withdrawn due to worsening of her condition after receiving 6 injections. Figure 1 depicts individual changes in vaginal bleeding.

Average rates of BA advancement decreased from 1.99 at baseline to 1.06 after 12 months of treatment, a difference of 0.93 ± 1.3 (95% CI -1.43, -0.43; p = 0.0007), when

Table 1 Baseline patient demographics (n = 30)

Mean age ± SD (range)	5.86 years ± 1.8 (1.7-8.5)
Ethnicity	
White	26 (87%)
Biracial	2 (7%)
Black	1 (3%)
Hispanic	1 (3%)
Polyostotic fibrous dysplasia (n)	21 (70.0%)
Café au lait spots (n)	24 (80.0%)
Confirmed Gsα mutation (n)	7 (23.3%)
Vaginal bleeding during 6 months pre-treatment (n)	23 (76.7%)
Median Tanner Stage for breasts (range)	III (I-IV)
Median Tanner Stage for pubic hair (range)	I (I-IV)
Mean growth velocity Z-score ± SD during 6 months prior to study	2.35 ± 3.3

SD-standard deviation.

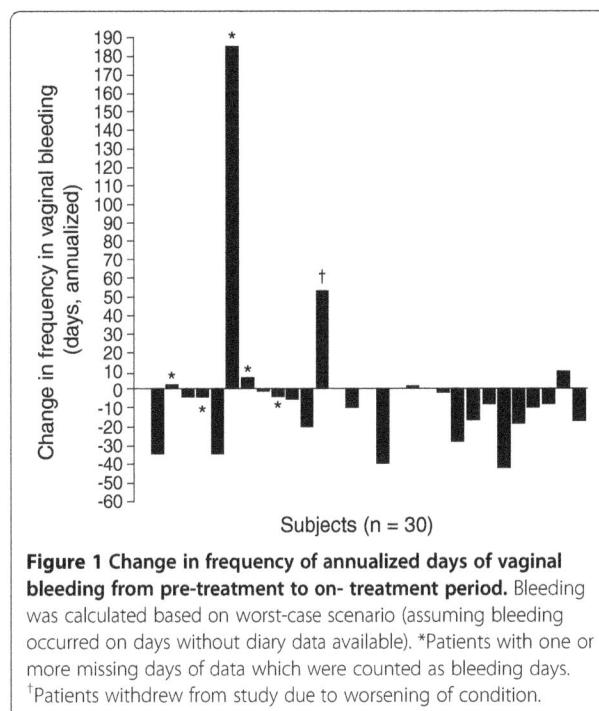

Figure 1 Change in frequency of annualized days of vaginal bleeding from pre-treatment to on- treatment period. Bleeding was calculated based on worst-case scenario (assuming bleeding occurred on days without diary data available). *Patients with one or more missing days of data which were counted as bleeding days. †Patients withdrew from study due to worsening of condition.

compared with the pre-treatment interval. Furthermore, this was progressive, as the mean BA advancement over the first 6 months of treatment decreased by 0.83 compared to pretreatment (95% CI -1.39, -0.26; p =0.005), while over the second 6 months, a more substantial decrease of 1.10 was seen (95% CI -1.63, -0.58; p = 0.0002). Individual changes in skeletal maturation are illustrated in Figure 2. No statistically significant difference was seen in mean growth velocity z-scores during treatment compared with the pre-treatment interval (mean change -1.14, 95% CI -2.67, 0.38; p = 0.135). Mean PAHs before and after treatment were equivalent (163.0 ± 6.9 cm vs. 163.5 ± 6.3 cm).

Hormone levels are presented in Table 2. Patients experienced a significant decrease in LH on treatment, with a median difference of 0.35 IU/L from baseline to 12 months (CI 0, 0.8; p < 0.005). No girls developed CPP during the study period. Mean uterine volume at baseline was 8.2 ± 5.0 ml, corresponding to a pubertal size. No significant difference was seen in uterine size during the 12 months of study. No significant changes in other hormones, Tanner staging, ovarian cysts, or ovarian volumes were seen throughout the study period.

Fulvestrant was generally well tolerated. Seven patients reported injection site reactions that were typically short lived, but recurred in over half of cases. These included mild hematoma and rash as well as mild-moderate inflammation. Vomiting and abdominal pain possibly related to fulvestrant were each reported in 1 patient. No serious treatment-related adverse events occurred

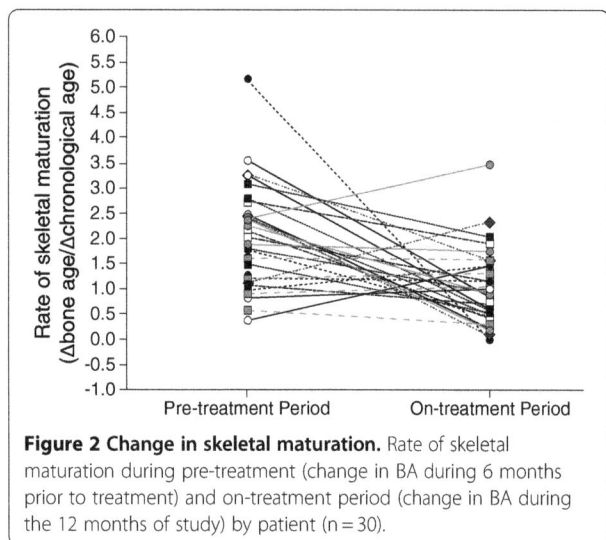

Figure 2 Change in skeletal maturation. Rate of skeletal maturation during pre-treatment (change in BA during 6 months prior to treatment) and on-treatment period (change in BA during the 12 months of study) by patient (n = 30).

and no patients discontinued the study secondary to adverse events. Of the 29 patients completing the study, 24 girls chose to enter the extension phase and continue treatment.

Discussion

The ideal treatment of PP in girls with MAS remains elusive. Medroxyprogesterone and cyproterone acetate can be effective for alleviation of vaginal bleeding, but have no effect on BA advancement [11,12]. Ketoconazole has been reported to result in cessation of bleeding and regression of secondary sexual characteristics in case studies, but lack of long-term data and concerns for risk

Table 2 Mean hormone levels

Hormone (units)	Visit	n	Mean ± SD	Median
Free thyroxine (pmol/L)	Screening	30	14.42 ± 2.53	14.65
Thyrotropin (mIU/L)	Screening	30	2.38 ± 3.30	1.53
Estradiol (pmol/L)	Screening	30	20.54 ± 25.59	9.18
	6 month visit	29	36.10 ± 104.95	9.18
	12 month visit	26	25.95 ± 30.72	9.55
LH (IU/L)*	Screening	30	0.84 ± 1.04	0.45
	6 month visit	29	0.10 ± 0.02	0.10
	12 month visit	28	0.11 ± 0.04	0.10
FSH (IU/L)	Screening	30	3.86 ± 5.42	1.95
	6 month visit	29	0.82 ± 0.78	0.50
	12 month visit	29	1.13 ± 1.02	0.60
Testosterone (nmol/L)	Screening	30	0.53 ± 0.19	0.48
	6 month visit	29	0.56 ± 0.24	0.45
	12 month visit	28	0.65 ± 0.27	0.66

Prepubertal normal ranges: free thyroxine 10.3-25.7 pmol/L; thyrotropin 0.7-6.4 mIU/L; estradiol < 73.4 pmol/L; LH 0.6-1.6 IU/L; FSH 0.7-6.7 IU/L; testosterone < 0.35-1.2 nmol/L.
* P < 0.005 for median change from baseline to month 12.

of adrenal insufficiency and hepatotoxicity have limited its use. Thus, recent interest has revolved around the use of antiestrogens [13-15].

Aromatase inhibitors (AIs) function by binding to the cytochrome P450 portion of aromatase, inhibiting the conversion of androgens to estrogens [16]. While this class of drugs initially showed promise in MAS, long-term studies of the first generation AI testolactone revealed no significant improvement in skeletal maturation [16-18]. Later generation agents with increased potency have similarly failed to indicate significant benefit in prospective trials, with the exception of letrozole [19-21]. While this third generation AI did have a positive effect on indices of PP in a small study, an increase in mean ovarian volumes and occurrence of ovarian torsion in one patient have raised concerns regarding the safety of this drug [21].

Tamoxifen, a selective estrogen receptor modulator widely used in breast cancer therapy, binds to the estrogen receptor and only partially triggers the normal activating sequence, thereby attenuating transcription [8]. While a prospective study of this medication in girls with MAS and PP demonstrated decreases in vaginal bleeding, growth velocities, and skeletal maturation, a progressive increase in uterine volume was observed during the treatment period [9]. Although the significance of this finding remains unknown, it is of concern given previous links to endometrial stromal tumor development in women undergoing tamoxifen therapy [22].

Fulvestrant was also developed as a treatment for breast cancer subsequent to its effects at the level of the estrogen receptor. Because of its purely antagonistic properties, the partial estrogen agonistic actions seen with tamoxifen should hypothetically be avoided [8]. This was supported by lack in changes in uterine or ovarian dimensions on treatment. To our knowledge, no previous reports utilizing fulvestrant in pediatric patients exist. This study demonstrated that fulvestrant significantly decreased vaginal bleeding and reduced rates of skeletal maturation to near normal in this population. However, complete cessation of vaginal bleeding occurred in only a third of subjects, and no significant change in growth velocity or PAH was seen. A progressive decrease in BA advancement with drug exposure supports that a longer treatment interval might improve these parameters. The etiology for the observed decrease in LH levels is unclear, but may have been temporally related to episodic autonomous ovarian activation, which would not be expected to be altered by fulvestrant.

There are several limitations to our study. Because of the rarity of MAS, each girl served as her own control. However, the inclusion of multiple centers enabled a reasonable sample size and generated statistically significant results. A conservative, worst-case scenario approach was applied to missing data for vaginal bleeding diaries that could potentially underestimate the benefits of treatment. Pre-treatment vaginal bleeding data was collected retrospectively and therefore may not have been as accurate as data collected during the treatment period. Conversely, concurrent MAS-related endocrinopathies and skeletal deformities resulting from fibrous dysplasia could have affected growth velocities, rates of skeletal maturation, and accuracy of height measurements. The lack of change in growth velocities and PAH could reflect an insufficient treatment interval or other aspects of MAS unrelated to PP.

Conclusion

In conclusion, fulvestrant was moderately effective in decreasing vaginal bleeding and rates of skeletal maturation in girls with progressive PP secondary to MAS over a 1 year period. The medication was well tolerated. Longer follow-up of patients receiving treatment will be necessary in order to confirm these results.

Abbreviations

PP: Precocious puberty; MAS: McCune-Albright Syndrome; CI: Confidence interval; Gsα: Alpha subunit of the heterotrimeric G-protein; BA: Bone age; CPP: Central precocious puberty; SD: Standard deviation; GnRHa: Gonadotropin-releasing hormone analog; INR: International normalized ratio; PAH: Predicted adult height; LH: Luteinizing hormone; FSH: Follicle stimulating hormone; AI: Aromatase inhibitor.

Competing interests

This study was supported by AstraZeneca and involves off-label use of fulvestrant for the treatment of precocious puberty in girls with McCune-Albright syndrome. The role of the sponsor involved an AstraZeneca statistician participating in analysis of the study data and approval of the final manuscript. EKS, FP and CS have no conflicts of interest to declare. EAE has served as a consultant for AstraZeneca, and reports this as a potential conflict of interest. SG is currently employed by AstraZeneca and FG is a former employee, and these authors report these roles as potential conflicts of interest.

Authors' contributions

EKS participated in analysis and interpretation of the data, wrote the first draft of the manuscript, revised the manuscript for intellectual content, and approved the final manuscript as submitted. SG analyzed the data, participated in the revision of the manuscript, and approved the final manuscript as submitted. FG participated in the design of the study and coordination of study results, analyzed the data, revised the manuscript for intellectual content, and approved the final manuscript as submitted. FP participated in interpretation of the data, revised the manuscript for intellectual content, and approved the final manuscript as submitted. CS participated in interpretation of the data, revised the manuscript for intellectual content, and approved the final manuscript as submitted. EAE participated in interpretation of the data, revised the manuscript for intellectual content, and approved the final manuscript as submitted. All authors read and approved the final manuscript.

Acknowledgments

The following investigators participated in this study: Professor Norbert Albers, M.D. (Kinderhospital, Osnabrueck, Germany); Professor Yong Bao (University of Miami, Miami, FL); Pascal Barat, M.D. (Hôpital des Enfants, Bordeaux cedex, France); Caroline Brain, M.D. (Great Ormond Street Hospital for Children, London, UK); Mohammed Didi, M.D. (Alder Hey Children's NHS Foundation Trust, Liverpool, UK); Professor Helmuth-Guenther Doerr, M.D. (Kinderk-und Jugendklinik der Universita et Erlangen-Nuernberg, Erlangen, Germany); Professor Carol Foster (University of Utah, Salt Lake City, UT); Adda Grimberg, M.D. (The Children's Hospital of Philadelphia, Philadelphia, PA); Muriel Houang, M.D. (Hôpital Armand Trousseau, Paris, France); Roberto Lala, M.D. (Ospedal Infantile Regina Margherita, Torino, Italy); Jefferson Lomenick, M.D. (University of Kentucky, Lexington, KY); Chantal Lutfallah, M.D. (Our Lady of the Lake Regional Medical Center, Baton Rouge, LA); Kenneth McCormick, M.D. (UAB, Birmingham, AL); Professor Marc Nicolino (Hôpital Mère-Enfant de Lyon, Bron Cedex, France); Professor Valentina Peterkova (Institute of Pediatric Endocrinology Research Center, Moscow, Russia); Professor Michel Polak (Hopital Arnaud de Villeneuvel, Montpellier, France); and Professor Ping Zhou (Children's Hospital at Montefiore Medical Center, Bronx, NY).

Author details

[1]Section of Pediatric Endocrinology/Diabetology, Riley Hospital for Children, Indiana University School of Medicine, 705 Riley Hospital Drive, Room 5960, Indianapolis, IN 46202, USA. [2]AstraZeneca, Macclesfield, United Kingdom. [3]Former-AstraZeneca, Wilmington, Delaware, USA. [4]Pediatric Gynecology and Endocrinology, University Hospital of Montpellier, Montpellier, France.

References

1. McCune D: Osteitis fibrosa cystica; the case of a nine year old girl who also exhibits precocious puberty, multiple pigmentation of the skin and hyperthyroidism. *Am J Dis Child* 1936, **52**:743–744.
2. Albright F, Butler AM, Hampton AO, Smith P: Syndrome characterized by osteitis fibrosa disseminata, areas of pigmentation and endocrine dysfunction, with precocious puberty in females: report of five cases. *N Engl J Med* 1937, **216**:727–776.
3. Weinstein LS, Shenker A, Gejman PV, Merino MJ, Friedman E, Spiegel AM: Activating mutations of the stimulatory G protein in the McCune-Albright syndrome. *N Engl J Med* 1991, **325**(24):1688–1695.
4. Happle R: The McCune-Albright syndrome: a lethal gene surviving by mosaicism. *Clin Genet* 1986, **29**(4):321–324.
5. Haddad N, Eugster E: An update on the treatment of precocious puberty in McCune-Albright syndrome and testotoxicosis. *J Pediatr Endocrinol Metab* 2007, **20**(6):653–661.
6. Foster CM, Feuillan P, Padmanabhan V, Pescovitz OH, Beitins IZ, Comite F, Shawker TH, Loriaux DL, Cutler GB Jr: Ovarian function in girls with McCune-Albright syndrome. *Pediatr Res* 1986, **20**(9):859–863.
7. Kaufman FR, Costin G, Reid BS: Autonomous ovarian hyperfunction followed by gonadotrophin-dependent puberty in McCune-Albright syndrome. *Clin Endocrinol (Oxf)* 1986, **24**(3):239–242.
8. Howell A, Osborne CK, Morris C, Wakeling AE: ICI 182,780 (Faslodex): development of a novel, "pure" antiestrogen. *Cancer* 2000, **89**(4):817–825.
9. Eugster EA, Rubin SD, Reiter EO, Plourde P, Jou HC, Pescovitz OH: Tamoxifen treatment for precocious puberty in McCune-Albright syndrome: a multicenter trial. *J Pediatr* 2003, **143**(1):60–66.
10. Osborne CK, Pippen J, Jones SE, Parker LM, Ellis M, Come S, Gertler SZ, May JT, Burton G, Dimery I, et al: Double-blind, randomized trial comparing the efficacy and tolerability of fulvestrant versus anastrozole in postmenopausal women with advanced breast cancer progressing on prior endocrine therapy: results of a North American trial. *J Clin Oncol* 2002, **20**(16):3386–3395.
11. Rao S, Colaco MP, Desai MP: McCune Albright Syndrome (MCAS): a case series. *Indian Pediatr* 2003, **40**(1):29–35.
12. Sorgo W, Kiraly E, Homoki J, Heinze E, Teller WM, Bierich JR, Moeller H, Ranke MB, Butenandt O, Knorr D: The effects of cyproterone acetate on statural growth in children with precocious puberty. *Acta Endocrinol (Copenh)* 1987, **115**(1):44–56.
13. Syed FA, Chalew SA: Ketoconazole treatment of gonadotropin independent precocious puberty in girls with McCune-Albright syndrome: a preliminary report. *J Pediatr Endocrinol Metab* 1999, **12**(1):81–83.
14. Janssen PA, Symoens JE: Hepatic reactions during ketoconazole treatment. *Am J Med* 1983, **74**(1B):80–85.
15. Sarver RG, Dalkin BL, Ahmann FR: Ketoconazole-induced adrenal crisis in a patient with metastatic prostatic adenocarcinoma: case report and review of the literature. *Urology* 1997, **49**(5):781–785.

16. Shulman DI, Francis GL, Palmert MR, Eugster EA: Use of aromatase inhibitors in children and adolescents with disorders of growth and adolescent development. *Pediatrics* 2008, **121**(4):e975–e983.

17. Feuillan PP, Foster CM, Pescovitz OH, Hench KD, Shawker T, Dwyer A, Malley JD, Barnes K, Loriaux DL, Cutler GB Jr: Treatment of precocious puberty in the McCune-Albright syndrome with the aromatase inhibitor testolactone. *N Engl J Med* 1986, **315**(18):1115–1119.

18. Feuillan PP, Jones J, Cutler GB Jr: Long-term testolactone therapy for precocious puberty in girls with the McCune-Albright syndrome. *J Clin Endocrinol Metab* 1993, **77**(3):647–651.

19. Nunez SB, Calis K, Cutler GB Jr, Jones J, Feuillan PP: Lack of efficacy of fadrozole in treating precocious puberty in girls with the McCune-Albright syndrome. *J Clin Endocrinol Metab* 2003, **88**(12):5730–5733.

20. Mieszczak J, Lowe ES, Plourde P, Eugster EA: The aromatase inhibitor anastrozole is ineffective in the treatment of precocious puberty in girls with McCune-Albright syndrome. *J Clin Endocrinol Metab* 2008, **93**(7):2751–2754.

21. Feuillan P, Calis K, Hill S, Shawker T, Robey PG, Collins MT: Letrozole treatment of precocious puberty in girls with the McCune-Albright syndrome: a pilot study. *J Clin Endocrinol Metab* 2007, **92**(6):2100–2106.

22. Treilleux T, Mignotte H, Clement-Chassagne C, Guastalla P, Bailly C: Tamoxifen and malignant epithelial-nonepithelial tumours of the endometrium: report of six cases and review of the literature. *Eur J Surg Oncol* 1999, **25**(5):477–482.

6

Prader-Willi syndrome: A primer for clinicians

Mary Cataletto[1*], Moris Angulo[1], Gila Hertz[2] and Barbara Whitman[3]

Abstract

The advent of sensitive genetic testing modalities for the diagnosis of Prader-Willi syndrome has helped to define not only the phenotypic features of the syndrome associated with the various genotypes but also to anticipate clinical and psychological problems that occur at each stage during the life span. With advances in hormone replacement therapy, particularly growth hormone children born in circumstances where therapy is available are expected to have an improved quality of life as compared to those born prior to growth hormone.

This manuscript was prepared as a primer for clinicians-to serve as a resource for those of you who care for children and adults with Prader-Willi syndrome on a daily basis in your practices. Appropriate and anticipatory interventions can make a difference.

Introduction

First described by Prader, Labhart and Willi in 1956 [1], this syndrome represents the most common genetic cause of obesity with an estimated incidence of 1:15,000 to 1:25,000 live births [2,3]. Reported prevalence rates vary among countries but both sexes appear to be equally affected. Prader-Willi syndrome (PWS) is the first human syndrome identified with genomic imprinting [4]. The original descriptions of this syndrome included short stature, hypotonia, hypogonadism and mental retardation [1]. As infants grow to age 2-4 years, failure to thrive related, at least in part, to poor muscle tone and poor suck are replaced by increased appetite and food intake resulting in obesity and its comorbidities. Early diagnosis and intervention to prevent obesity and the associated complications are critical.

Genetic testing and genetic counseling

Candidate genes for Prader-Willi syndrome have been located on the long arm of chromosome 15q11-q13. These genes are physiologically imprinted and silenced on the maternally inherited chromosome. PWS arises when the paternally derived genes are missing, defective or silenced. The frequencies of each are shown in Table 1.

High resolution chromosomal analysis (HRCA) is done along with the fluorescence *in situ* hybridization

(FISH) to detect deletions and translocation of chromosome 15 [5]. Deletion has been divided in type I (TI) and II (TII) according to the size. Studies indicate that individuals with the TI (~500 kb larger than TII) generally have more behavioral and psychological problems than individuals with the TII and UPD [6]. Negative FISH or karyotype analysis does not exclude the diagnosis and thus if done first should be followed by DNA methylation analysis. DNA methylation analysis is the only technique which can both confirm and reject the diagnosis of PWS, and therefore should typically be the investigation of choice. This is most commonly done using DNA methylation-specific techniques at the *SNURF-SNRPN* locus [7,8]. If DNA methylation analysis shows only a maternal pattern, then PWS is confirmed. Further methods may then be performed to determine the genetic subtype and allow appropriate genetic counseling. DNA methylation analysis has a sensitivity exceeding 99%; however, it does not differentiate between deletion, UPD and imprinting defect. In order to distinguish a maternal UPD from an imprinting defect, further DNA polymorphism analysis should be performed on the proband and parents [9,10].

Most cases of Prader-Willi syndrome occur sporadically. The overall recurrence risk is dependent on the type of molecular defect. In families where the proband has either maternal disomy or deletion, the recurrence risk is small (less than 1%). Patients with an imprinting defect warrant further investigation in a specialized laboratory to determine whether an imprinting center deletion is present. Those families with a child with an

* Correspondence: mcataletto@winthrop.org
[1]The Prader-Willi Syndrome Center at Winthrop University Hospital, 120 Mineola Blvd.-Suite 210, Mineola, N.Y. 11501, USA
Full list of author information is available at the end of the article

Table 1 Frequency of genetic subtypes associated with PWS

Subtype	Frequency
Paternal deletion of chromosome 15q11-q13 (type I or II)	75%
Maternal uniparental disomy (UPD)	24%
Imprinting center defects (ID)	1%
Translocation	< 1%

imprinting center deletion have a recurrence risk of up to 50% if the father of the child is a carrier for the imprinting center deletion [11]. When a deletion is the result of a translocation or structural rearrangement involving chromosome 15, then the recurrence risk can be high. The actual risk in individual families depends upon the rearrangement which they carry. Overall, the risk of recurrence in the case of chromosomal translocations has been estimated up to 15%.

In the future the methylation-specific multiplex ligation PCR amplification may be more widely used because it has the advantage of combining dosing and DNA methylation analysis in one assay, thus distinguishing different subtypes [12].

Clinical Presentation

Infants with Prader-Willi syndrome present with neonatal hypotonia, hypoplasia of the clitoris/labia minora in girls and small penis and undescended testis in boys. Their hypotonia is associated with poor suck and feeding, often resulting in failure to thrive. Mothers may report decreased fetal activity and infants are often found in the breech position at the time of delivery. Clinical features include increased neonatal head:chest circumference ratio, narrow bifrontal diameter, dolichocephaly, almond shaped eyes, downturned angles of the mouth with abundant and thick saliva, small hands and feet with straight borders of the ulnar side of the hands and inner side of the legs. The presence of some of these features associated with neonatal hypotonia should alert physicians for early diagnosis of PWS during infancy. These features may become more prominent by age 2-3 years (Figures 1 and 2). Excessive eating and obsession with food generally begins in the preschool age group and will lead to morbid obesity if not controlled.

As these individuals age, manifestations, such as obesity, short stature, hypogonadism, skin picking, learning disabilities, behavioral and psychiatric problems become more evident. Consensus criteria for the clinical diagnosis of PWS were first established in 1993 by Holm et al [13]. These criteria were used until the introduction of the highly sensitive genetic testing, described above. Currently, these criteria are used as a screening tool for determining the need for further PWS specific genetic

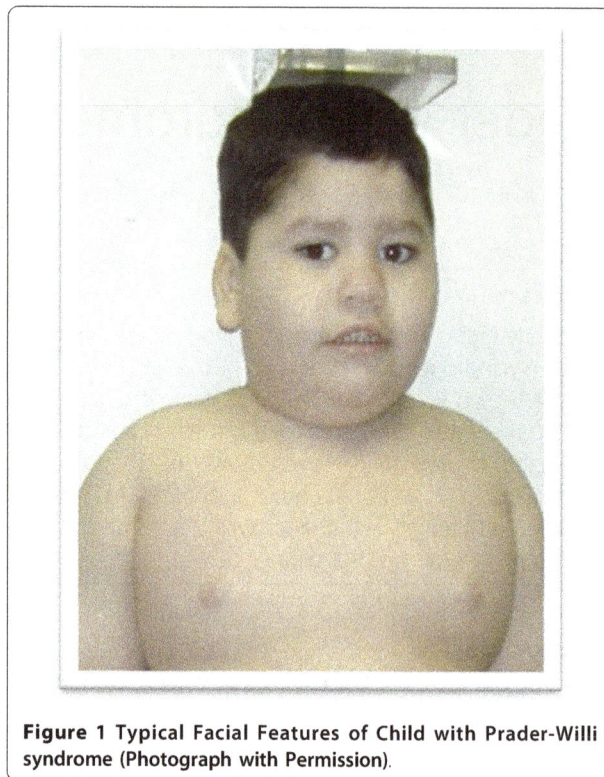

Figure 1 Typical Facial Features of Child with Prader-Willi syndrome (Photograph with Permission).

testing. In many infants poor cry and unexplained hypotonia may be the only clear clinical manifestations and indication for genetic testing.

As many as 16.7% of patients diagnosed with molecular testing do not meet these clinical diagnostic criteria, therefore a revised clinical criteria to help identify the appropriate patients for DNA testing was proposed in 2001 [14] and modified in 2008 [15]. See Table 2 for composite, including additional features suggested by authors.

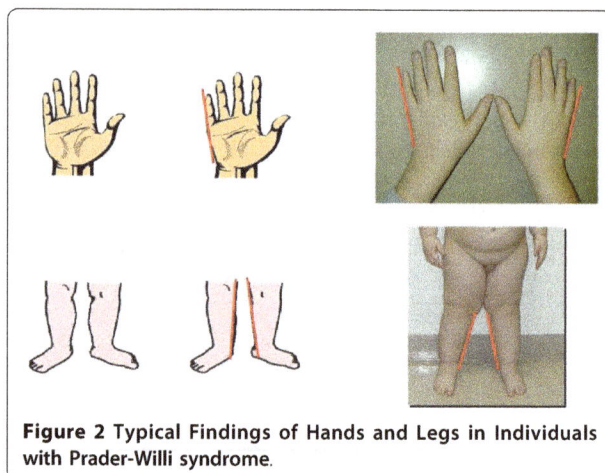

Figure 2 Typical Findings of Hands and Legs in Individuals with Prader-Willi syndrome.

Table 2 Indications for DNA testing

Age at assessment	Features sufficient to prompt DNA testing
Birth to 2 yr	Hypotonia with poor suck
2-6 yr	Hypotonia with a history of poor suck
	Global developmental delay
	Short stature and/or growth failure associated with accelerated weight gain
6-12 yr	Hypotonia with a history of poor suck (hypotonia often persists)
	Global developmental delay
	Excessive eating (hyperphagia, obsession with food) with central obesity if uncontrolled
	Short stature and/or decreased growth velocity*
13 yr through adulthood	Cognitive impairment, usually mild mental retardation
	Excessive eating (hyperphagia, obsession with food) with central obesity if uncontrolled
	Short stature and/or decreased growth velocity*
	Hypothalamic hypogonadism and/or typical behavior problems (including temper tantrums and obsessive-compulsive features)

*Features added by the authors

Endocrine Issues

Hypogonadism

Hypothalamic and pituitary dysfunction is most commonly manifested as hypogonadism, obesity and short stature. Hypogonadism with genital hypoplasia (cryptorchidism, scrotal or clitoral hypoplasia) can be identified in the newborn period. Cryptorchidism is present up to 86% of boys from birth [16,17] Undescended testes should be treated within the first year of life. There is evidence that early damage to the germ cells that produce sperm begins at this age. Scrotal hypoplasia and small penis however can make orchiopexy and circumcision difficult in infants with PWS. Repeat surgical interventions are frequently required, especially in those infants with underdeveloped scrotal sacs.

The most effective treatment for undescended testes is surgery. The Committee on Genetics, American Academy of Pediatrics however, recommends a therapeutic trial of human chorionic gonadotropin (hCG) for treatment of undescended testes before surgery, because avoidance of general anesthesia is desirable for infants with low muscle tone and potential for underlying respiratory compromise [18]. The precise mechanism of action in regards to testicular descent is unknown but benefits of a course of hCG may include increased scrotal size and partial normalization of phallus length, thereby improving surgical outcomes for undescended testes and facilitating later standing micturition.

Premature adrenarche (PA) is the precocious appearance of pubic and/or axillary hair and less commonly an apocrine odor, comedones, and acne without other signs of puberty or virilization. PA is usually seen before age 8 and 9 years, in girls and boys respectively. PA has been reported in 57% of children receiving GH therapy [19] but in general, pubertal development in PWS is characterized by normal adrenarche, pubertal arrest, and hypogonadism due to variable combinations of a unique primary gonadal defect and hypothalamic dysfunction [20,21].

At some stage almost all subjects will require sex hormone replacement therapy. Mental retardation should not be a contraindication to allow normal pubertal development or preclude sex hormone replacement at any age in those affected individuals. Regardless of body weight, patients with PWS have increased body fat content. Those individuals with low body weight or significant low sex hormone levels during adolescence and adulthood should be considered for sex hormone treatment. There is no consensus as to the most appropriate regimen for sex hormone replacement therapy in PWS. Intramuscular testosterone is given every 3 -4 weeks. Testosterone gel preparations can be useful in selected cases, although precautions must be taken to avoid cross-contamination. Whatever preparation is preferred, the initial dose should be one third to one half of the normally recommended androgen dose to prevent the aggressive behavior occasionally seen in some individuals. In females with PWS, the use of gonadal hormone replacement should be considered if there is amenorrhea/oligomenorrhea or decreased bone mineral density (BMD) in the presence of reduced estradiol levels. Hypogonadism is a common but not necessarily universal finding in adults with PWS [16,17]. Sexual counseling and contraceptive treatment should be used as appropriate, especially in the presence of complete sexual maturation, including regular menses. There are a few case reports of pregnancy in females with PWS [22,23]. Their cognitive dysfunction, social and emotional immaturity and the risk of Angelman syndrome in offspring of PWS deletion mothers prompt us to advise against pregnancy. At present there are no reports of paternity in PWS. Estrogen and androgen status should be monitored yearly during adolescence and adulthood and BMD assessed as indicated by dual-energy x-ray photon absorptiometry.

Adrenal insufficiency

When the pituitary begins to fail, there is generally a specific sequential failure of pituitary hormones, starting with growth hormone (GH), continuing through luteinizing (LH) and follicle stimulating hormone (FSH) deficiency, and culminating in the loss of thyrotropin stimulating hormone (TSH) and adrenocorticotropic hormone (ACTH). Generally ACTH is the last to be affected. Hypothalamic dysfunction is characteristic of individuals with PWS, therefore the clinical manifestations of pituitary hormone deficiency are expected. Short stature and hypogonadism, as a result of GH and gonadotropin (LH and FSH) deficiencies are seen in most individuals with this genetic syndrome. Under normal conditions the secretion of cortisol, the main adrenal glucocorticoid in humans is under the dominant control of pituitary ACTH. Clinical manifestations of adrenal insufficiency, however are uncommon in individuals with PWS.

The circadian peak serum cortisol usually occurs around 0800 hours. An extremely low basal serum cortisol at this time, below 100 nmol/liter (3.62 mcg/dl), may be assumed to demonstrate true cortisol deficiency [24]. However, levels at other times have little diagnostic utility. For this reason, various dynamic tests including insulin tolerance test (ITT), ACTH stimulation and metyrapone test have been devised to assess whether the patient can provide a stress-induced rise in cortisol similar to a normal person. The insulin tolerance test evaluates the integrity of the entire hypothalamic-pituitary axis (HPA) by inducing symptomatic and biochemical hypoglycemia, with cortisol then measured over 120 minutes. Peak cortisol values greater than 550 nmol/liter (19.75 mcg/dl) is considered a normal response. Under supervision by a nurse or physician, the ITT (0.15 U/kg administered intravenously (IV) is relatively safe [24]. The GH reserve can also be estimated with ITT.

Due to the relative inconvenience of the ITT, suggestions have been made to use a simpler and less invasive surrogate. The most widely performed is the short ACTH (Cortrosyn ™) stimulation test, where ACTH 0.25 mg is injected IV or IM and serum cortisol is measure at 0, 30 and 60 minutes. A peak cortisol is defined as normal if it is greater than 550 nmol/liter (19.75 mcg/dl) at any of these time points.

In 2008 a study using the overnight metyrapone test reported a 60% prevalence of central adrenal insufficiency (CAI) in children with PWS [25]. Based on the high prevalence of CAI, the authors suggested treatment with hydrocortisone during acute illness in patients with PWS unless CAI has recently been ruled out with a metyrapone test. ITT, as the gold standard dynamic test suggests that metyrapone test with an ACTH cut off of 33 pmol/l yields a high false positive rate. In our experience in the PWS center at Winthrop University Hospital, New York, we have not found any abnormal response to ITT or low cortisol levels during surgical stress of different natures. Three recent studies using a more sensitive stimulation and spontaneous acute stress in larger numbers of patients did not find high prevalence of central adrenal insufficiency in Prader-Willi syndrome [26-28]. Thus rather than common, CAI seems to be a rare event in children and adults with PWS, however, they should be evaluated and treated accordingly.

Growth & Growth hormone deficiency

Length in newborns with PWS is normal but there is significant decrease in growth velocity after age 2-3 years with final adult height ~ 2 standard deviations (SD) below the mean for the normal population [29-31]. Only a small percentage of children with PWS are GH sufficient, thus provocative testing is not required in the face of reduced growth velocity.

Multiple studies have documented the benefits of GH therapy in individuals with PWS including, but not limited to, improvements in lean body mass, decreased body fat, increased bone mineral density, and normalization of adult height [19,32-37]. The benefits of starting GH treatment as early as age 2 years are well established, but there is increasing evidence of additional benefit to starting therapy between ages 6-12 months, particularly in terms of motor development, muscle, head circumference, and possibly cognition [35-38].

It should be stressed that GH therapy should be used in conjunction with appropriate nutritional intake and physical activity. GH treatment should not be viewed as a substitute for diet and exercise. Treatment should commence using standard dose guidelines (0.18-0.3 mg/kg/week), given as a daily subcutaneous injection with careful monitoring of clinical status at regular intervals. Careful history and assessment of nutritional status, scoliosis, respiratory and sleep abnormalities should be evaluated prior to and during GH therapy.

Recent studies indicate that adults with Prader-Willi syndrome may also benefit from GH replacement therapy, with improvements in body composition, bone mineral density, exercise capacity, quality of life and well-being [39-45]. Treatment doses are typically started at 0.2 mg/day and increased by 0.2 mg increments as necessary to maintain IGF-1 levels within the normal range for age and gender. At the present time, documentation of GH deficiency by provocative testing is required for adults with PWS to receive insurance authorization for GH treatment in the United States. These patients should be monitored with IGF-1, glucose, insulin, lipid profile, BMD and cardiac evaluation during GH treatment [46].

Central hypothyroidism as a result of hypothalamic dysfunction can also be seen in individuals with PWS. Periodic monitoring of thyroid function, fasting plasma glucose and insulin level is strongly recommended regardless of growth hormone therapy.

Neurocognition and Behavior

Decreased intellectual functioning was among the four original defining characteristics of PWS [1]. Subsequent studies document a typical neurobehavioral profile that includes altered intellectual functioning and centrally driven maladaptive behaviors, including the hallmark hyperphagia that exists in the context of a more extensive food related behavioral constellation, an age related emotional and behavioral profile, altered sensory processing, social deficits and for many a predictable psychiatric profile [47-51].

Intellectual Functioning

Following the original description, early studies of intellectual development documented a wide range of intellectual abilities, although most affected individuals tested in the borderline to mildly slow IQ ranges. As more sensitive genetic testing has become available, the population of individuals with PWS has become more clearly defined. Table 3 highlights studies of individuals with PWS who had genetic confirmation of their diagnosis, and who received age appropriate and properly administered cognitive testing, supplemented with measures of adaptive functioning.

The Israeli data are notable for the number of individuals testing in a normal range, and represents a distribution of IQ scores that is quite different from the remaining four studies. The reasons for this are unclear. Setting aside the Israeli data and averaging across the

remaining studies, all with approximately the same number of participants, Full Scale IQ ranges are as follows: ≥ 70 in 21%; mild cognitive impairment in 47%; moderate cognitive impairment in 32% and severe to profound cognitive impairment in 2%. An earlier report by Curf and Fryns [56] reported a greater proportion of subjects both in the > 70 and in the mildly impaired range, however their population included many subjects for whom no genetic testing was available and thus may have included individuals who did not have PWS.

Separate from the overall range of functioning among an affected population is the question of subtype differences in intellectual functioning. Such differences may be relevant in understanding the role of various genes in the overall clinical features and phenotype of this disorder. While most studies have not found significant subtype differences in overall IQ scores, at least 2 studies have reported a greater number of UPD subjects with normal IQ scores when compared to those with deletion [57-59]. Indeed Torrado et al reported that 61.5% of those with UPD had a Full scale IQ > 70, while only 10.5% of the subjects with deletion scored in that range. However, the mean age of Torrado's subject population was 4.09 years (range 12 days-17 years), so that the significance and overall stability of the obtained IQ scores is open to question. Statistically significant subtype differences have been reported for overall Verbal vs. Performance IQ scores with at least 2 studies reporting that those with UPD have higher verbal IQ scores and those with a deletion subtype have higher performance IQ scores [49,54], although more recently Copet et al [54] found that only the greater performance IQ of the deletion group vs a disomy group was statistically significant. Keep in mind that even when subtype scores are statistically significant, in no case have those differences ever reached the level of 1 SD for the test in question. Thus, whether these statistical differences are reflected as clinically relevant functional differences between subtypes is a question that must be raised.

Table 3 Intelligence Quotient (IQ)

| Investigator | Year | Number enrolled | Mean Age* | Intelligence Quotient Degree of Mental Retardation (%) | | | |
				Normal -Borderline	Mild	Moderate	Severe
Einfeld[a] [47]	1999	46	17.7	21.6	64.9	13.5	0
Gross-Tsur[b] [51]	2001	18	14.3	73	27	0	0
Deschee-Maeker [52]	2002	55	14.1	25.4	27.3	40	7.3
Whittington [53]	2004	55	21.0	31	41.8	27.2	0
Copet [54]	2010	85	24.2	7	54	39	0
Roof [55]	2000	47	23.2	24	38	30	8

a. Only 1/2 of subjects genetically confirmed, most IQ's from records
b. Did not give a measure of adaptive functioning
*Age in Years

In addition to mild cognitive deficits which are seen in most individuals with PWS, the overall cognitive profile at all ages includes cognitive rigidity, attentional deficits, problems with short term memory, auditory processing, sequential processing, arithmetic and social cognition. Relative strengths include long term memory, visual spatial performance, simultaneous processing, unusual abilities with jigsaw puzzles, particularly in the deletion subtype and for some reading decoding (devoid of comprehension).

Neuro-behavioral Profile

While there are a number of clinical descriptions of a typical behavior profile among those with PWS, from the earliest efforts behavioral studies have primarily focused on describing and quantifying the development of problem behaviors and psychiatric difficulties. Despite calls to include investigations of strength and adaptive behaviors [60], these remain a rare study focus. Moreover many studies include such a wide age range, often including infants through late adulthood measured at a single point in time. Parceling out developmental aspects of the behavior profile requires a critical combination of clinical and empirical evidence. Nonetheless studies across time, taken together, yield a general behavior picture that is remarkably consistent across affected individuals, despite variation in severity and intensity across individuals and within the same individual across time. Foremost among these behaviors is the hyperphagia and associated food related behavior constellation. In addition, most clinical and empirical studies document the commonality of hoarding; cognitive rigidity along with the need for sameness, temper outbursts and emotional lability, repetitive and perseverative behaviors and skin-picking.

Hyperphagia remains the cardinal defining feature of PWS. Nonetheless, the hyperphagia is only one aspect of a larger food-related behavior constellation that included preoccupations surrounding food; food seeking/foraging; sneaking, hiding and hoarding food; eating unusual food-related items (sticks of butter, used cooking grease, decaying food, garbage), food flavored items, such as shampoos and for many, manipulative and sometimes illegal behaviors designed to acquire food. While hyperphagia is found in other genetic syndromes (e.g. WAGR syndrome, Bardet-Biedel syndrome), the development of the hyperphagia and eating patterns associated with PWS, distinguish the hyperphagia associated with PWS from other disorders. Primary among these is the relatively late age of emergence, the rapid escalation and intensification of the hyperphagia following several years of poor to relatively normal eating, often accompanied early on by failure to thrive. Additional distinguishing characteristics include the duration of eating, amount of food eaten and a delayed to absent deceleration of eating, leading to gorging when both physiologic satiation and volume induced discomfort should preclude additional intake.

In the daily run of life, this is reflected as constant talking about food and unrelenting requests and demands of parents and other caregivers for food, that when denied often precipitate a tantrum. This frequently happens at the grocery or while shopping in other stores that may also have food or candy aisles and at restaurants. The denial-related tantrums can be of such a nature that parents give in as a method of avoiding the behavior, thus creating a pattern that escalates in severity and intensity over time. In addition affected individuals display a constant preoccupation with food leading to extraordinary vigilance for detecting food anywhere in the environment often resulting in stealing other's lunches at school or work, food from teacher's desks or caregiver's purses, stealing food at home or in shopping areas, begging others for food, foraging in garbage cans, entering another's home in search of food and manipulating others to obtain food. It is a rare parent who has not received a call from the school or vocational site indicating that the affected individual has been obtaining extra food by convincing caregivers that parents are ill or haven't had time to feed them, often for an extended period of time.

The etiology of the hyperphagia remains elusive. Long attributed to a hypothalamically mediated failure of satiety control [61,62], current studies suggest a far more complex etiology than previously hypothesized, including, for many a theoretical reorientation that views the hyperphagia as reflecting a starvation syndrome rather than an obesity syndrome. From this vantage point, the obesity associated with PWS is seen as resulting from a physiologic signaling defect indicating that the body is in a constant state of starvation similar to that of malnourished infants, thus leading to the constant drive to obtain food.

To date there is no effective pharmacologic intervention. Management is environmental and behavioral, requiring restricted access to food in all environments, locks on cabinets and refrigerators, constant supervision, as well as measures to prevent obesity which include calorie restrictive diets, consistently scheduled meals and snacks and regularly scheduled physical activity. While simple in concept, the number of environments encountered in any given day, along with the cooperation needed from the individuals in those environments presents challenges that may be insurmountable for some families. Accounts from both parents and individuals with PWS support that strict limit setting with regard to foraging and food access is associated with reduced anxiety and a sense of safety [63].

Behavioral Disturbances

Separate from the food related behavioral issues, multiple studies document that affected individuals are more prone to behavioral disturbances including hoarding; inflexibility of thinking and behavior; repetitive and perseverative behaviors; the need for sameness; tantrums and emotional lability; and skin picking [62]. Furthermore, the overall rate, severity and chronicity of these disturbances are frequently more intense than those associated with comparable genetic disorders or cognitive impairments or other obese groups [43,64,65]. Like the hyperphagia, the behavioral patterns appear to evolve over time with predictable epochs. Most authors agree that, on the whole, infants and young toddlers with PWS are affectionate, placid and generally cheerful, largely compliant and usually cooperative. However as the hyperphagia emerges, a separate and distinctly negative behavioral shift is also observed including an emergence and escalation of both food and non food related tantrums, a shorter tolerance for frustration combined with an overreaction to frustration; repetitive and ritualistic behavior as well as becoming " stuck " or perseverating on issues both in thought and speech; and other behavior problems including increasing oppositional tendencies, a lessened ability to " go with the flow " along with a drive for sameness and " increasing stubbornness and rigidity ". Comparison studies indicate that typically developing children and other children with mental retardation also exhibit the emergence of such behaviors, but they occur only transiently, that is, the problem appears and then subsides. However the emergence of such behaviors in those with PWS not only is persistent, but appears to escalate with age, increasing in severity and intensity, independent of intellectual, language or motor abilities [66,67].

Chronic behavior disturbances, including emotional lability accompanied by unbridled displays of temper; repetitive, ritualistic and compulsive like behaviors and hoarding become particularly prevalent in adolescence and persist well into adulthood, distinguishing these individuals from both younger children and older individuals with PWS, as well as from typical adolescents. In addition there has recently been an increasing recognition of accompanying social cognition and social interaction deficits among affected individuals, including an inability to read facial expressions of emotion and difficulty interpreting visually presented social information, such as those inherent in any social interaction [68,69]. Indeed several authors sum up the behavioral profile of those with PWS as " egocentric " and who argue, lie, manipulate and confabulate to change rules, obtain their wishes or justify behavior. Their social judgement is poor, even considering their intellectual ability; and interpretations of visually presented social information is

on a level with children who have pervasive developmental disorder [62]. Although some behavioral modulation is often seen in later ages, nonetheless problematic behaviors still exceed those seen in other comparison groups.

The expression of this behavioral phenotype does appear to depend, at least to some degree, on genetic subtype, with hoarding and overt behavioral expressions of frustration, anger and aggression more common among those with a deletion, as is a greater likelihood of modulation in middle adulthood. Internalizing and autistic spectrum behaviors are more common among those with UPD, and appear to be unremitting with little age related modulation [70,71].

Sensory Issues in the form of an altered sensitivity to pain, failure to exhibit fevers when expected and high rates of skin picking and gouging other body areas are extremely problematic among this group of individuals. While little research has been done around the issues of pain and lack of fever when expected, nonetheless blunted pain sensitivity and lack of appropriate fever response and the inherent dangers these present are clinically well documented. In this same spectrum, skin picking and other similar self injurious behavior occurs with increased prevalence in PWS when compared to a general intellectually impaired population [67,72]. When looking specifically at a population of those with PWS, skin picking is ubiquitous and when quantified, is as prevalent and problematic and in some studies even more so than hyperphagia [47]. It is the source of significant behavior and medical concerns and management challenges. Management is directed towards minimizing both the occurrence and impact of the behavior. To this end, a recent survey of 67 affected children and adolescents documented skin picking in 96% of respondents, which were directly associated with measures of anxiety, inattention, oppositional behaviors, function and quality of life [73]. Thus separate from medical management, behavior management must be focused on decreasing anxiety and boredom while eliminating opportunities for picking.

A number of case series across time have alluded to a small subset of individuals for whom seizures were problematic; however, it was generally thought that these represented incidental findings rather than a risk associated with PWS. A recent report by Fan et al [74] documented seizure activity in 10 of 56 subjects between the ages of 1-37 years, with suspicion in yet another 6 subjects. Among the ten subjects with documented seizure, one youngster's seizure disorder was attributed to sequelae of a grade II intraventricular hemorrhage associated with an early pre-term birth. Among the other nine cases, eight occurred in those with a deletion subtype and the other in a subject whose etiology was a presumed imprinting center defect; none were found among those with a disomy. After reviewing prior studies in which seizures were reported, the authors conclude that the overall prevalence of seizures in PWS is 16 -17%. Further they suggest that among those with a deletion, the risk for seizure in a PWS population is three to four fold times greater than that expected in a general pediatric population.

Psychiatric Illness

For many, this wide ranging problematic, behavioral profile can become sufficiently impairing that hospitalization is needed, while for others it evolves into frank psychiatric difficulties. In fact, Cassidy found behavioral concerns to be the most frequent cause of hospitalization [75]. By late adolescence 15-17% will evidence a diagnosable mood disorder [76]. This appears to be especially true for those with UPD. Separate from a categorical psychiatric diagnosis, studies consistently document that the level of behavioral and thought psychopathology, such as delusions, paranoid ideation, common in adolescents and adults with PWS exceeds that of others with an intellectual disability of other origins or of a typical population [65,67], and is the primary source of residential and vocational failure and family stress among affected adolescents and adults. While pharmacologic intervention can be helpful and in the case of psychosis is mandatory, environmental restructuring and positive behavior support programs are even more critical for facilitating recovery and preventing further difficulties.

The proliferation of less invasive and more available brain imaging techniques during the past decade offers the possibility of new insights into the central origin of the behavioral picture associated with PWS. Mantoulan [77] compared MRI and PET scans in PWS and non-PWS individuals. MRI images did not show evidence of anatomic abnormalities. However the PET scans showed hypoperfused brain regions, particularly in the anterior cingulum and superior temporal regions. The authors went on to correlate regional cerebral blood flow (rCBF) in the hypoperfused regions with results from the Child Behavior Check list (CBCL) and identified significant correlations, which suggested that the functional consequences of these perfusion abnormalities in specific brain regions might help to explain the social and behavioral issues observed in PWS. Similarly, a number of studies looking at brain processing of food related concerns have yielded mixed findings [78-80]. Functional findings must be considered tentative as the technology is sufficiently challenging that few affected individuals can tolerate the technology nor cooperate with the necessary tasks. Nonetheless, as the technology evolves, the possibility for future studies holds great promise.

Sleep Disturbance
General Sleep Disturbances

Sleep disturbance is frequent in all patients with Prader-Willi syndrome independent of age and weight. PWS patients with normal weight have been shown to have multiple sleep disturbances including daytime sleepiness, disrupted sleep organization, prolonged nocturnal sleep and sleep disordered breathing (SDB). In infants, SDB consists primarily of central apneas and absent, reduced or delayed ventilatory responses and arousal to hypoxia and hypercapnia [81-84]. Adult individuals with PWS-related morbid obesity may have the preceding sleep disturbances as well as an obesity-hypoventilation syndrome and obstructive sleep apnea.

Clinical Features

Abnormal sleep-wake organization, daytime sleepiness and sleep disordered breathing are the most common sleep related complaints. Irregular REM cycle and sleep disordered breathing appear as early as during infancy [85-87].

Sleep wake organization

Early surveys of sleep in PWS reported long nocturnal sleep (> 8 hours) as a common finding [88]. Early morning awakenings and sleep fragmentation have also been reported [89].

The most consistent finding found in polysomnographic studies has been altered rhythm of REM sleep. Studies have shown a tendency towards shorter REM latency, increased number of REM periods and shorter intervals between REM cycles. Total percentage of REM sleep appears to be normal [90-92]. REM sleep alterations appear to be unrelated to the patient genotype [93].

Excessive daytime sleepiness

Excessive daytime sleepiness (EDS) is an almost universal characteristic of individuals with PWS [88,89,94]. Clarke et al [88] reported EDS in more than 90% of their surveyed patients. Those patients who reported EDS were more likely to exhibit temper tantrums during the day.

Early studies, using daytime polysomnographic recordings, confirmed the presence of pathologic sleepiness in > 95% of the patients studied [95]. Later studies employed the multiple sleep latency test (MSLT). This test, also called a " nap test " is used to measure the time elapsed to sleep onset. It consists of 4 or 5 nap opportunities during the day. The MSLT is the gold standard to quantify sleepiness and diagnose disorders of excessive sleepiness. Studies with MSLT in individuals with PWS have shown abnormally short sleep latencies and frequent sleep onset REM periods

(SOREMPs) [90,92,96]. Daytime sleepiness, as measured by MSLT, appears to be independent of the degree of sleep related breathing disorders [90,92,96-98], additionally suggesting that daytime sleepiness reflects a central, possibly hypothalamic hypoarousal.

EDS and the atypical REM sleep findings bear resemblance to features of narcolepsy. Indeed, preliminary evidence in a small number of patients showed that hypocretin deficiency, a characteristic finding in narcolepsy, was also found in individuals with PWS who were severely sleepy [99]. However, in a postmortem study, there was no significant difference in the number of hypothalamic hypocretin containing neurons between patients with PWS and age matched controls [100].

Several preliminary studies have suggested a link between EDS and disruptive behavior in PWS. Hertz et al [101] reported a significant correlation between daytime sleepiness and disruptive behavior as measured by care taker's ranking. Similarly, Richdale [89] reported increased behavioral disturbance in children and adolescents with PWS who also reported EDS. Finally, in Clarke et al's [88] survey, adult patients who reported EDS were more likely to exhibit temper tantrums during the day.

In contrast, Maas et al [94], reported no significant correlation between sleep disturbance and behavioral disturbance in a group of adults with PWS.

Sleep Disordered Breathing (SDB)

Infants with Prader-Willi syndrome, as young as 4 months old, already demonstrate evidence of sleep disordered breathing. The most frequent type of SDB in infants with PWS are central apneas and periodic breathing [85,86]. Hypotonia and central control abnormalities likely play an important role. As obesity develops, around age 2 years, sleep apnea of the obstructive type becomes more common. Obstructive sleep apnea in both children and adults is directly associated with the degree of obesity and is inversely associated with age [97]. Oxygen desaturation is commonly seen even when the Apnea-hypopnea index (AHI) is only mildly elevated. The degree of sleep related oxygen desaturation may be severe, especially during REM sleep related hypotonia. Its severity is significantly increased with greater body mass index (91).

Management of sleep disorders

A sleep evaluation of all patients with Prader-Willi syndrome should be routinely considered because of the high prevalence of sleep disturbances. Patients who are habitual snorers and/or sleepy during the day may require a polysomnogram to rule out sleep disordered breathing.

In recent years, as more patients are treated with growth hormone (GH), there has been a growing concern over the potentially adverse effects on sleep related breathing. GH may exacerbate OSA in PWS, especially in the presence of other respiratory complications [87]. Review of the death records from the French database of patients with PWS showed an association with respiratory tract infections in both GH and non GH treated patients, highlighting the need for added vigilance during these periods. In patients who were receiving GH treatment the concern for an adverse outcome of SDB and respiratory tract infection is particularly salient during the first nine months of treatment, more so among males [102]. Therefore, an overnight sleep study is recommended before GH therapy is instituted to rule out sleep disordered breathing.

The gold standard for the treatment of sleep apnea in adults is Continuous Positive Airways Pressure (CPAP) or BiPAP. In children adenoidectomy, tonsillectomy or adenotonsillectomy is often first line of treatment. Supplemental oxygen therapy may be added in the presence of obesity hypoventilation syndrome. The management of other sleep disturbances may include implementation of adequate sleep hygiene, sleep wake schedule regulation and even circadian rhythm modification.

In patients who present with excessive daytime sleepiness, a Multiple Sleep Latency Test (MSLT), is also indicated. Once diagnosed, daytime sleepiness can be managed pharmacologically or with behavioral intervention. The pharmacological management of daytime sleepiness has been controversial because of the potential side effects of stimulant medication. Additional research is needed to assess the effects of stimulant medication on daytime alertness, disruptive behavior and the general well being of the sleepy patient with PWS. Behavioral management of EDS focuses on improving nighttime sleep and scheduling daytime naps when needed.

Gastrointestinal Issues

Abnormal surges in ghrelin may precede the characteristic hyperphagia seen in PWS. Whether this causes or is the result of the lack of satiety in PWS is not clear. Left unchecked, lack of appetite control can lead to morbid obesity. Low calorie and well balanced diets with rigorous supervision and restriction of food access combined with regularly scheduled meals and activities are recommended [15]. Reduced energy requirements have been reported for children with PWS as compared to healthy, age matched controls [103-105]. Those initiating growth hormone replacement therapy may require increased caloric load during the initial muscle building phase, but once lean mass accretion has stabilized, a reduced caloric limit may again be needed.

Poor oromotor control, muscle hypotonia and voracious eating with a limited time for mastication of food may lead to choking episodes. Choking accounts for approximately 8% of all PWS deaths. Binge eating has been seen in both obese and lean individuals with PWS. Acute gastric distention with necrosis and death has been reported with and without binging behavior. While acute gastric distention is frequently accompanied by vomiting in the general population, individuals with PWS have a decreased ability to vomit and may be missed due to lack of this important finding. These issues may be further complicated by their increased tolerance to pain which may be in part responsible for delays in seeking medical attention related to these episodes.

Musculoskeletal Issues

The prevalence of scoliosis in PWS is high (30% before 10 yr of age; 80% after age 10 years) [106-109]. Many patients shows progression of scoliosis with age irrespective of the use of GH and therefore scoliosis should no longer be considered a contraindication for GH treatment in children with PWS.

Most published reports of scoliosis in children with PWS have been retrospective. Recent evaluation of concerns regarding worsening of scoliosis in patients currently receiving GH have not been substantiated [110,111]. Prospective studies however are warranted. Studies by Shim et al [111] showed a high prevalence of spinal deformity, limb malalignment and foot abnormalities. This group found correlations between various musculoskeletal abnormalities, independent of obesity, but noted that obesity may conceal some of these abnormalities, especially in the early stage. At this time annual musculoskeletal evaluations are recommended for scoliosis, hip dysplasia, foot abnormalities and lower limb malalignments [112].

Slipped femoral capital epiphysis is seen with increased frequency in otherwise healthy, obese children. This has not been reported with increased frequency in children with PWS.

Early work [113] compared gait strategies in patients with PWS with those of both obese and non obese healthy patients. Adults with PWS in their study were found to walk slower, with shorter stride length, lower cadence and longer stance phases compared to non PWS controls. Range of motion at the level of the knee and ankle and plantar-flexor activity were significantly reduced. Spatio-temporal gait parameters in adults with PWS were further evaluated. Using 3 D gait analysis in an attempt to develop rehabilitation therapies, Cimolin et al [113] found that participating adults with PWS showed cautious abnormal gait strategies characterized by longer stance duration, reduced anterior step length

and lower velocity of progression. Hip flexion with a forward pelvic tilt was present throughout the gait cycle. Investigators felt that this reflected an attempt to achieve balance and stability in the face of excessive body weight.

Prognosis

While there is no cure for Prader-Willi syndrome, major strides to improve quality of life have been made since the introduction of more sensitive genetic testing modalities which has allowed early diagnosis and intervention. The early use of GH has improved final adult height, body composition and muscle strength. Obesity and the consequences of obesity continue to be major risk factors for mortality in persons with PWS, even after correction for the effect associated with intellectual disability [114].

Consent

Written informed consent was obtained from the parent/guardian of the patient for publication of the accompanying image.

Author details

[1]The Prader-Willi Syndrome Center at Winthrop University Hospital, 120 Mineola Blvd.-Suite 210, Mineola, N.Y. 11501, USA. [2]Huntington Medical Group, PC, Sleep Disorders Center, 180 East Pulaski Rd., Huntington Station, N.Y. 11746, USA. [3]Saint Louis University School of Medicine, 1465 S. Grand, St. Louis, Mo. 63104, USA.

Authors' contributions

All authors contributed to the development and writing of this manuscript and each has many years of clinical experience in the care of individuals with Prader-Willi syndrome. All authors read and approved the final manuscript.

Competing interests

The authors declare that they have no competing interests.

References

1. Prader A, Labhart A, Willi H: **Ein syndrome von adipositas, kleinwuchs, kryptorchismus und oligophrenie nach myotonierartigem zustand im neugeborenenalter.** *Schweiz Med Wochen* 1956, **86**:1260-1261.
2. Vogels A, Van Den Ende J, Keymolen K, Mortier G, Devriendt K, Legius E, Fryns JP: **Minimum prevalence, birth incidence and cause of death for Prader-Willi syndrome in Flanders.** *Eur J Hum Genet* 2004, **12(3)**:238-240.
3. Whittington JE, Holland AJ, Webb T, Butler J, Clarke D, Boer H: **Population prevalence and estimated birth incidence and mortality rate for people with Prader-Willi syndrome in one UK Health region.** *J Med Genet* 2001, **38(11)**:792-798.
4. Nicholls RD, Knoll JH, Butler MG, Karam S, Lalande M: **Genetic imprinting suggested by maternal heterodisomy in nondeletion Prader-Willi syndrome.** *Nature* 1989, **342**:281-285.
5. Butler MG: **High resolution chromosome analysis and fluorescence in situ hybridization in patient referred for Prader-Willi or Angelman syndrome.** *Am J Med Genet* 1995, **56(4)**:420-422.
6. Butler MG, Bittel DC, Kibiryeva N, Talebizadeh Z, Thompson T: **Behavioral differences among subjects with Prader_Willi syndrome and type I or type II deletion and maternal disomy.** *Pediatrics Mar* 2004, **113**:565-573.

7. Glenn CC, Saitoh S, Jong MT, Filbrandt MM, Surti U, Driscoll DJ, Nicholl RD: Gene structure, DNA methylation and imprinted expression of the human SNRPN gene. *Am J Hum Genet* 1996, 58(2):335-346.

8. Chotai KA, Payne SJ: A rapid PCR based test for differential molecular diagnosis of Prader-Willi syndrome and Angelman syndromes. *J Med Genet* 1998, 35(6):472-475.

9. Glenn CC, Nicholls RD, Robinson WP, Saitoh S, Niikawa N, Schinzel A, Horsthemke B, Driscoll DJ: Modification of 15q11-q13 DNA methylation imprints in unique Angelman and Prader-Willi patients. *Hum Mol Genet* 1993, 2(9):1377-1382.

10. Reis A, Dittrich B, Greger V, Buiting K, Lalande M, Gillessen-Kaesbach G, Anvret M, Horsthemke B: Imprinting mutation suggested by abnormal DNA methylation patterns in familial Angelman and Prader-Willi syndromes. *Am J Hum Genet* 1994, 54(5):733-40.

11. Buiting K, Saitoh S, Gross S, Dittrich B, Schwartz S, Nicholls RD, Horsthemke B: Inherited microdeletions in the Angelman and Prader-Will syndromes define an imprinting centre on human chromosome 15. *Nat Genet* 1995, 9(4):395-400.

12. Procter M, Chou LS, Tang W, Jama M, Mao R: Molecular diagnosis of Prader-Willi and Angelman syndroems by methylation specific melting analysis and methylation-specfic multiplex ligation-dependent probe amplification. *Clin Chem* 2006, 52(7):1276-1283.

13. Holm VA, Cassidy SB, Butler MG, Hanchett JM, Greenswag LR, Whitman BY, Greenberg F: Prader-Willi syndrome: consensus diagnostic criteria. *Pediatrics* 1993, 91(2):398-402.

14. Gunay-Aygun M, Schwartz S, Heeger S, O'Riordan MA, Cassidy SB: The changing purpose of Prader-Willi syndrome clinical diagnostic criteria and proposed revised criteria. *Pediatrics* 2001, 108(5):E92.

15. Goldstone AP, Holland AK, Hauffa BO, Hokken-Koelega AC, Tauber M: Recommendations for the Diagnosis and Management of Prader-Willi syndrome. *J Clin Endocrinol Metabol* 2008, 93:4183-97.

16. Crino A, Schiaffini R, Ciampalini P, Spera S, Beccaria L, Benzi F, Bosio L, Corrias A, gargantini L, Salvatoni A, Tonini G, Trifiro G, Livieri C: Genetic Obesity Study Group of the Italian Society of Pediatric Endocrinology and Diabetology (SIEDP), Hypogonadism and pubertal development in Prader-Willi syndrome. *Eur J Pediatr* 2003, 162(5):327-333.

17. Eiholzer U, l'Allemand D, Rousson V, Schlumpf M, Gasser T, Girard J, Gruters A, Simoni M: Hypothalamic and gonadal components of hypogonadism in boys with Prader-Labhart-Willi syndrome. *J Clin Endocrinol Metab* 2006, 9(3):892-898.

18. McCandless S: the Committee on Genetics, Health Supervision for Children With Prader-Willi Syndrome. *Pediatrics* 2011, 127:195-204.

19. Angulo MA, Castro-Magana M, Lamerson M, Arguello R, Accachia S, Khan A: Final adult height I children with Prader-Willi syndrome with and without human growth hormone treatment. *Am J Med Genet A* 2007, 143A(13):1456-61.

20. Eldar-Geva T, Hirsch HJ, Benarroch F, Rubinstein O, Gross-Tsur V: Hypogonadism in females with Prader-Willi syndrome from infancy to adulthood: variable combinations of a primary gonadal defect and hypothalamic dysfunction. *Eur J Endocrinol* 2010, 162(2):377-84.

21. Eiholzer U, l'Allemand D, Rousson V, Schlumpf M, Gasser T, Girard J, Grüters A, Simoni M: Hypothalamic and Gonadal Components of Hypogonadism in Boys with Prader-Labhart-Willi Syndrome. *J Clin Endocrinol Metab* 2006, 91:892-898.

22. Akefeldt A, Tornhage CJ, Gillberg C: A woman with Prader-Willi syndrome gives birth to a healthy baby girl. *Dev Med Child Neurol* 1999, 41(11):789-790.

23. Schulze A, Mogensen H, Hamborg-Petersen B, Graem N, Ostergaard JR, Brondum-Nielsen K: Fertility in Prader-Willi syndrome: a case report with Angelman syndrome in the offspring. *Acta Paediatr* 2001, 90(4):455-459.

24. Grossman AB: The Diagnosis and Management of Central Hypoadrenalism. *J Clin Endocrinol Metab* 2010, 95(11):4855-4863.

25. de Lind van Wijngaarden RF, Otten BJ, Festen DA, Joosten KF, de Jong Fh, Sweep FC, Hokken-Koelega AC: High prevalence of central adrenal insufficiency in patients with Prader-Willi syndrome. *J Clin Endocrinol Metab* 2008, 93(5):1649-1654.

26. Connell NA, Paterson WF, Wallace AM, Donaldson MD: Adrenal function and mortality in children and adolescents with Prader-Willi syndrome attending a single centre from 1991-2009. *Clin Endocrinol (Oxf)* 2010, 73(5):686-8.

27. Nyunt O, Cotterill AM, Archbold SM, Wu JY, Leong GM, Verge CF, Crock PA, Amble GR, Hofman P, Harris M: Normal Cortisol Response on Low-dose synacthen (1 μg) test in children with Prader-Willi syndrome. *J Clin Endocrinol Metab* 2010, 95(12):E464-467E.

28. Farholt S, Sode-Carlsen R, Christiansen JS, Ostergaard JR, Hoybye C: Normal cortisol response to high dose synacthen and insulin tolerance test in children and adults with Prader-Willi syndrome. *J Clin Endocrinol Metabol* 2011, 96(1):E173-180.

29. Holm VA, Nuget JK: 1982 Growth in the Prader-Willi syndrome. *Birth Defects Orig Artic Ser* 1982, 18(3B):93-100.

30. Bray GA, Dahms WT, Swerdloff RS, Fiser RH, Atkinson RL, Carrel RE: The Prader-Willi syndrome: a study of 40 patients and a review of the literature. *Medicine (Baltimore)* 1983, 62(2):59-80.

31. Butler MG, Meaney FJ: Standards for selected anthropometric measurements in Prader-Willi syndrome. *Pediatrics* 1991, 88(4):853-860.

32. Lee PDK: In *Endocrine and metabolic aspects of Prader-Willi Syndrome*. Edited by: Greenswag LR, Alexander RC. Management of Prader-Willi syndrome, second edition, Springer-Verlag, New York; 1995:32-60.

33. Carrel AL, Myers SE, Whitman BY, Allen DB: Benefits of long term GH therapy in Prader-Willi syndrome: A four year study. *J Clin Endocrinol Metab* 2002, 87(4):1581-5.

34. Haqq AM, Stadler DD, Jackson RH, Rosenfeld RG, Purnell JQ, LaFranchi SH: Effects of Growth hormone on pulmonary function, sleep quality, behavior, cognition, growth velocity, body composition and resting energy expenditure in Prader-Willi syndrome. *J Clin Endocrinol Metab* 2003, 88(5):2206-12.

35. Festen DA, Wevers M, Lindgren AC, Bohm B, Otten BJ, Wit JM, Duivenvoorden HJ, Hokken-Koelega AC: Mental and motor development before and after growth hormone treatment in infants and toddlers with Prader-Willi syndrome. *Clin Endocrinol (Oxf)* 2008, 68(6):919-25.

36. Festen DA, Wevers M, Lindgren AC, Bohm B, Otten BJ, Wit JM, Duivenvoorden HJ, Hokken-Koelega AC: Mental and motor development before and during growth hormone treatment in infants and toddlers with Prader-Willi syndrome. *Clin Endocrinol (Oxf)* 2008, 68:991-925.

37. Myers SE, Whitman BY, Carrel AL, Moerchen V, Bekx MT, Allen Db: Two years of growth hormone therapy in young children with Prader-Willi syndrome: physical and neurodevelopmental benefits. *Am J Med Genet A* 2007, 143(5):443-8.

38. Carrel AL, Moerchen V, Myers SE, Bekx MT, Whitman BY, Allen DB: Growth hormone improves mobility and body composition in infants and toddlers with Prader-Willi syndrome. *J Pediatr* 2004, 145(6):744-749.

39. Lindgren AC, Lindberg A: Growth hormone treatment completely normalizes adult height and improves body composition in Prader-Willi syndrome: Experience from KIGS (Pfizer International Growth Database). *Horm Res* 2008, 70(3):182-7.

40. Mogul HR, Lee PD, Whitman BY, Zipf WB, Frey M, Myers S, Cahan M, Pinyerd B, Southren AL: Growth hormone treatment of adults with Prader-Willi syndrome and growth hormone deficiency improves lean body mass, fractional body fat and serum triiodothyronine without glucose impairment: results from the United States multicenter trial. *J Clin Endocrinol Metab* 2008, 93(4):1238-45.

41. Hoybye C: Five year Growth Hormone treatment in adults with Prader-Willi syndrome. *Acta Pediatr* 2007, 96(3):410-3.

42. Sode-Carlsen R, Farholt S, Rabben KF, Bollerslev J, Schreiner T, Jurik AG, Christiansen JS, Höybye C: One year Growth hormone treatment in adults with Prader-Willi syndrome improves body composition: results from a randomized, placebo controlled study. *J Clin Endocrinol Metab* 2010, 95(11):4943-4950.

43. Akefeldt A, Gillberg C: Behavior and personality characteristics of children and young adults with Prader-Willi syndrome: a controlled study. *J Am Acad Child and Adoles Psychiatry* 1999, 38(6):761-769.

44. Gondoni LA, Vismara L, Marzullo P, Vettor R, Liuzzi A, Grugni G: Growth hormone therapy improves exercise capacity in adult patients with Prader-Willi syndrome. *J Endocrinol Invest* 2008, 31(9):765-72.

45. Bertella L, Mori I, Grugni G, Pignatti R, Ceriani F, Molinari E, Ceccarelli A, Sartorio A, Vettor R, Semenza C: Quality of life and psychological well-being in GH-treated, adult PWS patients: a longitudinal study. *J Intellect Disabil Res* 2007, 51(Pt 4):302-11.

46. Marzullo P, Marcassa C, Campini R, Eleuteri E, Minocci A, Sartorio A, Vettor R, ALiuzzi A, Grugni G: Conditional Cardiovascular Response to

Growth Hormone Therapy in Adult Patients with Prader-Willi Syndrome. *J Clin Endocrinol Metab* 2007, **92**:1364-1371.

47. Einfeld SL, Smith A, Durvasula S, Florio T, Tonge BJ: **Behavior and emotional disturbances in Prader-Willi syndrome.** *Am J Med Genet* 1999, **82**(2):123-7.

48. Milner KM, Craig EE, Thompson RJ, Veltman MW, Thomas NS, Roberts S, Bellamy M, Curran SR, Sporikou CM, Bolton PF: **Prader-Willi syndrome: intellectual abilities and behavioral features by genetic subtype.** *J Child Psychol Psychiatry* 2005, **46**(10):1089-1096.

49. Grugni G, Crino A, Bosio L, Corrias A, Cuttini M, De Toni T, Di Battista E, Franzese A, Gargantini L, Greggio N, Iughetti L, Livieri C, Naselli A, Pagano C, Pozzan G, Ragusa L, Salvatoni A, Trifirò G, Beccaria L, Bellizzi M, Bellone J, Brunani A, Cappa M, Caselli G, Cerioni V, Delvecchio M, Giardino D, Iannì F, Memo L, Pilotta A, Pomara C, Radetti G, Sacco M, Sanzari A, Sartorio A, Tonini G, Vettor R, Zaglia F, Chiumello G, Genetic Obesity Study Group of Italian Society of Pediatric Endocrinology and Diabetology (ISPED): **The Italian National Survey for Prader-Willi syndrome: An Epidemiologic Study.** *Am J Med Genet A* 2008, **146**(7):861-872.

50. Cassidy SB, Driscoll DJ: **Prader-Willi syndrome.** *Eur J of Hum Genet* 2009, **17**(1):3-13.

51. Gross-Tsur V, Landau YE, Benarroch F, Wertman-Elad R, Shalev R: **Cognition, attention and behavior in Prader-Willi syndrome.** *J Child Neurol* 2001, **16**(4):288-290.

52. Descheemaeker M, Vogels A, Govers V, Borghgraef M, Willekens D, Swillen A, Verhoeven W, Fryns JP: **Prader-Willi Syndrome: new insights in the behavioral and psychiatric spectrum.** *J Intellect Disabil Res* 2002, **46**(Pt 1):41-50.

53. Whittington JE, Holland A, Webb T, Butler J, Clarke D, Boer H: **Cognitive abilities and genotype in a population based sample of people with Prader-Willi syndrome.** *J Intellect Disabil Res* 2004, **48**(Pt 2):172-187.

54. Copet P, Jauregi J, Laurier V, Ehlinger V, Arnaud C, Cobo AM, Molinas C, Taber M, Thuilleaux D: **Cognitive profile in a large French cohort of adults with Prader-Willi syndrome: differences between genotypes.** *J Intellect Disabil Res* 2010, **54**(3):204-215.

55. Roof E, Stone W, MacLean W, Feuer ID, Thompson T, Butler MG: **Intellectual characteristics of Prader-Willi syndrome: comparison of genetic subtypes.** *J Intellect Disabil Res* 2000, **44**(Pt 1):25-30.

56. Curfs LM, Fryns JP: **Prader-Willi syndrome: a review with special attention to the cognitive and behavioral profile.** *Birth Defects Orig Artic Ser* 1992, **28**(1):99-104.

57. Dykens EM, Cassidy SB, King BH: **Maladaptive behavior differences in Prader-Willi syndrome due to paternal deletion versus uniparental disomy.** *Am J Ment Retard* 1999, **104**(1):67-77.

58. Torrado M, Araoz V, Baialardo E, Abraldes K, Mazza C, Krochik G, Ozuna B, Leske V, Caino S, Fano V, Chertkoff L: **An interdisciplinary Study. Clinical-etiologic correlation in children with Prader-Willi syndrome(PWS).** *Am J Med Genet A* 2007, **143**(5):460-468.

59. Dykens EM, Hodapp RM, Walsh K, Nash J: **Adaptive and maladaptive behavior in Prader-Willi syndrome.** *J Am Acad Child Adolesc Psychiatry* 1992, **31**(6):1131-1136.

60. Holland AJ, Treasure J, Coskeran P, Dallow J, Milton N, Hillhouse E: **Measurement of excessive appetite and metabolic changes in Prader-Willi syndrome.** *Int J Obes Relat Metab Disord* 1993, **17**(9):527-532.

61. Goldstone A: **Prader-Willi syndrome Advances in genetics, pathophysiology and treatment.** *Trends Endocrinol Metab* 2004, **15**(1):12-20.

62. Benarroch F, Hirsch HJ, Genstil L, Landau YE, Gross-Tsur V: **Prader-Willi syndrome: Medical prevention and behavioral challenges.** *Child Adolesc Psychiatr Clin N Am* 2007, **16**(3):695-708.

63. Whitman B, Jackson K: **Tools for Psychological and Behavioral Mangement.** In *Management of Prader-Willi syndrome. Volume 324..* 3 edition. Edited by: Butler MG, Lee PDK and Whitman B. NY: Springer Publishing; 2006.

64. Holland AJ, Whittington JE, Butler J, Webb T, Boer H, Clarke D: **Behavioral phenotypes associated with specific genetic disorders: evidence from a population-based study of people with Prader-Willi syndrome.** *Psychol Med* 2003, **33**(1):141-153.

65. Reddy LA, Pfeiffer S: **Behavior and emotional symptoms of children and adolescents with Prader-Willi syndrome.** *J Autism Dev Disord* 2007, **37**(5):830-839.

66. Dimitropoulos A, Feurer ID, Butler MG, Thompson T: **Emergence of compulsive behavior and tantrums in children with Prader-Willi syndrome.** *Am J Ment Retard* 2001, **106**(1):39-51.

67. Kim JW, Yoo HJ, Cho SC, Hong K, Kim BN: **Behavioral Characteristics of Prader-Willi syndrome in Korea: Comparison with children with mental retardation and normal controls.** *J Child Neurol* 2005, **20**(2):134-138.

68. Koenig K, Klin A, Schultz R: **Deficits in social attribution ability in Prader-Willi syndrome.** *J Autism Dev Disord* 2004, **34**(5):573-582.

69. Whittington J, Holland T: **Recognition of emotion in facial expression by people with Prader-Willi syndrome.** *J Intellect Disabil Res* 2011, **54**(1):75-85.

70. Dykens EM, Roof E: **Behavior in Prader-Willi syndrome: relationship to genetic subtypes and age.** *J Child Psychol Psychiatry* 2008, **49**(9):1001-8.

71. Hartley SL, Maclean WE, Butler MG, Zarcone J, Thompson T: **Maladaptive behaviors and risk factors among genetic subtypes of Prader-Willi syndrome.** *Am J Med Genet* 2005, **136**(2):140-145.

72. Arron K, Oliver C, Moss J, Berg K: **Burbidge. The prevalence and phenomenology of self injurious and aggressive behavior in genetic syndromes.** *J Intellect Disabil Res* 2011, **55**(2):109-120.

73. Morgan JR, Storch EA, Woods DA, Bodzin D, Lewin AB, Murphy TK: **A Preliminary Analysis of the phenomenology of skin picking in Prader-Willi syndrome.** *Child Psychiatry Hum Dev* 2010, **41**(4):448-463.

74. Fan Z, Greenwood R, Fisher A, Pendyal S, Powell CM: **Characteristics and frequency of seizure disorder in 56 patients with Prader-Willi syndrome.** *Am J Med Genet A* 2009, **149A**(7):1581-1584.

75. Cassidy SB, Devi A, Mukaida C: **Aging in Prader-Willi syndrome: 22 patients over age 30 years.** *Proc Greenwood Genet Cent* 1994, **13**:102-103.

76. Vogels A, De Hert M, Descheemaeker MJ, Govers V, Devriendt K, Legius E, Prinzie P, Fryns JP: **Psychotic disorders in Prader-Willi syndrome.** *Am J Med Genet A* 2004, **127A**(3):238-243.

77. Mantoulan C, Payoux P, Diene G, Glattard M, Roge B, Molinas C, Sevely A, Zilbovicius M, Celsis P, Tauber M: **PET scan perfusion imaging in the Prader-Willi syndrome: new insights into the psychiatric and social disturbances.** *J Cereb Blood Flow Metab* 2011, **31**(1):275-82.

78. Shapira NA, Lessing MC, He AG, James GA, Driscoll DJ, Liu Y: **Satiety dysfunction in Prader-Willi syndrome demonstrated by f MRI.** *J Neurol Neurosurg Psychiatry* 2005, **76**(2):260-262.

79. Holsen LM, Zarcone JR, Chambers R, Butler MG, Bittel DC, Brooks WM, Thompson T, Savage CR: **Genetic subtype differences in neural circuitry of food motivation in Prader-Willi syndrome.** *Int J Obes (Lond)* 2009, **33**(2):273-283.

80. Miller JL, James GA, Goldstone AP, Couch J, He G, Driscoll DJ, Liu Y: **Enhanced activation of reward mediating prefrontal regions in response to food stimuli in Prader-Willi syndrome.** *J Neurol Neurosurg Psychiatry* 2007, **78**(6):615-619.

81. Arens R, Gozal D, Omlin KJ, Livingston FR, Liu J, Keens TG, Ward SL: **Hypoxic and hypercapneic ventilatory responses in Prader-Willi syndrome.** *J Appl Physiol* 1994, **77**(5):2224-30.

82. Arens R, Gozal D, Burrell BC, Bailey SL, Bautista DB, Keens TJ, Ward SI: **Arousal and cardiorespiratory responses to hypoxemia in Prader-Willi syndrome.** *Am J Respir Crit Care Med* 1996, **153**(1):283-7.

83. Livingston FR, Arens R, Bailey SL, Keen TG, Ward SL: **Hypercapnic arousal responses in Prader-Willi syndrome.** *Chest* 1995, **108**(6):1627-31.

84. Menendez AA: **Abnormal ventilatory responses in patients with Prader-Willi syndrome.** *Eur J Pediatr* 1999, **158**(11):941-2.

85. Festen DA, Wevers M, DeWeerd AW, VandenBossche RA, Duivenvorden HJ, Otten BJ, Wit JM, Hokken-Koelega AC: **Psychomotor development in infants with Prader-Willi syndrome and association with sleep related breathing disorders.** *Pediatr Res* 2007, **62**:221-224.

86. Cataletto M, Hertz G, Angulo M: **Sleep in Infants with Prader-Willi syndrome: analysis of sleep patterns and early identification of sleep disordered breathing.** *Rom J Rare Dis* 2010, **1**(1).

87. Miller J: **Sleep Disordered breathing in Infants with Prader-Willi syndrome during the first 6 weeks of Growth hormone therapy: A pilot study.** *J Clin Sleep Med* 2009, **5**(5).

88. Clarke DJ, Water J, Corbett JA: **Adults with Prader-Willi syndrome: abnormalities of sleep and behaviours.** *JR Soc Med* 1989, **82**(1):21-4.

89. Richdale AL, Cotton S, Hibbit K: **sleep and behavior disturbance in Prader-Willi syndrome: a questionnaire study.** *J Intellect Disabil Res* 1999, **43**(Pt 5):380-92.

90. Hertz G, Cataletto M, Feinsilver S, Angulo M: **REM sleep abnormalities in Prader-Willi syndrome: A genetic link.** *Neurology* 1993, **43**(4):56.

91. Hertz G, Cataletto M, Feinsilver S, Angulo M: **Sleep and breathing patterns in patients with Prader-Willi syndrome (PWS): effect of age and gender** Sleep. 1993, **16**:366-71.

92. Vgontzas AN, Bixler EO, Kales A, Centurione A, Rogan PK, Mascari M, Vela Bueno A: **Daytime sleepiness and REM abnormalities in Prader-Willi syndrome: evidence of generalized hyperarousal.** *Int J Neurosci* 1996, **87**(3):127-39.

93. Vgontzas AN, Kales A, Seip J, Mascari MJ, Bixler EO, Myers DC, Vela-Bueno AV, Rogan PK: **Relationship of sleep abnormalities to patient genotype in Prader-Willi syndrome.** *Am J Med Genet* 1996, **67**(5):478-83.

94. Maas AP, Sinnema M, Didden R, Maaskant MA, Smits MG, Schrander-Stumpel CT, Curfs LM: **Sleep disturbances and behavioural problems in adults with Prader-Willi syndrome.** *J Intellect Disabil Res* 2010, **54**(10):906-17.

95. Helbing-Zwanenberg B, Kamphuisen HA, Mourtazaev MS: **The origin of excessive daytime sleepiness in the Prader-Willi syndrome.** *J Intellect Disabil Res* 1993, **37**:533-41.

96. Manni R, Politini L, Nobili L, Ferrillo F, Liveri C, Veneselli E, Bianchieri R, Martinetti M, Tartara A: **Hypersomnia in the Prader-Willi syndrome: clinical-electrophysiological features and underlying factors.** *Clin Neurophysiol* 2001, **112**(5):800-805.

97. Hertz G, Cataletto M, Feinsilver S: **Angulo, Developmental Trends in Sleep and breathing patterns in patients with Prader-Willi syndrome.** *Am J Med Genet* 1995, **56**:188-190.

98. Caffermann D, McEvoy ED, O'Donoghue F, Lushington K: **Prader-Willi syndrome and Excessive Daytime Sleepiness.** *Sleep Med Rev* 2008, **12**(1):65-75.

99. Nevsimalova S, Vankova J, Stepanova I, Seemanova E, Mignot E, Nishino S: **Hypocretin deficiency in Prader-Willi syndrome.** *Eur J Neuro* 2005, **12**(1):70-72.

100. Fronczek R, Lammers GJ, Balesar R, Unmehopa UA, Swaab DF: **The number of hypothalamic hypocretin (orexin) neurons is not affected in Prader-Willi syndrome.** *J Clin Endocrinol Metab* 2005, **90**(9):5466-70.

101. Hertz G, McGrath A, Cataletto M: **excessive daytime sleepiness in Prader-Willi syndrome: behavioral and cognitive measures.** *Sleep* 1999, **22**(Suppl 1):319.

102. Tauber M, Diene G, Molinas C, Hebert M: **Review of 64 cases of death in children with Prader-Willi syndrome(PWS).** *Am J Med Genet A* 2008, **146**(7):881-7.

103. Schoeller DA, Levetsky LI, Bandini LG, Dietz WW, Walcak A: **Energy expenditure and body composition in Prader-Willi syndrome.** *Metabolism* 1988, **37**:115-120.

104. Butler MG, Theodore MF, Bittel DC, Donnelly JE: **Energy Expenditure and physical activity in Prader-Willi syndrome: comparison with obese subjects.** *AM J Med Genet* 2007, **143**:449-59.

105. Lindemark M, Trygg K, Giltvedt K, Kolset S: **Nutrient intake of young children with Prader-Willi syndrome.** *Food and Nutrition Research* 2010, **54**:2112.

106. de Lind van Wijngaarden RF, de Klerk LW, Festen DA: **Hokken-Koelega AC 2008 Scoliosis in Prader-Willi syndrome: prevalence, effects of age, gender, body mass index, lean body mass and genotype.** *Arch Dis Child* **93**:1012-1016.

107. Nagai T, Obata K, Ogata T, Murakami N, Katada Y, Yoshino A, Sakazume S, Tomita Y, Sakuta R, Niikawa N: **Growth hormone therapy and scoliosis in patients with Prader-Willi syndrome.** *Am J Med Genet A* 2006, **140**:1623-1627.

108. Odent T, Accadbled F, Koureas G, Cournot M, Moine A, Diene G, Molinas C, Pinto G, Tauber M, Gomes B, de Gauzy JS, Glorion C: **Scoliosis in patients with Prader-Willi syndrome.** *Pediatrics* 2008, **122**:499-503.

109. Greggi T, Martikos K, Lolli F, Bakaloudia G, DiSilvestre M, Cioni A, Barbanti Brodaom G, Nagai T, Obata K, Ogata T, *et al*: **Growth hormone therapy and scoliosis in patients with Prader-Willi syndrome.** *Am J Med Genet* 2006, **140**:1623-27.

110. Odent T, Accadbled F, Koureas G, Cournot M, Moine A, Diene G, Molinas C, Pinto G, Tauber M, Gomes B, de Gauzy JS, Glorion C: **Scoliosis in patients with Prader-Willi syndrome.** *Pediatr* 2008, **122**:e 499-503.

111. Shim JS, Lee SH, Seo SW, Koo KH, Jin DK: **The Musculoskeletal manifestations of Prader-Willi syndrome.** *J Pediatr Orthop* 2010, **30**(4):390-395.

112. Vismara L, Romei M, Galli M, Montesano A, Baccalaro G, *et al*: **Clinical implications of gait analysis in the rehabilitation of adult patients with Prader-Willi syndrome: a cross sectional comparative study.** *J Neuroeng Rehabil* 2007, **4**:14.

113. Cimolin V, Galli M, Grugni G, Vismara L, Albertini G, Rigoldi C, Capodaglio P: **Gait patterns in Prader-Willi and Down syndrome patients.** *J Neuroeng Rehabil* 2010, **7**:28.

114. Einfeld SL, Kavanaugh SJ, Smith A, Evans EJ, Tonge BJ, Taffe J: **Mortality in Prader-Willi syndrome.** *Am J Ment Retard* 2006, **111**(3):193-8.

7

Lower A1c among adolescents with lower perceived A1c goal: a cross-sectional survey

Scott A Clements[1*], Matthew D Anger[2], Franziska K Bishop[3], Kim K McFann[4], Georgeanna J Klingensmith[3], David M Maahs[3] and R. Paul Wadwa[3]

Abstract

Background: The International Society for Pediatric and Adolescent Diabetes (ISPAD) and the American Diabetes Association (ADA) have established a hemoglobin A1c (A1c) target of less than 7.5% for adolescents with type 1 diabetes (T1D). However, many adolescents are unaware of their A1c target, and little data exist on how knowledge of this A1c target affects the actual A1c they achieve. We sought to evaluate the relationship between awareness of the A1c target and the actual A1c achieved in adolescents with T1D.

Methods: In a cohort of 240 adolescents with T1D age 13–19 years, we measured A1c and administered a questionnaire to assess their knowledge of the ISPAD guideline for A1c target.

Results: Of the total cohort, 42 subjects (18%) had an A1c below target and 198 subjects (82%) had an A1c above target. Almost all subjects (98%) reported that they were told their A1c target by a healthcare provider, and most of those (88%) claimed to know their A1c target, but few (8%) were correct. More subjects with actual A1c below 7.5% thought their A1c goal was lower than the ISPAD target, compared to subjects with A1c above target (75% vs. 59%, $p = 0.07$), although this did not achieve statistical significance.

Conclusion: In this cohort of adolescents with T1D, there was a trend toward a lower achieved A1c in those with a lower perceived A1c goal. Further studies should focus on identification of factors influencing an adolescent's ability to achieve a lower A1c.

Keywords: Type 1 diabetes, Hemoglobin A1c, Adolescents

Background

Hemoglobin A1c (A1c) is a widely used measure of glycemic control for patients with type 1 diabetes (T1D). Elevated A1c is associated with increased risk of developing microvascular and macrovascular complications, whereas an A1c less than 7.5% is associated with increased hypoglycemia [1-3]. Debate exists regarding the optimal A1c target for adolescents with T1D. Seeking to minimize long-term complications of diabetes, while also minimizing hypoglycemia, the International Society for Pediatric and Adolescent Diabetes (ISPAD) has established an A1c target of less than 7.5% for all children and adolescents with T1D [4]. However, scant data exist on how well adolescents can identify their A1c target or how knowledge of this A1c target relates to the actual A1c achieved by adolescents [5,6].

One determinant of achieving the A1c target in adolescents may be awareness of this target. If adolescents are aware of the A1c target, they may be more likely to work toward achieving that goal. If they are able to achieve a lower A1c, their risk of developing long-term complications of diabetes decreases. The purpose of this analysis was to determine the relationship between awareness of the A1c target and achievement of that target in a cohort of adolescents with T1D. We hypothesized that subjects who were aware of the A1c target would be more likely to achieve a lower A1c compared to those not aware of the target.

* Correspondence: scott.clements@hsc.utah.edu
[1]Utah Diabetes & Endocrinology Center, University of Utah School of Medicine, 615 Arapeen Dr, Suite 100, Salt Lake City, UT 84108, USA
Full list of author information is available at the end of the article

Methods

Participants

Data were obtained from a cohort of 240 subjects, age 13–19 years with T1D for a minimum of 5 years, from April 2008 through June 2010 [7]. Each subject was managed by a pediatric endocrinologist and the diabetes team at the Barbara Davis Center for Childhood Diabetes. There were an additional 60 subjects in the cohort age 12 years who were excluded from this analysis due to potential confusion between American Diabetes Association (<8%) and ISPAD (<7.5%) A1c targets for this age. Study participants with T1D were diagnosed by islet cell antibody and/or by provider clinical diagnosis. The study was approved by the Colorado Multiple Institution Review Board, and informed consent and assent (for subjects <18 years) were obtained from all subjects.

All subjects were followed in a pediatric diabetes subspecialty clinic by a team including pediatric endocrinologists, nurses, dieticians, and social workers. Subjects were generally seen every 3 months, with an A1c obtained at every visit. Diabetes providers in general review the target A1c of less than 7.5% with patients and families at every visit. On rare occasions, a provider may have suggested a higher A1c goal to avoid hypoglycemia or as a step towards better glycemic control in an adolescent in poor control, but these situations do not occur frequently.

Study visit

All subjects fasted overnight (≥8 hours). Medical history was obtained with standardized questionnaires, including method of insulin administration (injections versus insulin pump). As part of a survey regarding cardiovascular health, subjects were asked questions about awareness of their A1c target. Blood pressure measurements were obtained after subjects had been laying supine for a minimum of 5 minutes. Height was measured to the nearest 0.1 cm with shoes removed using a wall-mounted stadiometer, and weight was measured to the nearest 0.1 kg using a Detecto scale. Tanner Stage was assessed by a pediatric endocrinologist, except in 29 subjects who refused assessment of pubertal status by a provider.

Laboratory assays

A1c was measured on the DCA Advantage by Siemens (Princeton, New Jersey) at the Children's Hospital Colorado main clinical lab. Total cholesterol, high-density lipoprotein cholesterol (HDL-c), and triglycerides were performed in the Clinical Translational Research Core (CTRC) lab using an Olympus AU400e Chemistry (Olympus, Brea, California). Low-density lipoprotein cholesterol (LDL-c) was calculated using the Friedwald formula.

Categorization

The A1c target recommended by ISPAD of less than 7.5% for adolescents with T1D was used as the correct target. Those subjects who stated they knew their A1c target were asked to identify that target. Subjects were initially divided into 3 categories based on their responses: stated A1c target was correct, stated A1c target was below the ISPAD recommendation, and stated A1c target was above the ISPAD recommendation. However, some subjects stated an A1c range as the target, rather than a discrete number. If their stated A1c range was below the ISPAD recommendation of less than 7.5% (e.g. 6–7%), then they were included with the group whose stated A1c target was below the ISPAD recommendation. If their stated A1c range was above the ISPAD recommendation of less than 7.5% (e.g. 8–10%), then they were included with the group whose stated A1c target was above the ISPAD recommendation. If their stated A1c range included the ISPAD recommendation of less than 7.5% (e.g. 7–8%), then their responses were considered as a fourth category and were analyzed separately.

Statistical analysis

Continuous variables were checked for the distributional assumption of normality. Because the majority of variables exhibited a skewed distribution, Wilcoxon Sign Rank test was used to test for differences between those who achieved their A1c target and those who did not. Chi-square test of independence or Fisher's exact tests were used to test differences among categorical variables. Fisher's exact test was used when there were fewer than 5 subjects in a group. Descriptive statistics are reported as mean ± standard deviation or frequency and %. A p-value of <0.05 was considered significant. SAS version 9.3 was used to perform statistical tests.

Results

Of the 240 adolescent subjects with T1D who were surveyed, 52% were male, 78% were non-Hispanic white (11% were Hispanic, 4.2% were black, 1.3% were American Indian or Alaska Native, 0.8% were Hawaiian or Pacific Islander, 0.4% were Asian, and 3.8% were mixed race), mean age was 16.1 ± 1.8 years, diabetes duration was 9.0 ± 3.1 years (range 5.0–17.8 years), and mean A1c was 9.0% ± 1.7% (range 5.7%–14%). Clinical characteristics stratified by A1c below or above target are shown in Table 1. A graph of the actual A1c values by target A1c category is shown in Figure 1. There were 42 subjects (18%) with A1c below target and 198 subjects (82%) with A1c above target.

Almost all subjects (98%, n = 237) reported that they had been told their A1c target by a healthcare provider. Most of those (88%, n = 212) claimed to know their A1c target. Of the 212, only a small portion (8%, n = 18) were correct, 11% stated a target above the recommended target, and 70%

Table 1 Characteristics of subjects with A1c below target compared to those with A1c above target

		A1c below target (N = 42)	A1c above target (N = 198)	P-value
Age (years)		15.9 ± 1.8	16.1 ± 1.8	0.33
Hemoglobin A1c,%		7.0 ± 0.5	9.5 ± 1.5	< 0.0001
Sex, n (% male)		24 (57.1%)	101 (51.0%)	0.70
BMI z-score		0.56 ± 0.71	0.70 ± 0.84	0.62
Ethnicity:				0.03
	Non-Hispanic White	39 (92.9%)	149 (75.3%)	
	Hispanic	3 (7.1%)	36 (18.2%)	
	Other	0 (0%)	13 (6.6%)	
Insulin pump use		28 (67%)	109 (55%)	0.16
Categorization:				
	Stated Target Correct	0 (0%)	18 (9.1%)	0.05*
	Stated Target Incorrect	42 (100%)	180 (90.9%)	
Stated Target Above vs. Other		3 (7.1%)	20 (10.1%)	0.24*
Stated Target Below vs. Other		31 (73.8%)	117 (59.1%)	0.07
Stated Target Included vs. Other		4 (9.5%)	19 (9.6%)	0.99*
No Stated Target Given vs. Other		4 (9.5%)	24 (12.1%)	0.79*
Systolic BP (mm Hg)		114 ± 9	115 ± 9	0.56
Diastolic BP (mm Hg)		67 ± 6	70 ± 7	0.02
Total Cholesterol (mg/dl)		144 ± 25	160 ± 38	0.007
LDL-c (mg/dl)		81 ± 21	91 ± 29	0.04
HDL-c (mg/dl)		48 ± 8	51 ± 11	0.50
Triglycerides (mg/dl)		70 ± 28	90 ± 53	0.02
Tanner Stage Pubic Hair:				0.76
	1–3	5 (11.9%)	20 (10.1%)	
	4–5	31 (73.8%)	155 (78.3%)	
	Not assessed by provider	6 (14.3%)	23 (11.6%)	

*Fisher's Exact.

stated a target below the recommended target. There were 42 subjects that stated the A1c target as a range, of which 18 (43%) gave a range that was completely below the correct A1c target (e.g. 6–7%) and are included in the below target group, 1 (2%) gave a range that was completely above the correct A1c target (e.g. 8–10%) and is included in the above target group, and 23 (55%) gave a range that included the correct A1c target (e.g. 7–8%) and were analyzed separately.

Mean measured A1c in the 42 subjects below the ISPAD target (<7.5%) was significantly lower compared to the 198 subjects with A1c above target (7.0% vs. 9.5%, p < 0.0001). Among subjects with A1c below 7.5%, 74% thought their A1c target was lower than the actual target, compared to 59% of subjects above target (p = 0.07). Interestingly, among subjects with A1c below 7.5%, none stated the correct A1c target, whereas 18 subjects (9%) with an A1c above 7.5% knew the correct A1c target.

Age at diabetes diagnosis had no effect on perceived A1c target (p = 0.23).

Those subjects with an insulin pump (n = 137) had an average A1c of 8.6% ± 1.3%, whereas those using insulin by injection (n = 103) had an average A1c of 9.7% ± 1.9% (p = <0.0001). Of the 137 subjects using an insulin pump, 28 had an A1c below 7.5%, compared to 14 of the 103 using insulin by injection (20% vs. 14%, p = 0.16). Subjects who achieved A1c levels below 7.5% had lower total cholesterol, LDL-c, triglycerides, and diastolic blood pressure (p < 0.05 for all). There was no difference in distribution by Tanner stage among those with A1c below target versus those with A1c above target (Table 1, p = 0.76).

Discussion

In this cohort of adolescents with T1D, the mean A1c of 9.0% was significantly higher than the ISPAD goal of less

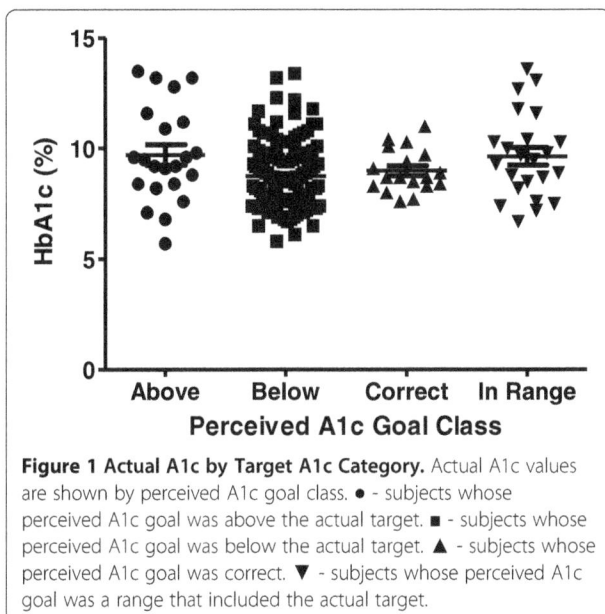

Figure 1 Actual A1c by Target A1c Category. Actual A1c values are shown by perceived A1c goal class. ● - subjects whose perceived A1c goal was above the actual target. ■ - subjects whose perceived A1c goal was below the actual target. ▲ - subjects whose perceived A1c goal was correct. ▼ - subjects whose perceived A1c goal was a range that included the actual target.

than 7.5%. This is similar to glycemic control observed in the T1D Exchange adolescent cohort (mean A1c 8.8%) and slightly higher than a cohort of adolescents with T1D in the SEARCH for Diabetes in Youth study (mean A1c 8.3%) [8,9]. We also found lower cardiovascular disease risk factors (total cholesterol, LDL-c, triglycerides, and diastolic blood pressure) in those subjects with A1c below target compared to those with A1c above target, which is also consistent with the SEARCH adolescent cohort [10,11].

In this cohort, nearly all subjects claimed to know their A1c target, but few were able to accurately identify the A1c target of less than 7.5%. These data suggest that few adolescents with T1D for 5 years or more are aware of their A1c target, despite having diabetes for a mean of almost 10 years. Furthermore, the adolescents in this cohort are all cared for at a large diabetes specialty center by a team including a pediatric endocrinologist and diabetes educators, where diabetes education and A1c goals are reviewed frequently. One would expect these subjects to have a better understanding of diabetes than other adolescents not seen at a diabetes specialty clinic. There was a large number of pateints on insulin pumps, suggesting a higher level of sophisticated diabetes care. However, subjects on insulin pumps gave similar incorrect answers as those adolescents treated with insulin injections.

Among those who believed their A1c goal was lower than the actual A1c target, more subjects had A1c below target than above target. The general trend suggests that those who perceived their A1c goal to be lower than the actual target were more likely to achieve an A1c below the actual target, although this difference did not reach statistical significance. While causality cannot be confirmed from our data, it would follow logically that adolescents who perceive their A1c goal to be lower than the actual target are more likely to strive to achieve that lower goal.

Thus, lowering the A1c target for adolescents could potentially lead to improved A1c levels and decreased long-term complications of diabetes. However, lowering the A1c target could also lead to an increased frequency of hypoglycemia. Data from the Diabetes Control and Complications Trial (DCCT) suggested that more intensive therapy led to significantly higher rates of severe hypoglycemia [3]. Although the DCCT was carried out before the availability of current insulin analogs, the risk for more frequent hypoglycemia should be considered when determining A1c targets for this age group. It is also possible that lowering the A1c target could lead to greater disappointment at not achieving that goal, which could result in unanticipated anxiety and frustration in adolescents with type 1 diabetes. However, evidence regarding adolescent reactions to A1c goals is lacking.

ISPAD has set an A1c target of less than 7.5% for children and adolescents with T1D [4]. This recommendation is based on adolescent and adult data from the DCCT, which showed that an elevated A1c was associated with increased risk for development of microvascular and macrovascular complications and that a lower A1c was associated with increased hypoglycemia [1-3]. The ISPAD A1c target of less than 7.5% represents a balance between decreasing long-term complications of diabetes and minimizing acute episodes of hypoglycemia.

An adult study has shown that when patients know their A1c, they are more likely to report better diabetes care [12]. Similarly, a study in adolescents showed that setting glycemic goals has a strong influence on A1c outcomes [6]. However, another study in children and adolescents has shown that there is a significant lack of knowledge concerning the A1c test and the long-term complications of an elevated A1c [5]. Our data are consistent with these studies in that few adolescents (8%) correctly identified their A1c target.

One of the main limitations of our study is that 42 subjects stated their A1c target as a range, rather than identifying a discrete value. Of those, 23 subjects stated an A1c target range that included the true A1c target of less than 7.5%, many of whom stated their A1c target as 7–8%. If they had been required to give a discrete value as an A1c target, it is unclear if they would have stated less than 7%, 7.5%, or 8%. Thus, their responses required separate analysis, rather than contributing to the analysis of the entire cohort. Another limitation of our study is that we do not have subject-specific data on what education subjects received at each clinic visit. It is possible that some providers may have suggested a higher A1c goal for certain adolescents to avoid hypoglycemia or as a step towards better glycemic control for those in poor control. While we do not have recorded data on how many study participants were given interim targets to pursue improved glycemic control, we do know that all patients were seen at a specialized diabetes clinic where the recommended goals are generally considered to be standard of care and are included in teaching materials provided to all families [13]. An additional limitation of our study is that some subjects may have been seen for a study visit shortly after turning age 13 years, but had not yet been seen at the diabetes clinic to discuss their A1c target.

The prevalence of T1D is increasing in the U.S., and adolescents make up a significant portion of those with T1D [14,15]. Adolescence is a time of cognitive development and increasing autonomy. As adolescents become more independent and more mature, they begin to take more responsibility for the management of their diabetes. This transfer of responsibility often occurs in the early teenage years, and there are a number of factors that can influence their ability to manage their diabetes. One important factor that may influence how well adolescents manage their diabetes is an awareness of treatment goals. Our data suggest that adolescents who think their A1c goal is lower than the ISPAD target may be more likely to achieve a lower A1c.

Conclusions

In this cohort of adolescents with T1D, we found a general trend that a lower perceived A1c goal was associated with a lower achieved A1c. As adolescents become more responsible for their diabetes care, a discussion of treatment goals should be a consideration. It is important for them to know their A1c target and understand how their actual A1c compares to that target. Further studies should focus on identification of other factors influencing an adolescent's ability to achieve a lower A1c without excessive hypoglycemia.

Abbreviations
A1c: Hemoglobin A1c; DCCT: Diabetes Control and Complications Trial; HDL-c: high-density lipoprotein cholesterol; ISPAD: International Society for Pediatric and Adolescent Diabetes; LDL-c: Low-density lipoprotein cholesterol; T1D: Type 1 diabetes.

Competing interests
The authors declare that they have no competing interests.

Authors' contributions
SAC compiled the data and wrote the manuscript. MDA helped compile the data and write the manuscript. FKB collected the data, compiled the data, and edited the manuscript. KKM analyzed the data and performed the statistical analysis. GJK participated in the design of the study and edited the manuscript. DMM participated in the design of the study, collected the data, and edited the manuscript. RPW participated in the design of the study, compiled the data, analyzed the data, and edited the manuscript. All authors read and approved the final manuscript.

Acknowledgements
We would like to thank the study participants and their families as well as the staff of the Barbara Davis Center for Childhood Diabetes. Dr. Clements was supported by an NIH training grant (T32DK063687), Dr. McFann by NIH/NCRR Colorado CTSI Grant Number UL1 RR025780, Dr. Maahs by a grant from NIDDK (DK075360), and Dr. Wadwa by an early career award from the Juvenile Diabetes Research Foundation (11-2007-694). This project was supported by NIH/NCRR Colorado CTSI Grant Number UL1 TR000154. Preliminary data from this cohort was presented in part in an abstract for the ADA 70th Scientific Sessions in 2010. Its contents are the authors' sole responsibility and do not represent official NIH, ADA, or JDRF views.

Author details
[1]Utah Diabetes & Endocrinology Center, University of Utah School of Medicine, 615 Arapeen Dr, Suite 100, Salt Lake City, UT 84108, USA. [2]University of Colorado School of Medicine, 13001 E 17th Place, N4223, Aurora, CO 80045, USA. [3]Barbara Davis Center for Childhood Diabetes, University of Colorado School of Medicine, 1775 Aurora Ct, A140, Aurora, CO 80045, USA. [4]University of Colorado School of Public Health, 13001 E 17th Place, B119, Aurora, CO 80045, USA.

References
1. Effect of intensive diabetes treatment on the development and progression of long-term complications in adolescents with insulin-dependent diabetes mellitus: Diabetes Control and Complications Trial. Diabetes Control and Complications Trial Research Group. J Pediatr 1994, 125:177–188.
2. Nathan DM, Cleary PA, Backlund JY, Genuth SM, Lachin JM, Orchard TJ, Raskin P, Zinman B: Intensive diabetes treatment and cardiovascular disease in patients with type 1 diabetes. N Engl J Med 2005, 353:2643–2653.
3. Hypoglycemia in the Diabetes Control and Complications Trial. The Diabetes Control and Complications Trial Research Group. Diabetes 1997, 46:271–286.
4. Rewers M, Pihoker C, Donaghue K, Hanas R, Swift P, Klingensmith GJ: Assessment and monitoring of glycemic control in children and adolescents with diabetes. Pediatr Diabetes 2009, 10(Suppl 12):71–81.
5. Patiño-Fernández AM, Eidson M, Sanchez J, Delamater AM: What do youth with type 1 diabetes know about the HbA1c test? Child Health Care 2010, 38:157–167.
6. Swift PG, Skinner TC, de Beaufort CE, Cameron FJ, Aman J, Aanstoot HJ, Castaño L, Chiarelli F, Daneman D, Danne T, et al: Target setting in intensive insulin management is associated with metabolic control: the Hvidoere childhood diabetes study group centre differences study 2005. Pediatr Diabetes 2010, 11:271–278.
7. Specht BJ, Wadwa RP, Snell-Bergeon JK, Nadeau KJ, Bishop FK, Maahs DM: Estimated insulin sensitivity and cardiovascular disease risk factors in adolescents with and without type 1 diabetes. J Pediatr 2013, 162:297–301.
8. Beck RW, Tamborlane WV, Bergenstal RM, Miller KM, DuBose SN, Hall CA: The T1D Exchange clinic registry. J Clin Endocrinol Metab 2012, 97:4383–4389.
9. Wadwa RP, Urbina EM, Anderson AM, Hamman RF, Dolan LM, Rodriguez BL, Daniels SR, Dabelea D: Measures of arterial stiffness in youth with type 1 and type 2 diabetes: the SEARCH for diabetes in youth study. Diabetes Care 2010, 33:881–886.
10. Rodriguez BL, Fujimoto WY, Mayer-Davis EJ, Imperatore G, Williams DE, Bell RA, Wadwa RP, Palla SL, Liu LL, Kershnar A, et al: Prevalence of cardiovascular disease risk factors in U.S. children and adolescents with diabetes: the SEARCH for diabetes in youth study. Diabetes Care 2006, 29:1891–1896.
11. Urbina EM, Wadwa RP, Davis C, Snively BM, Dolan LM, Daniels SR, Hamman RF, Dabelea D: Prevalence of increased arterial stiffness in children with type 1 diabetes mellitus differs by measurement site and sex: the SEARCH for diabetes in Youth Study. J Pediatr 2010, 156:731–737. 737.e731.
12. Heisler M, Piette JD, Spencer M, Kieffer E, Vijan S: The relationship between knowledge of recent HbA1c values and diabetes care understanding and self-management. Diabetes Care 2005, 28:816–822.

8

A single sample GnRHa stimulation test in the diagnosis of precocious puberty

Parvin Yazdani[1*], Yuezhen Lin[1], Vandana Raman[2] and Morey Haymond[3]

Abstract

Context: Gonadotropin-releasing hormone (GnRH) has been the standard test for diagnosing central precocious puberty. Because GnRH is no longer available, GnRH analogues (GnRHa) are now used. Random LH concentration, measured by the third-generation immunochemiluminometric assay, is a useful screening tool for central precocious puberty. However, GnRHa stimulation test should be considered, when a basal LH measurement is inconclusive. However optimal sampling times for luteinizing hormone (LH) have yet to be established.

Purpose: To determine the appropriate sampling time for LH post leuprolide challenge.

Methods: A retrospective analysis of multi-sample GnRHa stimulation tests performed in 155 children (aged 1–9 years) referred for precocious puberty to Texas Children's Hospital.
After 20 mcg/kg of SQ leuprolide acetate, samples were obtained at 0, 1, 3, and 6 hours.

Results: Of 71 children with clinical evidence of central precocious puberty, fifty nine children had a peak LH >5 mIU/mL. 52 (88%) of these responders had positive responses at 1 hour (95% CI is 80–96%), whereas all 59 children (100%) had a peak LH response >5 mIU/mL at 3 hours (95% CI is 94-100%), P = 0.005.

Conclusions: A single serum LH sample collected 3 hours post GnRHa challenge is the optimal sample to establish the diagnosis of central precocious puberty.

Keywords: Central precocious puberty, Luteinizing hormone, Gonadotropin releasing hormone analogue

Background

Central precocious puberty is the early onset of pubertal development as a result of gonadotropin release by the pituitary gland. Precocious puberty in a child can be associated with adverse consequences including compromised final adult height and psychosocial problems. Establishing the diagnosis of central precocious puberty requires documenting pubertal physical findings and measuring luteinizing hormone (LH) concentration, which is the key biochemical assessment of pubertal status. Gonadotropin-releasing hormone (GnRH)-stimulated plasma LH concentrations have been the mainstay for establishing the diagnosis of precocious puberty, but it is no longer available in the United States. GnRH analogue (leuprolide acetate) administered subcutaneously is a suitable substitute for GnRH in the diagnosis of central precocious puberty [1-5]. Ibanez et al.

reported that a peak serum LH response >8 IU/L occurred in patients with progressive puberty and in patients with Tanner stage II puberty 3 hours post leuprolide acetate challenge [3]. The LH concentrations declined progressively from 3 to 6 hours post-stimulation. In patients with non-progressive puberty and in pre-pubertal controls, the LH peak occurred between 3 and 6 hours after injection [3].

Rosenfield et al. measured gonadotropin levels at 0, 2, 4, 8, 16, and 24 hours post leuprolide acetate injection in a dose–response study comparing acute hormonal responses of the GnRHa leuprolide acetate to GnRH in 15 women and 15 men [6]. They reported peak plasma LH concentration at 1 and 4 hours in men and women, respectively. Other investigators using alternative sampling times demonstrated peak sample at 1 hour following leuprolide administration [2]. A previous study by Houk et al. demonstrated that a single LH measurement obtained 30 minutes post GnRHa stimulation provided adequate information to ascertain pubertal status in

* Correspondence: pyaz777@gmail.com
[1]Pediatric Endocrinology, Baylor College of Medicine, Houston 77030, TX, USA
Full list of author information is available at the end of the article

girls. However, they examined GnRHa stimulation testing with single 30-minute post-stimulus gonadotropin measurements, and none of the patients in their study had slowly progressive puberty [7]. Thus, despite the evidence of the efficacy of subcutaneous leuprolide acetate in the diagnosis of central precocious puberty, the optimal sampling times for LH post leuprolide challenge has not yet been determined based on the published results. The objective of our study is to re-evaluate optimal sampling time for LH post leuprolide acetate challenge in a cohort of patients presenting with signs of early pubertal development.

Materials and Methods

We conducted a retrospective analysis of the results of leuprolide acetate stimulation tests in children referred for possible precocious puberty to Texas Children's Hospital from January 2003-December 2006. During this time, we utilized a multiple sampling protocol as described below.

Children of both genders and all ethnicities (aged 1–9 yrs) were identified who had undergone this multi-sample leuprolide acetate (20 mcg/kg SQ) stimulation tests for the suspected diagnosis of central precocious puberty [2]. Serum luteinizing hormone (LH) and follicle stimulating hormone (FSH) concentrations were measured at 0, 1, 3 and 6 h post-injection. Serum estradiol and testosterone concentrations were measured at 0 and 6 h. Of the 155 subjects identified, one subject did not have a blood sample taken at 6 hours; the data from this subject was included since the analysis of the overall data including or excluding these data did not affect the results or conclusions and the primary comparisons were between 1 and 3-hour samples.

The diagnosis of central precocious puberty was established based on the clinical history of onset of pubertal changes (girls <8y, boys <9y), physical examination suggesting puberty based on Tanner-stage breast and pubic hair development in girls, testicular volume in boys, growth velocity over at least 6 months and bone age.

Based on these criteria and a follow up of at least 6 months with the exception of a few cases in which thelarche resolved after 4 months, the subjects were divided into three groups: A. Non-progressive puberty with thelarche, B. Non-progressive puberty with adrenarche, and C. Central precocious puberty.

Gonadotropin and sex steroid assays

The serum LH and FSH concentrations were analyzed at our clinical laboratory using the ADVIA Centaur immunoanalyzer (a two-site sandwich immunoassay) and direct chemiluminometric technique (ICMA, third-generation assay). The sensitivity of the FSH and LH assays were 0.3 mIU/mL and 0.07 mIU/mL, respectively. The published per cent coefficient of variation for replicate analysis were <4% for both assays in the 0.3-200 mIU/ml for FSH and 0.07-200 mIU/mL for LH, and the precision accuracy of assay was validated according to CAP laboratory accreditation standards. Serum estradiol and testosterone were measured by LCMS at Esoterix, Calabasas Laboratory.

Statistical analysis

All data are provided as mean ± SEM. An LH value < 0.1 mIU/mL was assumed to be 0.1mIU/ml for purposes of calculations. The generalized estimating equations method for the binomial distribution and logit link function (SPSS 18.0) was used to estimate and compare the percent with LH >5 at each time point while accounting for repeated measures collected longitudinally on each subject. Time was treated as fixed, AR1 was assumed for the correlation structure, and Fisher's LSD was used in the pairwise comparison of time points 1 vs 3, 1 vs 6, and 3 vs 6. Correlations of basal and GnRHa-stimulated peak serum LH values were analyzed by Spearman's rank correlation.

Subjects

Of the 155 subjects identified with premature sexual development who had undergone a leuprolide stimulation test, 48 were excluded. Thirty eight (38) had inadequate follow-up, 3 were diagnosed with organic disorders of hypothalamic-pituitary axis and 7 had peripheral puberty e.g. congenital adrenal hyperplasia, testotoxicosis and McCune Albright syndrome. Thus the total number of subjects included for analyses were 107. There were 21 girls in Group A with non-progressive puberty with thelarche. Group B, non-progressive puberty with adrenarche, had 15 subjects of which 12 were girls and 3 were boys. Finally, Group C with central progressive puberty included 71 children (58 girls & 13 boys) (Table 1).

Table 1 Patient Characteristics

	Premature Thelarche	Premature Adrenarche	Central Precocious Puberty
Patients#	21 (girls)	15 (12 girls, 3 boys)	71 (58 girls, 13 boys)
Chronological Age	5.04 ± 0.46 **	6.0 ± 0.55 *	7.78 ± 0.18
Bone Age	6.73 ± 0.57 **	8.64 ± 0.57	10.46 ± 0.25

Values represent "Mean ± SEM".
*P <0.05 (compared to puberty group), **P < 0.005 (compared to puberty group).

Baseline hormone concentrations

Group A (Premature thelarche)

Basal serum LH concentrations were 0.1 ± 0.0 mIU/ml. None had a basal LH concentration > 0.1 mIU/mL. Mean basal serum FSH was 2.18 ± 0.3 mIU/ml. All 21 girls had a basal LH/FSH ratio < 1. The basal serum concentrations of estradiol were 0.37 ± 0.15 ng/dL (pre-pubertal < 1.5 ng/dL). Serum testosterone was not measured in this group.

Group B (Premature adrenarche)

Basal serum LH concentrations were 0.1 ± 0.0 mIU/ml whereas basal FSH concentrations were 1.48 ± 0.31 mIU/ml (Figure 1). All 15 subjects with premature adrenarche had a basal LH/FSH ratio < 1. The basal estradiol concentration in the girls (n = 12) was 0.51 ± 0.17 ng/dL. Although the mean basal estradiol concentration was slightly higher than the patients with premature thelarche, it was statistically insignificant (P = 0.38). Additionally, their estradiol levels were in the pre-pubertal range and clinical follow up confirmed the diagnosis of premature adrenarche. Mean testosterone concentrations in the boys (n = 3) was 2.05 ± 0.34 ng/dL (pre-pubertal < 10 ng/dL) (Figure 2).

Group C (true central precocious puberty)

The basal LH and FSH concentrations were 1.96 ± 0.26 and 3.68 ± 0.31 mIU/mL, respectively (Figure 1). Both were higher than in either the children with premature thelarche or premature adrenarche (p < 0.005). Of the 58 female subjects with true puberty, fifteen (26%) had a basal LH value < 0.1 mIU/mL. All 13 of male subjects had a basal LH value > 0.1 mIU/mL (ranged from 0.5-5.3 mIU/mL). Basal estradiol concentrations of the 58 female subjects were 2.59 ± 0.46 ng/dl, and basal testosterone concentrations of the 13 male subjects were 187.69 ± 41.84 ng/dl (Figure 2).

Leuprolide - Stimulated Hormonal Concentrations

Group A (premature thelarche)

All 21 girls with a clinical diagnosis of premature thelarche had a peak stimulated LH concentration < 5 mIU/mL (Figure 1). Of these, 3 had a peak LH concentration at 1 h (14%), 18 at 3 h (86%), 0 at 6 h (Figure 3). Two girls had values at 1 and 3 h which were identical. Plasma FSH concentrations increased and peaked at 3 hr and decreased slightly by 6 h. All of these girls had stimulated LH/FSH ratios of < 1 at 1, 3 and 6 hours. Mean stimulated estradiol concentrations of these 21 girls at 6 hours was 2.00 ± 0.5 ng/dL (Figure 2).

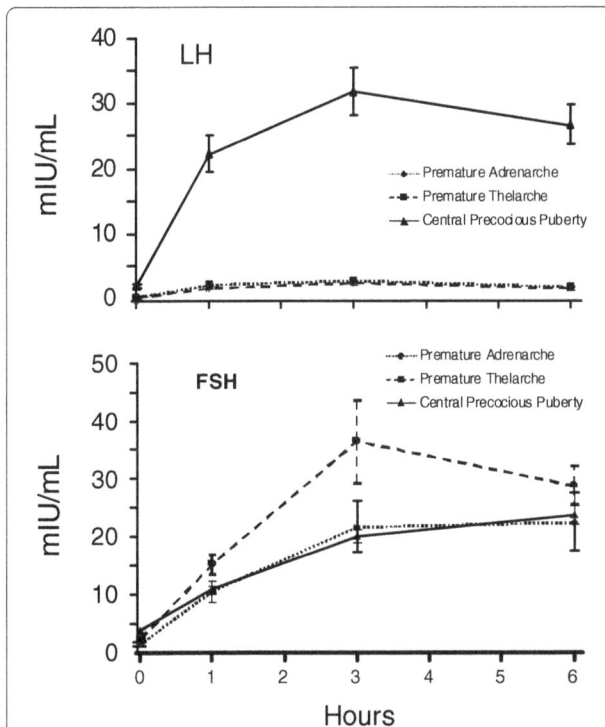

Figure 1 Baseline and peak stimulated serum LH (upper panel) and FSH (lower panel) concentrations (mean ± SEM) at 1, 3, and 6 hours after leuprolide injection. LH concentrations in central precocious puberty were significantly higher than in either the children with premature thelarche or premature adrenarche (P< 0.005).

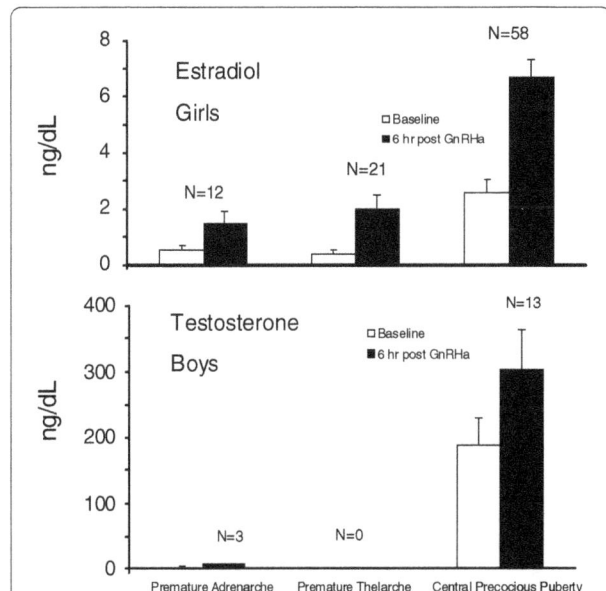

Figure 2 Baseline and peak stimulated serum Estradiol (upper panel) and Testosterone (lower panel) concentrations (mean ± SEM) at baseline and 6 hours after leuprolide injection. Estradiol and Testosterone concentrations in central precocious puberty were significantly higher than in either the children with premature thelarche or premature adrenarche (P< 0.005).

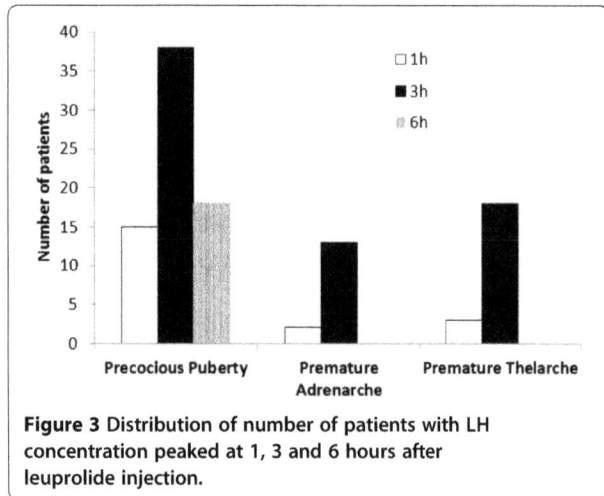

Figure 3 Distribution of number of patients with LH concentration peaked at 1, 3 and 6 hours after leuprolide injection.

Group B (premature adrenarche)

Of the 15 children with premature adrenarche (Figure 1) only 1 girl had a stimulated LH concentration > 5 mIU/ mL; the child had a baseline LH = 0.1 mIU/mL and peak stimulated plasma LH concentrations of 5.3 and 5.2 mIU/mL at 3 and 6 h, respectively. Clinically, her diagnosis remained premature adrenarche after 23 months follow up. Among these 15 children, two had a peak stimulated LH at 1 h (13%), 13 at 3 h (87%), none at 6 hr (Figure 3). One child had values of LH that were equal at 1 and 3 h. All had a stimulated LH/FSH ratio < 1 at 1, 3 and 6 hours. It was surprisingly observed that children with premature adrenarche had an FSH-predominant response in our cohort. Their plasma FSH concentrations increased following leuprolide injection and peaked at 3 h but the peak concentrations were significantly less than those of the girls with premature thelarche. We noted that two of the patients in this cohort who were significantly younger (15 months and 3 years) than most patients had a significant FSH–predominant response, but our clinical observation confirmed the diagnosis of premature adrenarche. The mean stimulated serum estradiol of the 12 girls was 1.46 ± 0.42 ng/dl at 6 h and the mean stimulated serum testosterone of the 3 boys was 6.6 ± 1.23 ng/dL at 6 hours (Figure 2).

Group C (central precocious puberty)
Group C Overall Results

Of the 71 children with central precocious puberty (Figure 1) 15 subjects had a maximum plasma concentrations of LH at 1 h (21%), 38 at 3 h (54%), 18 at 6 h (25%) and 2 subjects had a maximum concentration at both 3 & 6 hours (Figure 3). The plasma LH concentrations were higher than in either the children with premature thelarche or premature adrenarche (p < 0.005).

The mean stimulated FSH concentrations of girls with premature thelarche (Group A) were higher than children with central precocious puberty or premature adrenarche at both 1 and 3 h, but not at 6 h. Maximal FSH responses were detected 3 hours post stimulation in children with premature adrenarche and thelarche but at 6 h in children with central precocious puberty (Figure 1).

All 13 boys with central precocious puberty had a stimulated LH/FSH ratio > 1 at 1 & 3 hours. In contrast, only 32 (70%) girls with central precocious puberty, and a stimulated LH > 5 mIU/mL, had a stimulated LH/FSH ratio > 1 at 1 and 3 hours.

Mean Stimulated testosterone concentrations of 13 male subjects with central precocious puberty (302 ± 61.3) were higher than the boys with premature adrenarche (6.6 ± 1.2 ng/dl) at 6 h, (P < 0.005). The mean stimulated plasma estradiol concentrations of the 58 girls with central precocious puberty (6.68 ± 0.64 ng/ dL) were higher than those of the girls in Groups A and B at 6 h (p < 0.005) (Figure 2).

Concordant and Discordant Stimulated LH with Clinical Precocious Puberty

Pubertal subjects were divided in two groups based on their responses to leuprolide challenge:

a. With a concordant response for the leuprolide challenge (LH > 5 mIU/mL)

Out of 71 children with clinical evidence of progressive puberty, 59 subjects (83%) had a pubertal response to leuprolide challenge (13 boys and 46 girls). Among these 59 subjects, 52 (88%) had a peak LH > 5 mIU/mL at 1 h (95% CI: 80-96%), but all 59 children (100%) had a peak LH > 5 mIU/mL at 3 h (95% CI: 94-100%), P = 0.005 (Figure 3). All 13 boys had clinical evidence of true puberty, and a pubertal response (LH > 5mIU/mL) at 1, 3 and 6 h. Out of these 13 boys, 11 had a maximum concentration of LH at 3 h. Eleven (11) boys (85%) and 32 girls (70%) were treated with GnRHa.

b. With a discordant response for the leuprolide challenge (LH < 5 mIU/mL)

Among 71 children with clinical evidence of true puberty, 12 girls (17%) had a pre-pubertal response (LH < 5 mIU/mL) to Leuprolide challenge despite pubertal progression. Among these 12 subjects, the peak stimulated LH concentrations ranged from 0.9 to 4.6 mIU/mL regardless of the sampling time but had a predominant FSH response, such that we know that the leuprolide was in fact administered. Their stimulated estradiol concentrations at 6 h were not different from groups A and B (data not shown).

Diagnostic values of the measured hormones in the evaluation of central precocious puberty

Although not the primary purpose of this study, we evaluated and compared the relative diagnostic values of different parameters including basal LH, estradiol and testosterone, stimulated LH, LH/FSH ratio in the prediction of pubertal status. Our data demonstrates that in boys basal LH (>0.1 mIU/mL), testosterone concentrations (≥ 10 ng/dL), basal and stimulated LH/FSH ratios (at 1 and 3 h) have excellent sensitivity and specificity all to be 100% (Table 2). However, in girls basal LH > 0.1 mIU/ml, basal and stimulated LH/FSH ratios and basal estradiol (≥ 1.5 ng/dL) have low sensitivity though excellent specificity (Table 2). When serial potential predictors were combined, the sensitivities were reduced even though specificities were improved (Table 2). Compared to stimulated LH concentration at 1 h, the LH concentration > 5 mIU/ml at 3 h had better sensitivity (83% vs 73%) without compromising specificity (97% vs 100%). This cut off also has optimal sensitivity (83%) and specificity (97%) when compared to a lower cut off of 3mIU/ml or a higher cut off of 7mIU/ml (Table 2).

Table 2 Diagnostic values of basal LH, Estradiol, Testosterone, stimulated LH and the ratio of LH/FSH for Puberty

Predictors of puberty	Sensitivity	Specificity	PPV	NPV
Basal LH > 0.1 mIU/ml (M)	100%	100%	100%	100%
Basal LH > 0.1 mIU/ml (F)	67%	100%	100%	63%
Basal Estradiol ≥ 1.5 ng/dL	50%	94%	94%	52%
Basal Testosterone ≥ 10 ng/dL	100%	100%	100%	100%
LH at 1 h ≥ 5 mIU/ml	73%	100%	100%	80%
LH at 3 h ≥ 5 mIU/ml	83%	97%	98%	74%
LH at 3 h ≥ 3 mIU/ml	92%	75%	88%	82%
LH at 3 h ≥ 7 mIU/ml	80%	100%	100%	71%
Basal LH/FSH >1 (M)	100%	100%	100%	100%
Basal LH/FSH >1 (F)	10%	100%	100%	39%
LH/FSH at 1 h >1(M)	100%	100%	100%	100%
LH/FSH at 1 h >1(F)	50%	100%	100%	53%
LH/FSH at 3 h >1(M)	100%	100%	100%	100%
LH/FSH at 3 h >1(F)	45%	100%	100%	51%
LH at 1 h ≥ 5 mIU/ml and basal LH/FSH >1	61%	100%	100%	56%
LH at 3 h ≥ 5 mIU/ml and basal LH/FSH >1	16%	100%	100%	38%
LH at 3 h ≥ 5 mIU/ml and LH/FSH at 1 h >1	59%	100%	100%	56%

M – Male; F- Female; PPV – Positive predictive value; NPV – Negative predictive value.

Discussion

In the early phase of central sexual precocious puberty, laboratory confirmation is important to provide an accurate diagnosis and appropriate therapy. When random plasma LH concentrations are low in the presence of physical findings suggestive of precocious puberty, GnRHa stimulation testing is recommended to determine activation of hypothalamic-pituitary-gonadal axis. Despite wide utilization of the GnRHa stimulation test, the timing of blood sampling remains controversial if a single sample protocol is used. In our present study, the peak LH response occurred 3 hours post leuprolide stimulation test in those with true central precocious puberty. However, only 59 of 71 of the children with true central precocious puberty had an LH concentration > 5 mIU/mL at 3 hours. When compared to the 1 h value, the 3 h value was higher ($p < 0.005$) and had better sensitivity in diagnosing central precocious puberty. We recommend that a 3 h sample should be considered for those cases in which clinical presentation and base line laboratory values are not conclusive, despite the practical difficulties posed by a prolonged test protocol, particularly for those families traveling at a distance.

Girls with central precocious puberty in the early phase of activation of the hypothalamic-pituitary-gonadal axis are capable of clinically relevant estradiol production, which may occur in the face of low LH secretion and low LH/FSH ratios [2]. This observation is puzzling and one speculation is that endocrine or paracrine factors other than LH and FSH may play an important role in amplifying the effects of gonadotropins on ovarian E2 secretion in the early phase of sexual precocity [2]. Among our subjects with clinical evidence of precocious puberty, 12 girls with Tanner stage II-III breast development had a pre-pubertal response to leuprolide challenge (LH < 5 mIU/mL), a predominant FSH response and therefore a low LH/FSH ratio. Their laboratory findings were indistinguishable from those of subjects with proven premature thelarche and adrenarche. Interestingly, 10 out of these 12 subjects had both breast and pubic hair development at initial presentation, and only 2 subjects presented with just thelarche. Only one of these 12 girls with discordant response required GnRHa treatment. She was 6.5 y of age at presentation with Tanner III breast and pubic hair, a bone age of 10 y and a normal brain MRI. Her baseline LH was 0.1 mIU/mL, peak stimulated LH 3.9 mIU/mL at 3 h and estradiol concentration of 5.2 ng/dl at 6 h despite continued pubertal development. Therefore, clinical judgment and follow up continues to be of great importance in the evaluation of precocious puberty.

In our study, the basal plasma LH concentration differentiated the pubertal and pre-pubertal boys, without overlap, and is entirely consistent with the findings of

Resende et al. in normal male subjects [8]. However, this was not true for the girls. Twenty six percent of the girls ultimately diagnosed with central precocious puberty (Tanner breast stage II-III at presentation) and pubertal responses to leuprolide had basal serum LH concentrations in the pre-pubertal range (LH <0.1 mIU/mL).

Basal LH concentrations in excess of 0.1 mIU/mL were strongly correlated with a pubertal stimulated LH concentrations (>5 mIU/mL at 3 h) in pubertal subjects (r = 0.842, P, 0.0001) (data not shown). This finding is in agreement with others [9]. Thus, a random LH concentration measured by third-generation assays such as immunochemiluminometric assay is a useful tool in screening for central precocious puberty. However, our experience suggests that a GnRHa stimulation test should be considered when a basal serum LH is inconclusive or does not fit with the clinical presentation. This conclusion is further strengthened in that none of our children with either premature thelarche or premature adrenarche had a random serum LH > 0.1 mIU/mL.

Although mean spontaneous serum FSH concentrations were greater in children with central precocious puberty (p < 0.005) and provided fair sensitivity and specificity, subjects in groups A and B had predominant FSH responses to leuprolide challenge and mean stimulated serum FSH concentrations in girls with premature thelarche were higher than pubertal children at both 1 and 3 h (P < 0.005). These observations further strengthen the findings of others [9] that the stimulated FSH is of limited utility in partitioning the children with central precocious puberty from those without central stimulation. We also demonstrate that both basal LH/FSH > 1 and the stimulated LH/FSH ratio >1 at 1 and 3 hours are excellent predictors in diagnosing central precocious puberty in boys. This was not true for girls however (Table 2).

Conclusion

This is the largest group of children reported who have undergone a 6 h leuprolide acetate stimulation test for the evaluation of central precocious puberty. We conclude that in our study a single basal LH measurement using third-generation assays was adequate to diagnose central precocious puberty in boys. In addition, basal LH is adequate to diagnose central precocious puberty in most but not all girls, indicating the need for GnRHa test when a basal LH is inconclusive. Basal testosterone (measured by LCMS) in conjunction with clinical correlation is diagnostic of central precocious puberty in boys. In contrast, a basal estradiol (measured by LCMS) is helpful in most girls, but not all. However, when a GnRHa stimulation test is undertaken, our data demonstrates that a single sample at 3 h is superior in sensitivity and specificity to that of the 1 h sampling time in diagnosing central precocious puberty in girls, and provides the optimal sample to ascertain a diagnosis of central precocious puberty. Obviously, clinical judgment and follow up continues to be essential in that a quarter of our girls with central precocious puberty had discordant clinical findings with those of either the basal or stimulated LH values.

Abbreviations

GnRH, Gonadotropin-releasing hormone; LH, Luteinizing hormone; FSH, Follicle stimulating hormone; GnRHa, Gonadotropin-releasing hormone analogue; ICMA, Immunochemiluminometric assay; SQ, Subcutaneous.

Acknowledgments

We would like to thank E. O'Brian Smith, PhD for his statistical help and Arman Sadeghpour PhD, Andrea Balazs, MD, and Rachel Edelen, MD for their support in the development of this protocol.

Financial disclosure

The authors have no financial relationship relevant to disclose regarding this article.

Author details

[1]Pediatric Endocrinology, Baylor College of Medicine, Houston 77030, TX, USA. [2]University of Utah, Salt Lake City, UT, USA. [3]Baylor College of Medicine, Children's Nutritional Research Center, Houston, TX, USA.

References

1. Carel JC, Eugster EA, Rogol A, Ghizzoni L, Palmert MR, Antoniazzi F, Berenbaum S, Bourguignon JP, Chrousos GP, Coste J, et al: Consensus statement on the use of gonadotropin-releasing hormone analogs in children. Pediatrics 2009, 123(4):e752–e762.
2. Garibaldi LR, Aceto T Jr, Weber C, Pang S: The relationship between luteinizing hormone and estradiol secretion in female precocious puberty: evaluation by sensitive gonadotropin assays and the leuprolide stimulation test. J Clin Endocrinol Metab 1993, 76(4):851–856.
3. Ibanez L, Potau N, Zampolli M, Virdis R, Gussinye M, Carrascosa A, Saenger P, Vicens-Calvet E: Use of leuprolide acetate response patterns in the early diagnosis of pubertal disorders: comparison with the gonadotropinreleasing hormone test. J Clin Endocrinol Metab 1994, 78(1):30–35.
4. Sathasivam A, Garibaldi L, Shapiro S, Godbold J, Rapaport R: Leuprolide stimulation testing for the evaluation of early female sexual maturation. Clin Endocrinol (Oxf) 2010, 73(3):375–381.
5. Potau N, Ibanez L, Sentis M, Carrascosa A: Sexual dimorphism in the maturation of the pituitary-gonadal axis, assessed by GnRH agonist challenge. Eur J Endocrinol 1999, 141(1):27–34.
6. Rosenfield RL, Perovic N, Ehrmann DA, Barnes RB: Acute hormonal responses to the gonadotropin releasing hormone agonist leuprolide: dose–response studies and comparison to nafarelin--a clinical research center study. J Clin Endocrinol Metab 1996, 81(9):3408–341. 1.
7. Houk CP, Kunselman AR, Lee PA: The diagnostic value of a brief GnRH analogue stimulation test in girls with central precocious puberty: a single 30-minute post-stimulation LH sample is adequate. J Pediatr Endocrinol Metab 2008, 21(12):1113–1118.
8. Resende EA, Lara BH, Reis JD, Ferreira BP, Pereira GA, Borges MF: Assessment of basal and gonadotropin-releasing hormone-stimulated gonadotropins by immunochemiluminometric and immunofluorometric assays in normal children. J Clin Endocrinol Metab 2007, 92(4):1424–1429.
9. Neely EK, Wilson DM, Lee PA, Stene M, Hintz RL: Spontaneous serum gonadotropin concentrations in the evaluation of precocious puberty. J Pediatr 1995, 127(1):47–52.

9

Higher prevalence of obesity and overweight without an adverse metabolic profile in girls with central precocious puberty compared to girls with early puberty, regardless of GnRH analogue treatment

Ana Colmenares[1][*], Peter Gunczler[2] and Roberto Lanes[2]

Abstract

Objectives: 1. To determine BMI, obesity/overweight rates, glucose and lipids at baseline, during GnRHa treatment and shortly after therapy discontinuation in female children with CPP and EP. 2. To compare this response to that seen in a similar group of untreated patients.

Methods: A retrospective analysis of 71 children with either CPP (n = 37) or EP (n = 34) was undertaken. Forty three were treated with a GnRHa for at least 2 years, while 28 were followed without treatment.

Results: At the time of diagnosis, a higher BMI (z-score of 1.1 ± 0.8 vs. 0.6 ± 0.7, p = 0.004) and a higher prevalence of obesity/overweight (72.9 vs. 35.3%, p = 0.001) was observed in subjects with CPP when compared to those with EP. Children with EP had higher fasting glucose and total cholesterol than those with CPP. BMI z-score, obesity/overweight rates, fasting glucose and lipids did not change significantly in girls with CPP or EP during 3 yrs of follow up, regardless of treatment. Weight z-scores were higher at 3 years in treated than in untreated girls with CPP (p = 0.02), while it was higher in untreated than in GnRHa-treated patients with EP at baseline, 1, 2 and 3 years (p = 0.007, p = 0.002, p = 0.02 and p = 0.04, respectively) and remained so shortly after stopping therapy (p = 0.03).

Conclusions: There is a high prevalence of obesity/overweight in girls with CPP and EP at diagnosis. However, this risk is greater in CPP than in EP girls. BMI, Obesity/overweight rates, fasting glucose and lipids remained stable in CPP and EP girls regardless of therapy. Weight z-scores were found to be higher in treated CPP girls and in untreated girls with EP.

Keywords: Central precocious puberty, Early puberty, GnRHa, BMI, Overweight and obesity rates, Glucose, Lipids

Introduction

Central precocious puberty (CPP) and early puberty (EP) may be associated with an increased body mass index (BMI), adiposity, and with an increased prevalence of obesity before, during and after discontinuing GnRH analog (GnRHa) treatment when compared with age- and sex-matched reference values of the same population [1-4]. Until 2012, around 20 studies had addressed the

BMI outcome and the prevalence of obesity in children with CPP or EP treated with a GnRHa [1-3,5-17]. Of these only two studies analyzed patients with EP separately [18,19]. Additionally only two previous publications reported on the evolution of glucose and lipids during GnRHa therapy [4,20]. The consensus statement on the use of GnRHa in children [21] highlighted the need for studies regarding body composition, fat distribution or metabolic syndrome in this population.

Data in the literature concerning the influence of GnRHa therapy on the evolution of BMI and the rate of obesity-overweight in children with CPP and EP remain

* Correspondence: acolmena62@hotmail.com
[1]Department of Pediatrics, Hospital Dr. Patrocinio Peñuela-IVSS, San Cristobal, Táchira 5001, Venezuela
Full list of author information is available at the end of the article

controversial. In some studies, obesity in patients with CPP seems to be unrelated to GnRHa administration [1,6] and girls treated in childhood with a GnRHa have been found to have a normal BMI and body composition in early adulthood [17]. However in other reports a positive correlation between BMI before GnRHa administration and BMI after this treatment has been shown [7,22] and an increase in BMI, total body fat, and in insulin resistance has been described in some GnRHa-treated CPP subjects [4,15,23]. Only one publication documented a reduction of BMI z-score and of the obesity rate in girls with CPP during GnRHa treatment [11].

In this unicenter study we assessed BMI, rate of obesity and overweight, as well as fasting glucose and lipid profiles at the time of diagnosis, during at least 2 years of GnRHa therapy and shortly after treatment discontinuation in a group of 71 girls affected by CPP or by EP. We compared results at these time periods between CPP and EP patients with a similar group of untreated patients.

Subjects and methods

The medical records of 130 girls with a diagnosis of early or precocious puberty from the Pediatric Endocrine Unit of the Hospital de Clínicas Caracas were screened. Of these we selected only those records (n = 71) that met the following inclusion criteria: 1. Confirmed CPP or EP: a) onset of breast development (stage B2 or above according to Tanner) before a chronological age of 9 yrs, b) pubertal LH response (>7 IU/liter) to a GnRH stimulation test, c) advancement of bone age over chronological age by at least 1 yr, d) pubertal uterine and ovarian volume at pelvic ultrasonography [24]. 2. No evidence of hypothalamic-pituitary organic lesions following magnetic resonance imaging. 3. Absence of other conditions that might affect the onset of puberty and the BMI (e.g. GH deficiency, congenital adrenal hyperplasia, hypothyroidism). 4. Regular follow up during at least 2 years. 5. Measurement of lipid and glucose levels once a year during at least 2 years of follow up. 6. Compliance with the GnRHa treatment during the period of follow up. 7. Confirmed gonadotropin suppression throughout the period of GnRHa administration.

According to criteria previously established, we excluded all patients with isolated thelarche, non progressive forms of puberty, normal puberty, non confirmed laboratory tests suggestive of advanced puberty at diagnosis, incomplete medical records, irregular follow up, absence of lipid and glucose measurements at baseline or at follow, less than 2 years of follow up and no treatment compliance.

Patients were diagnosed with CPP (n = 37) if clinically and biochemically confirmed puberty presented at less than 8 yrs of age and they were diagnosed with EP (n = 34) if puberty was confirmed between the ages of 8–9 yrs. Based on the therapeutic policy of our Pediatric Endocrine

Unit at that time, gonadotropin-suppressive therapy was offered to all the girls after an observation period of 1 to 3 months in order to rule out transient or slowly progressive forms of puberty, which do not require treatment. Therapy was offered on the basis of either: 1. A diagnosis of a rapidly progressive form of CPP, regardless of stature, 2. A rapidly progressive form of EP associated with emotional difficulties or a low predict adult height. Of the CPP girls, 29 accepted treatment, 5 had a slowly progressive form of CPP and were therefore not treated and 3 refused therapy. Of the EP girls, 20 were followed without therapy, while 14 were treated. Those who had a slowly progressive form of CPP and EP or refused therapy were included in the study as controls.

GnRHa treatment consisted of depot-triptorelin, 3.75 mg im every 28 days. During treatment, gonadotropin suppression was regularly confirmed clinically and by prepubertal levels of LH following acute iv LHRH stimulation (LH <2 mIU/ml). Therapy was discontinued at a bone age of 11.5 to 12.5 yrs. The duration of GnRHa-therapy was 2–4 yrs.

Patients with an elevated BMI at every evaluation were recommended to increase physical activity and to improve nutritional habits (to eat more fruits, grains and vegetables and to decrease their caloric intake). The number of patients in each group that were recommended to diet and to increase physical activity was not significantly different (CPP: 79.3 vs. 50%, p = 0.17 and EP: 29 vs. 40%, p = 0.71, for treated vs. untreated patients respectively).

Methods

A retrospective analysis of the medical records of these patients was undertaken. All patients had been evaluated every 3–4 months by the same pediatric endocrinologist. Body weight was measured with an electronic scale to the nearest 0.1 kg. Height was measured with a Harpender stadiometer to the nearest millimeter. BMI was calculated as weight (kilograms)/height (meter square) and was expressed as Z-score (z-scores) for chronological age according to the CDC reference range [25]. Using Venezuelan BMI percentile cut-off values, we defined overweight as above the 90th percentile and obesity as above the 97th percentile [26]. Centile curves were drawn so that at age 18 years they passed through the widely used cut off points of 25 and 30 kg/m(2) for adult overweight and obesity.

Laboratory evaluation included measurement of LH, FSH, estradiol, fasting glucose and lipid levels (total cholesterol, high density lipoprotein cholesterol (HDL-C), and triglycerides). According to hospital policy blood samples were obtained early in the morning in the fasting state in all patients and with the proper parental approval. Serum LH, FSH, and estradiol levels were measured by chemoluminescence in an Immulite autoanalyzer using reagents from Diagnostic Product Corporation (DPC, Los Angeles, USA). The intra- and interassay coefficients of variation (CVs) were 5.7-6.1% and 5.3-6.5% for LH and FSH and 6.3%-6.4% for estradiol, respectively. Serum glucose, total cholesterol, HDL-C and triglycerides where measured by enzymatic methods with a Technicon autoanalyzer (Boehringer Mannheim Diagnostics). LDL-C was estimated using the Friedewald formula (LDL-C = TC − Tg/5 + HDL-C) [27]. The triglyceride/HDL-C ratio was calculated [28]. All assays were performed in the clinical biochemistry laboratory of the Hospital. Total cholesterol and triglyceride levels were compared to equivalent Venezuelan reference data [26].

The data shown at baseline corresponds to the start of treatment in GnRHa treated patients and the time of confirmed diagnosis in non-treated patients. This means that all patients had the same short period of follow up between the first visit and the inclusion into the study. We did not observe any significant difference in the BMI of our patients during this short period of observation. In the analysis we also include the clinical data from 9 patients shortly after discontinuation of GnRHa therapy (6–12 months; mean of 9 ± 3 months). These patients had previously received GnRHa treatment for at least 2 years and therefore, all of them were included in the 2 year analysis of the GnRHa treated group.

The institutional review board of the hospital approved the study, and informed consent for inclusion into the study was obtained from all adolescents and their parents.

Statistical analysis

All values are expressed as mean ± SDS unless otherwise stated. Differences in categorical variables between the groups were tested by the paired Fisher's exact test. Differences in the continuous variables comprised a non parametric paired Wilcoxon signed rank test to assess the changes between baseline values and all other time points within the groups (intragroup comparison). Differences between GnRHa treated and non treated patients (intergroup comparison) were assessed by the non-paired non parametric Mann–Whitney sign rank tests. Statistical significance was set at 5%. All statistical analyses were performed by the SPSS computer program, version 17.0 software for Windows (SPSS Inc., Chicago, IL, USA).

Results

Baseline characteristics of CPP and EP girls are summarized in Table 1. All patients were in Tanner stage 2–3 of puberty. The CPP girls were younger (p = <0.001), had a higher BMI (1.1 ± 0.8 vs. 0.6 ± 0.7 yr, p = 0.004) and a higher prevalence of obesity and overweight (72.9 vs. 35.3%, p = 0.001) than the EP patients. Fasting glucose

Table 1 Baseline characteristics of patients with CPP and EP

	CPP	EP	p value
n	37	34	-
Treated/Untreated	29/8	14/20	-
Clinical characteristics			-
Chronological age (yr)	7.4 ± 1.3	8.8 ± 0.6	**0.001**
Bone age (yr)	8.7 ± 2.1	9.3 ± 1.3	NS
Weight (Kg)	32.1 ± 6.7	32.6 ± 4.4	NS
Weight (z-score)	1.4 ± 0.8	1.9 ± 1.2	**0.001**
Height (SDS)	2.8 ± 1.2	1.3 ± 1.1	**0.001**
BMI (Kg/m2)	18.8 ± 2.4	18.2 ± 2	NS
BMI (z-score)	1.1 ± 0.8	0.6 ± 0.7	**0.004**
Obesity/Overweight n(%)	27 (72.9)	12 (35.3)	**0.001**
Obesity n(%)	9 (24.3)	3 (8.8)	NS
Overweight n(%)	18 (48.6)	9 (26.5)	0.054
Predict adult height (SDS) (SDS) (SDS)	0.3 ± 2.3	1.5 ± 1.2	**0.04**
Height velocity (SDS)	1.6 ± 2.1	1.8 ± 1.8	NS
Hormonal evaluation			
DHEAS (ng/ml)	51.1 ± 34.2	52.8 ± 23.7	NS
LH peak (IU/L)	10.9 ± 7.3	6.1 ± 4.5	**0.01**
LH to FSH stimulated ratio	1.1 ± 0.7	1.1 ± 1.7	NS
Estradiol (pg/ml)	22.3 ± 17	14 ± 11.8	**0.01**
Ovarian volume (ml)	1.7 ± 0.7	1.8 ± 0.5	NS
Uterine length (cm)	3.7 ± 1.2	3.4 ± 1	NS
Metabolic profile			
Fasting glucose (mg/dl)	73.3 ± 8.5	80.2 ± 10.2	**0.04**
Total Cholesterol (mg/dl)	158.6 ± 31.9	185.6 ± 35.7	**0.02**
LDL-C (mg/dl)	97 ± 35.1	113.2 ± 17.6	NS
HDL-C (mg/dl)	45 ± 8.9	53 ± 9.1	NS
TGR (mg/dl)	89.8 ± 46.7	104.8 ± 48.8	NS
TGR/HDL-C ratio	2.2 ± 0.9	1.5 ± 0.5	NS

Data are displayed as mean (± SDS). BMI, body mass index; DHEAS, dehydroepiandrosterone sulfate; LH, luteinizing hormone; FSH, follicle-stimulating hormone; LDL-C, low-density lipoprotein cholesterol; HDL-C, high-density lipoprotein cholesterol; TGR, Triglycerides.

and lipids were in the normal range for age and sex according to Venezuelan reference values in all girls [26]. Mean total cholesterol levels at baseline, were however, 185.6 ± 35.7 mg/dl (in the 90th percentile) in EP patients. The EP girls had higher fasting glucose (80.2 ± 10.2 vs. 73.3 ± 8.5 mg/dl, p = 0.04) and total cholesterol levels (185.6 ± 35.7 vs. 158.6 ± 31.9 mg/dl, p = 0.02) than CPP girls.

Tables 2 and 3 describe clinical and laboratory characteristics of GnRHa treated and untreated females with CPP and EP, respectively, during 3 years of follow up.

Table 2 Three years evolution in GnRHa treated and untreated patients with CPP

	Baseline		1 yr		2 yrs		3 yrs		
	Treated	Untreated	Treated	Untreated	Treated	Untreated	Treated	Untreated	After Tx
CA (yr)	7.3 ± 1.5	7.7 ± 0.7	8.3 ± 1.5	8.7 ± 0.9	9.2 ± 1.5	9.6 ± 0.7	10.1 ± 1.5	10.7 ± 1.2	11.04 ± 0.4
Weight (z-score)	1.4 ± 0.7	1.2 ± 0.8	1.4 ± 0.6	1.3 ± 0.8	1.3 ± 0.9	1.2 ± 0.7	**1.6 ± 0.6***	**0.9 ± 0.5**	0.8 ± 0.9
BMI (z-score)	1.2 ± 0.9	1 ± 0.8	1.2 ± 0.7	1.1 ± 0.8	1.1 ± 1	1 ± 0.7	1.3 ± 0.8	0.7 ± 0.5	0.7 ± 0.9
Ob/over (%)	79.3	50	65.4	50	65.4	50	81.8	40	40
Obesity (%)	24.1	25	26.9	25	23.1	25	45.5	0	20
Overweight (%)	55.2	25	38.5	25	42.3	25	36.4	40	20
Glycemia (mg/dl)	73.1 ± 9.1	74 ± 7.6	79.6 ± 8.9	88.6 ± 6.5	76 ± 10.1	84.3 ± 11.7	84.4 ± 5.3	80 ± 2.6	81 ± 18.4
Total-C (mg/dl)	156 ± 31.5	167.6 ± 35.7	172.1 ± 34.8	146.5 ± 42.3	152.8 ± 38.6	177.3 ± 23.9	159.2 ± 26.5	171.7 ± 39.1	167.3 ± 19.4
LDL-C (mg/dl)	96.6 ± 38.1	99.5 ± 16.3	108.1 ± 19.1	71.3 ± 24.1	92.9 ± 30.5	112.5 ± 7.8	100.2 ± 22.8	128.8 ± 13.9	122.5 ± 2.1
HDL-C (mg/dl)	43.8 ± 9	52 ± 7.1	35 ± 10.1	37.3 ± 9	48.5 ± 12.8	37 ± 4.2	43.8 ± 14	45.5 ± 2.1	44.5 ± 14.9
TRG (mg/dl)	83.3 ± 36.2	115.8 ± 78.5	80.9 ± 30.7	90.8 ± 33.7	79.9 ± 46.5	117 ± 66.8	83.3 ± 52.7	98.5 ± 37.5	64 ± 31.1
TRG/HDL-C ratio	2.1 ± 0.8	3 ± 1.5	2.5 ± 1	2.4 ± 0.5	1.7 ± 1.2	2.9 ± 2.2	1.9 ± 1.3	2.2 ± 0.9	2 ± 0.8

Data are expressed as mean ± SDS. SDS denotes the standard-deviation score for age and sex.
After Tx, after treatment; CA, Chronological age; BMI, body mass index; Ob/Over, obesity and overweight rate; Total-C, total cholesterol; LDL-C, Low density lipoprotein cholesterol; HDL-C, High density lipoprotein cholesterol; TGR, Triglycerides.
*p 0.02, treated vs. untreated at 3 years of follow up.

Central Precocious Puberty patients (CPP)

Weight and BMI z-scores remained unchanged over the first 2 years in both GnRHa-treated and untreated subjects. However, at 3 years of follow up, weight z-scores were higher in GnRHa-treated than in untreated patients (p = 0.02) and BMI z-scores followed this same trend, but did not reach significance (p = 0.06). A decreasing trend in weight and BMI z-scores was also detected in GnRHa-treated patients shortly after stopping therapy, but did not reach significance (n = 37, see Table 2).

At the time of diagnosis, both GnRHa-treated and untreated patients had a high prevalence of obesity and overweight. During 3 years of follow up, the prevalence of obesity and overweight remained unchanged in both groups of patients. In GnRHa treated patients who stopped treatment following at least 2 years of therapy, the rate of obesity and overweight showed a decreasing,

Table 3 Three years evolution of GnRHa treated and untreated patients with EP

	Baseline		1 yr		2 yrs		3 yrs		
	Treated	Untreated	Treated	Untreated	Treated	Untreated	Treated	Untreated	After Tx
CA (yr)	8.9 ± 0.6	8.8 ± 0.5	9.9 ± 0.6	9.8 ± 0.6	10.8 ± 0.7	10.7 ± 0.6	11.6 ± 0.7	11.5 ± 0.5	11.8 ± 0.4
Weight (z-score)	0.3 ± 0.7*	0.9 ± 0.6	0.1 ± 08*	0.9 ± 0.3	0.2 ± 0.9*	0.9 ± 0.4	0.1 ± 0.9*	0.9 ± 0.5**	−0.1 ± 1.1
BMI (z-score)	0.4 ± 0.7	0.9 ± 0.6	0.3 ± 0.8	0.8 ± 0.5	0.4 ± 0.9	0.7 ± 0.6	0.3 ± 1.2	0.8 ± 0.6	0 ± 0.8
Ob/over (%)	29	40	14	15	33	32	28.6	27	0
Obesity (%)	0	15	0	5	0	0	0	9	0
Overweight (%)	29	25	14	10	33	32	28.6	18	0
Glycemia (mg/dl)	79 ± 9.9	81.3 ± 11.1	89 ± 15.3	83.3 ± 9.7	84.3 ± 6.1	81.2 ± 8.6	84 ± 5.7	83 ± 6.4	83
Total-C (mg/dl)	195 ± 36.4	178.3 ± 35.5	184.8 ± 37.1	183.5 ± 33.8	186.8 ± 25	187.7 ± 41.8	133.5 ± 0.7	139.4 ± 37.6	123
LDL-C (mg/dl)	125 ± 38.4	113.2 ± 17.6	117.5 ± 42.8	131.5 ± 28.4	89.6 ± 66	105.8 ± 21.8	70.8 ± 5.1	83.7 ± 6.5	N.A
HDL-C (mg/dl)	50.6 ± 1.8	53 ± 9.1	51.3 ± 4.8	42.1 ± 7.4	47.7 ± 2.5	56 ± 24.3	49 ± 1.4	34.3 ± 4	N.A
TGR (mg/dl)	92.5 ± 30.9	113.4 ± 58.3	110 ± 43	73.9 ± 18	88 ± 18.5	85 ± 36	68.5 ± 14.9	96.5 ± 36.6	N.A.
TGR/HDL-C ratio	1.8 ± 0.6	1.5 ± 0.5	2.2 ± 1.3	1.9 ± 0.5	1.8 ± 0.3	1.5 ± 1	1.4 ± 0.3	2 ± 0.5	N.A.

Data are expressed as mean ± SDS. SDS denotes the standard-deviation score for age and sex.
After Tx, after treatment; CA, Chronological age; BMI, body mass index; Ob/Over, obesity and overweight rate; Total-C, total cholesterol; LDL-C, Low density lipoprotein cholesterol; HDL-C, High density lipoprotein cholesterol; TGR, Triglycerides.
*p <0.05 treated vs. untreated patients.
**p 0.03 untreated vs. patients after stop treatment.

although non significant trend (p = 0.2). Therefore, at 3 years of follow up the prevalence of obesity and overweight were similar between groups, but tended to be lower in untreated patients and in treated girls shortly after GnRHa discontinuation. Fasting glucose, total cholesterol, LDL, HDL-cholesterol, triglycerides and the triglyceride/HDL-cholesterol ratio, remained unchanged over the 3-year period, regardless of whether patients were treated or not. We found no differences between treated and untreated children for fasting glucose and lipids at baseline and during 3 years of follow up.

Early Puberty patients (EP)

Weight and BMI z-scores remained unchanged over 3 years in both GnRHa-treated and untreated subjects. However, during the 3 year follow up period, weight z-scores were higher in untreated than in GnRHa-treated patients (p = 0.007, p = 0.002, p = 0.02, p = 0.04 at baseline, 1, 2 and 3 years, respectively); a similar trend was observed in BMI z-scores, but the differences were not significant. Weight z-scores were also significantly higher in untreated subjects than in treated subjects shortly after stopping therapy (p = 0.03) (n = 34, see Table 3).

Prevalence of obesity-overweight remained unchanged over 3 years of follow up regardless of whether patients were treated or not. A decreasing tendency was, however, noted in GnRHa-treated girls shortly after therapy discontinuation. Fasting glucose, total cholesterol, LDL, HDL-cholesterol, triglycerides and the triglyceride/HDL-cholesterol ratio, remained unchanged over the 3-year period, regardless of whether patients were treated or not. We found no differences between treated and untreated children for fasting glucose and lipids at baseline and during 3 years of follow up.

Discussion

Our study confirms the high prevalence of obesity and overweight in girls with CPP and EP at the time of diagnosis. However, CPP girls presented with a higher BMI z-score and a higher prevalence of obesity and overweight than EP patients at baseline. The reason why so many subjects with CPP and EP have a BMI SDS above the 90th percentile for chronological age is unclear. Whether the hormonal changes of puberty trigger an increase in BMI or whether a preexisting increased in BMI contributes to the onset of puberty at an earlier age is still not clear [29,30].

However, our study showed no difference in the BMI z-score and the obesity/overweight rates over the 3-year period of follow up, regardless of whether patients with CPP or EP were treated or not. This finding is confirmed by previous studies [1,14] that reported no significant change in BMI or obesity/overweight prevalence after GnRHa therapy in subjects with CPP or EP.

An interesting finding emerging at 3 years of follow from our study is the higher weight z-score noted in GnRHa treated than in untreated girls with CPP, with a similar trend being observed for the BMI z-score. This finding would suggest a negative influence of GnRHa treatment on body weight after 3 years of follow up in CPP girls. Furthermore, both our patients with CPP or EP showed a decreasing trend in BMI z-scores and in the obesity/overweight rate following GnRHa treatment discontinuation. Accordingly, some previous studies have demonstrated that the mean BMI z-score returned to pre-treatment values after therapy withdrawal [2,9,19].

The administration of GnRHa to girls with EP has been associated with greater BMI z-score at the end of therapy [19]. However in our cohort of EP patients, it is of interest to note that non-treated girls had a significantly higher weight z-scores than treated patients at baseline and that this difference remained unchanged over the three year follow-up, despite GnRHa treatment.

Sorensen et al. [20] observed higher fasting insulin, triglycerides, and LDL-cholesterol levels compared with controls in 23 girls with CPP and EP at the time of diagnosis. In our cohort of girls with CPP and EP, glucose, triglycerides, LDL- and HDL-cholesterol and the triglyceride/HDL-C ratio were in the normal range at the time of diagnosis and remained unchanged at 1, 2 and 3 years of follow up, regardless of whether they were treated or not. An unexpected finding are the higher fasting glucose and total cholesterol levels noted in EP than in CPP patients at the time of diagnosis, despite the higher BMI and obesity/overweight prevalence in the latter group. Even though we cannot explain this finding, it lead us to suggest that the higher prevalence of obesity/overweight in CPP patients could be an artifact due to the shift of the SD curve in puberty that is now applied on younger children.

A limitation of this study is the small sample of girls with CPP or EP, especially after therapy withdrawal, which could limit the statistical power of the analysis. As to insulin measurements, the blood sample we had was small and did not allow us to measure this parameter in our analysis. Data regarding the parental weight is lacking in different studies, including ours, and increased weight in parents certainly increases the risk of being overweight in childhood [31].

In summary, there is a high prevalence of obesity and overweight among girls with CPP and EP at diagnosis. This risk is greater in CPP than in EP girls. BMI z-scores and obesity/overweight rates remain stable during GnRHa therapy in girls with CPP and EP, but tend to decrease in GnRHa treated patients once therapy is discontinued for several months. Weight z-scores were higher at 3 years in GnRHa treated than in untreated girls with CPP, while they were higher in untreated subjects with EP during the whole three year follow up period. Fasting glucose and lipids, however, were in the normal reference ranges at the time of diagnosis and remained stable during the 3 year period of follow up, regardless of whether patients were treated or not, so that the metabolic profile of CPP and EP patients does not seem to be adversely affected by GnRHa therapy.

Therefore, physicians treating patients with CPP and EP must be aware of the increased BMI and obesity-overweight prevalence rates seen at the moment of diagnosis in these children and consider that these parameters could persist or even increase further during GnRHa treatment.

Abbreviations
CPP: Central precocious puberty; EP: Early puberty; GnRHa: Gonadotropin releasing hormone analog; BMI: Body mass index.

Competing interests
The authors declare that they have no competing interests.

Authors' contributions
AC participated in the design of the study, recollected the data, performed the statistical analysis and drafted the manuscript. RL conceived of the study, participated in the design and coordination of the study, contributed part of the study population and helped draft the manuscript. PG participated in the design of the study and contributed part of the study population. All authors read and approved the final manuscript.

Acknowledgement
The authors thank all patients and their parents for participating in this study.

Author details
[1]Department of Pediatrics, Hospital Dr. Patrocinio Peñuela-IVSS, San Cristobal, Táchira 5001, Venezuela. [2]Pediatric Endocrine Unit, Hospital de Clínicas Caracas, Caracas, Venezuela.

References
1. Palmert MR, Mansfield MJ, Crowley WF Jr, Crigler JF Jr, Crawford JD, Boepple PA: Is obesity an outcome of gonadotropin-releasing hormone agonist administration? Analysis of growth and body composition in 110 patients with central precocious puberty. *J Clin Endocrinol Metab* 1999, **84**(12):4480–4488.
2. Paterson WF, McNeill E, Young D, Donaldson MD: Auxological outcome and time to menarche following long-acting goserelin therapy in girls with central precocious or early puberty. *Clin Endocrinol (Oxf)* 2004, **61**(5):626–634.
3. Traggiai C, Perucchin PP, Zerbini K, Gastaldi R, De Biasio P, Lorini R: Outcome after depot gonadotrophin-releasing hormone agonist treatment for central precocious puberty: effects on body mass index and final height. *Eur J Endocrinol* 2005, **153**(3):463–464.
4. Tascilar ME, Bilir P, Akinci A, Kose K, Akcora D, Inceoglu D, Fitöz SO: The effect of gonadotropin-releasing hormone analog treatment (leuprolide) on body fat distribution in idiopathic central precocious puberty. *Turk J Pediatr* 2011, **53**(1):27–33.
5. Lazar L, Padoa A, Phillip M: Growth pattern and final height after cessation of gonadotropin-suppressive therapy in girls with central sexual precocity. *J Clin Endocrinol Metab* 2007, **92**(9):3483–3489.
6. Heger S, Partsch CJ, Sippell WG: Long-term outcome after depot gonadotropin-releasing hormone agonist treatment of central precocious puberty: final height, body proportions, body composition, bone mineral density, and reproductive function. *J Clin Endocrinol Metab* 1999, **84**(12):4583–4590.
7. Pasquino AM, Pucarelli I, Accardo F, Demiraj V, Segni M, Di Nardo R: Long-term observation of 87 girls with idiopathic central precocious puberty treated with gonadotropin-releasing hormone analogs: impact on adult height, body mass index, bone mineral content, and reproductive function. *J Clin Endocrinol Metab* 2008, **93**(1):190–195.
8. Feuillan PP, Jones JV, Barnes K, Oerter-Klein K, Cutler GB Jr: Reproductive axis after discontinuation of gonadotropin-releasing hormone analog treatment of girls with precocious puberty: long term follow-up comparing girls with hypothalamic hamartoma to those with idiopathic precocious puberty. *J Clin Endocrinol Metab* 1999, **84**(1):44–49.
9. Van der Sluis IM, Boot AM, Krenning EP, Drop SL, de Muinck Keizer-Schrama SM: Longitudinal follow-up of bone density and body composition in children with precocious or early puberty before, during and after cessation of GnRH agonist therapy. *J Clin Endocrinol Metab* 2002, **87**(2):506–512.
10. Antoniazzi F, Arrigo T, Cisternino M, Galluzzi F, Bertelloni S, Pasquino AM, Borrelli P, Osio D, Mengarda F, De Luca F, Tatò L: End results in central precocious puberty with GnRH analog treatment: the data of the Italian Study Group for Physiopathology of Puberty. *J Pediatr Endocrinol Metab* 2000, **13**(Suppl 1):773–780.
11. Arrigo T, De Luca F, Antoniazzi F, Galluzzi F, Segni M, Rosano M, Messina MF, Lombardo F: Reduction of baseline body mass index under gonadotropin-suppressive therapy in girls with idiopathic precocious puberty. *Eur J Endocrinol* 2004, **150**(4):533–537.
12. Messaaoui A, Massa G, Tenoutasse S, Heinrichs C: [Treatment of central precocious puberty with Gonadotropin-Releasing Hormone agonist (triptorelin) in girls: breast development, skeletal maturation, height and weight evolution during and after treatment]. *Rev Med Brux* 2005, **26**(1):27–32.
13. Aguiar AL, Couto-Silva AC, Vicente EJ, Freitas IC, Cruz T, Adan L: Weight evolution in girls treated for idiopathic central precocious puberty with GnRH analogues. *J Pediatr Endocrinol Metab* 2006, **19**(11):1327–1334.
14. Glab E, Barg E, Wikiera B, Grabowski M, Noczynska A: Influence of GnRH analog therapy on body mass in central precocious puberty. *Pediatr Endocrinol Diabetes Metab* 2009, **15**(1):7–11.
15. Chiocca E, Dati E, Baroncelli GI, Mora S, Parrini D, Erba P, Bertelloni S: Body mass index and body composition in adolescents treated with gonadotropin-releasing hormone analogue triptorelin depot for central precocious puberty: data at near final height. *Neuroendocrinology* 2009, **89**(4):441–447.
16. Ko JH, Lee HS, Lim JS, Kim SM, Hwang JS: Changes in bone mineral density and body composition in children with central precocious puberty and early puberty before and after one year of treatment with GnRH agonist. *Horm Res Paediatr* 2011, **75**(3):174–179.
17. Magiakou MA, Manousaki D, Papadaki M, Hadjidakis D, Levidou G, Vakaki M, Papaefstathiou A, Lalioti N, Kanaka-Gantenbein C, Piaditis G, Chrousos GP, Dacou-Voutetakis C: The efficacy and safety of gonadotropin-releasing hormone analog treatment in childhood and adolescence: a single center, long-term follow-up study. *J Clin Endocrinol Metab* 2010, **95**(1):109–117.
18. Chiavaroli V, Liberati M, D'Antonio F, Masuccio F, Capanna R, Verrotti A, Chiarelli F, Mohn A: GNRH analog therapy in girls with early puberty is associated with the achievement of predicted final height but also with increased risk of polycystic ovary syndrome. *Eur J Endocrinol* 2010, **163**(1):55–62.
19. Lazar L, Kauli R, Pertzelan A, Phillip M: Gonadotropin-suppressive therapy in girls with early and fast puberty affects the pace of puberty but not total pubertal growth or final height. *J Clin Endocrinol Metab* 2002, **87**(5):2090–2094.
20. Sorensen K, Mouritsen A, Mogensen SS, Aksglaede L, Juul A: Insulin sensitivity and lipid profiles in girls with central precocious puberty before and during gonadal suppression. *J Clin Endocrinol Metab* 2010, **95**(8):3736–3744.
21. Carel JC, Eugster EA, Rogol A, Ghizzoni L, Palmert MR, Antoniazzi F, Berenbaum S, Bourguignon JP, Chrousos GP, Coste J, Deal S, de vries L, Foster C, Heger S, Holland J, Jahnukainen K, Juul A, Kaplowitz P, Lahlou N, Lee MM, Lee P, Merke DP, Neely EK, Oostdijk W, Phillip M, Rosenfield RL, Shulman D, Styne D, Tauber M, Wit JM, *et al*: Consensus statement on the use of gonadotropin-releasing hormone analogs in children. *Pediatrics* 2009, **123**(4):e752–e762.
22. Chen SK, Fan X, Tang Q: [Impact of gonadotropin-releasing hormone analogs treatment on final height in girls with central precocious puberty]. *Zhongguo Dang Dai Er Ke Za Zhi* 2009, **11**(5):374–376.

Higher prevalence of obesity and overweight without an adverse metabolic profile in girls...

71

23. Boot AM, De Muinck K-SS, Pols HA, Krenning EP, Drop SL: **Bone mineral density and body composition before and during treatment with gonadotropin-releasing hormone agonist in children with central precocious and early puberty.** *J Clin Endocrinol Metab* 1998, **83**(2):370–373.

24. Bridges NA, Cooke A, Healy MJ, Hindmarsh PC, Brook CG: **Standards for ovarian volume in childhood and puberty.** *Fertil Steril* 1993, **60**(3):456–460.

25. National Center for Health Statistics and National Center for Chronic Disease Prevention and Health promotion: **CDC Growth chart.** 2000.

26. Mendez Castellano H, López M, Benaim G, Maza D, González I: *Estudio nacional de crecimiento y desarrollo humano de la Republica de Venezuela , Proyecto Venezuela.* Fundacredesa; 1996.

27. Friedewald WT, Levy RI, Fredrickson DS: **Estimation of the concentration of low-density lipoprotein cholesterol in plasma, without use of the preparative ultracentrifuge.** *Clin Chem* 1972, **18**(6):499–502.

28. Quijada Z, Paoli M, Zerpa Y, Camacho N, Cichetti R, Villarroel V, Arata-Bellabarba G, Lanes R, Arata-Bellabarba G, Lanes R: **The triglyceride/HDL-cholesterol ratio as a marker of cardiovascular risk in obese children; association with traditional and emergent risk factors.** *Pediatr Diabetes* 2008, **9**(5):464–71.

29. Lee JM, Appugliese D, Kaciroti N, Corwyn RF, Bradley RH, Lumeng JC: **Weight status in young girls and the onset of puberty.** *Pediatrics* 2007, **119**(3):e624–30.

30. Davison KK, Susman EJ, Birch LL: **Percent body fat at age 5 predicts earlier pubertal development among girls at age 9.** *Pediatrics* 2003, **111**(4 Pt 1):815–21.

31. Whitaker RC, Wright JA, Pepe MS, Seidel KD, Dietz WH: **Predicting obesity in young adulthood from childhood and parental obesity.** *N Engl J Med* 1997, **337**(13):869–73.

10

Altered glucose disposition and insulin sensitivity in peri-pubertal first-degree relatives of women with polycystic ovary syndrome

Nouhad Raissouni[1], Andrey Kolesnikov[1], Radhika Purushothaman[1], Sunil Sinha[1], Sonal Bhandari[1], Amrit Bhangoo[1], Shahid Malik[1], Revi Mathew[2], Jean-Patrice Baillargeon[3], Maria Isabel Hernandez[4], Michael Rosenbaum[5], Svetlana Ten[1*] and David Geller[6]

Abstract

Background: First-degree relatives (FDRs) of women with PCOS are at increased risk for impaired insulin sensitivity and diabetes mellitus. Glucose tolerant FDR have evidence of insulin resistance and hyperinsulinemia prior to emergence of frank PCOS.

Aim: To study insulin dynamics parameters in the early adolescent FDR of women with PCOS.

Methods: This is a cross-sectional study involving 18 adolescents whose mothers or sisters had been diagnosed with PCOS and 21 healthy, age-matched control adolescents without FDR. Subjects underwent anthropometric measurements, steroid profiling and frequently sampled Intravenous Glucose Tolerance Test (IVGTT), Homeostasis Model Assessment (HOMA) index, Glucose Disposal Index (GDI), Acute Insulin Response (AIR) and Quantitative insulin sensitivity check index (QUICKI) were derived from IVGTT results.

Results: FDRs showed significantly higher mean HOMA and lower GDI. There were no differences in mean age or BMI Z-score between the cohorts. No differences in sex steroids or AIR were identified between groups.

Conclusion: Female adolescent FDR of women with PCOS have higher HOMA index and lower QUICKI, reflecting altered insulin sensitivity and lower GDI reflecting poorer beta-cell function. The presence of multiple risk factors for type 2 diabetes suggests that aggressive screening of the early adolescent FDR of women with PCOS is indicated.

Keywords: PCOS, Insulin resistance, Insulin sensitivity, Anovulation, Hyperandrogenemia, Premature pubarche, Diabetes mellitus, Beta cell function

Introduction

POLYCYSTIC OVARY SYNDROME (PCOS) is an endocrine-metabolic disorder, which is highly prevalent (5–10%) in reproductive-age women [1-3]. PCOS is characterized by hyperandrogenism [4,5]. The phenotypic characterization is heterogeneous; PCOS can manifest in the prepubertal years as premature pubarche [6]; hirsutism, acne and anovulatory cycles may remain clinically silent until late adolescence. Peripheral insulin resistance plays a key role in the pathogenesis of this syndrome. It has been suggested that insulin excess facilitates ovarian and/or adrenal hyperandrogenism [7-10]. Insulin resistance in PCOS women has long-term health consequences, predisposing to type 2 diabetes mellitus, cardiovascular disease and pregnancy-associated disorders like infertility, miscarriage, premature labor and gestational diabetes [11-15].

Female first-degree relatives (FDRs) of PCOS-affected women are at higher risk for developing PCOS symptoms [16]. FDRs are also at higher risk of developing the endocrine and metabolic co-morbidities of PCOS, such as obesity, insulin resistance and impaired insulin sensitivity, hyperlipidemia and metabolic syndrome[17-21]. An abundant literature supports familial clustering of hyperandrogenemia in PCOS women, consistent with a

* Correspondence: Tenlana@aol.com
[1]Division of Pediatric Endocrinology at Infants and Children's Hospital of Brooklyn at Maimonides & SUNY Downstate Medical Center, 1068 48th St, Brooklyn, NY 11219, USA
Full list of author information is available at the end of the article

genetic contribution to the disease [16,22]. Recent studies have shown an increased prevalence of hyperandrogenism and insulin resistance in adult FDRs of PCOS [16].

Despite the alarming increase in the prevalence of type 2 diabetes in children, and efforts to identify risk factors for the development of this disease in children studies of glucose homeostasis in pediatric FDRs of PCOS, have not been performed. In the present study we assessed the insulin secretion (β-cell function), insulin sensitivity, adrenal and ovarian steroid levels in peri-pubertal daughters and sisters of women diagnosed with PCOS. Our purpose was to determine the presence of early biochemical changes in females at risk of PCOS before clinical manifestations occurred and to evaluate whether insulin resistance or hyperandrogenemia occurs before in FDRs of PCOS women. We performed IVGTT to more comprehensively study the insulin dynamics in this cohort, and compared the results with those of an age- and weight-matched group of controls who were daughters or sisters of women without PCOS. The short version of IVGTT provides enough testing points to calculate indexes to assess insulin sensitivity and β-cell function. We also compared the steroid levels in both groups to evaluate the existence of the hormonal imbalance in FDRs. We hypothesized that being an FDR of a PCOS conveys an independent risk for the development of type 2 diabetes independent of other biochemical or clinical evidence of PCOS.

Subjects and methods

Study subjects

We studied 18 healthy premenarchal girls (mean age of 11.6 ± 1.1 years, range 8–14) whose mothers or sisters had been diagnosed with PCOS and were followed in adult and pediatric endocrinology clinics at Maimonides Medical Center, University of Sherbooke, University of Chile, Vanderbilt University and Cedars-Sinai Medical Center. All had been diagnosed with PCOS based upon the National Institute of Child Health and Human Development criteria for PCOS [23], including history of documented chronic oligomenorrhea or amenorrhea and hyperandrogenism, with the exclusion of secondary causes. The anthropometric, insulin dynamics and steroid data of FDR subjects was determined for NIH K23 HD040325, "Insulin Resistance in Adolescents at High Risk for Polycystic Ovary Syndrome".

The control group consisted of 21 healthy premenarchal girls (mean age of 12.1 ± 0.4 years, range 8–14) whose mothers had no history of irregular menstrual cycles or hirsutism. Children were recruited from a school-based study that is part of Reduce Obesity and Diabetes (ROAD) Project, a collaborative project between Maimonides Medical Center and Columbia University Medical Center,

Cohen Children's Medical Center, Mount Sinai Medical Center, Winthrop University Hospital and New York City public schools. This ongoing project is supported by Academy for Medical Development and Collaboration (AMDeC). These children had no personal history of diabetes or family history of irregular menstruation, diabetes or hirsutism.

First-degree relatives of PCOS women were recruited and tested following approval from the Institutional Review Boards at Cedars-Sinai Medical Center (Los Angeles), Sherbrooke University (Sherbrooke, Canada), University of Chile (Santiago, Chile), Vanderbilt University (Nashville, TN), and Maimonides Medical Center (Brooklyn, New York). The ROAD Project study was approved by the Institutional Review Board for each participating hospital, school boards and the Department of Health and Education. Written informed consent was obtained from all parents and assent from the peri-adolescent study subjects.

Study protocol

Assessment

All study subjects were either tested at Maimonides Medical Center Clinic (MMCC), ROAD school based study or at Cedars-Sinai Medical Center, Vanderbilt University, University of Sherbrooke or University of Chile. Enrollees presented after an overnight fast. A comprehensive medical assessment and medical history were obtained, including a personal and family history of type 2 diabetes, metabolic syndrome or heart disease. Anthropometric measurements included weight, height, body mass index (BMI), and waist circumference (waist: midway between the lower rib margin and the iliac crest). Age- and sex-specific BMI z-scores were calculated by using National Center for Health Statistics (NCHS) data [24]. Body fat composition was determined by bioelectrical impedance (Body Fat Analyzer, Model HBF-306, Omron, Gays Mills, WI). A Tanner stage was assigned to each study subject based on levels of both DHEAS and E2. No participants in the study were taking medications known to affect either sex steroids or carbohydrate metabolism.

IVGTT

Rapid frequently sampled intravenous glucose tolerance testing (IVGTT) was performed on all FDRs [25]. Each subject was given IV 25% Dextrose at 2 ml/Kg (max 25gm of Dextrose) delivered over 1 min, and blood was drawn through the same butterfly needle for measurements of serum glucose and insulin at 2, 3, 4 and 5 min after glucose administration. Short version of IVGTT (5 point over 5 minutes versus 3 hr classic IVGTT) had been chosen in control group because it was less time consuming in the school-based study.

Hormonal assay

Additional baseline blood samples were obtained for determination of DHEAS and Estradiol (E2).

Serum glucose was determined by the glucose hexokinase procedure from Raichem. The intra- and interassay coefficient of variation of this method was less than 3%. Serum insulin was determined by a solid phase sandwich immunoassay developed by Wallace/Perkin-Elmer. The intra-assay coefficient of variation of this method is 3-6%. Serum assays for DHEAS and E2 were performed by Labcorp Institute (Burlington, NC). Assay sensitivities for DHEAS and E2 were 1.7 ng/dl, 10 pg/ml, respectively. Intra- and interassay coefficients of variation were 7.9-9.8% for DHEAS and 97% for E2.

Calculations

Insulin resistance was estimated by the Homeostasis Model Assessment for Insulin Resistance (HOMA-IR), calculated as [fasting insulin (μU/ml) x fasting glucose (mg/dl)]/405] [26] and insulin sensitivity was estimated by Quantitative Insulin Sensitivity Check Index (QUICKI), calculated as [1/(log fasting insulin μU/ml) + log (fasting glucose mg/dl)] [27]. The acute insulin response (AIRg) was calculated as mean incremental rise in plasma insulin at 3 and 5 min after IV glucose. Pancreatic β-cell function was assessed by calculating the Glucose Disposal index as [$\log_{10}$ (AIRg x fasting glucose concentration/fasting insulin concentration)] [25,28].

Statistical methods and analysis

Data are expressed as mean ± SD. Freidman's repeated measures ANOVA was used to compare variables (age, BMI Z-score, HOMA, QUICKI, GDI, DHEAS, etc.) within the same group. Comparisons of means between the PCOS affected first-degree relatives group (PCOS-FDR) and the control group were performed using the Unequal Variance, Unequal Sample Size t-test. Regression analysis and Spearman correlations were used to evaluate the relationship between the variables of interest. Statistical analysis was performed using SPSS Statistics 17.0.

Results

Anthropometry and hormonal assay

There were no significant differences between the PCOS-FDR and the control groups with respect to age, BMI, BMI Z score, waist circumference or percent of body fat (Table 1). There were no significant differences in serum DHEA-S between groups. E_2 levels were significantly higher in PCOS-FDR group comparing to the control group. Both groups had similar Tanner stage distributions, as a function of DHEA-S and E2 levels.

Table 1 Anthropometric characteristic of PCOS FDR and Control Daughters (Cd)

	FDR-PCOS (n = 18)	Cd group (n = 21)
Age (yr)	11.6 ± 1.4	12. ± 0.8
BMI (kg/m^2)	21.5 ± 3.5	21.5 ± 3.2
BMI Z Score	1.01 ± 0.85	0.93 ± 0.9
Waist Circumference (cm)	72 ± 10.9	76 ± 8.7
Body Fat %	25 ± 2.5	25.76 ± 3.2

Data are presented as the mean ± SD. *P value < 0.05.

IVGTT

The HOMA-IR ratio was significantly higher, and both the QUICKI and GDI parameters were significantly lower in the PCOS-FDR group compared to the control group (Table 2). The HOMA-IR ratio findings were unchanged even after segregating the PCOS-FDR and control groups according to Tanner stage. AIR was not significantly different between groups.

Discussion

The major findings of this study are that both decreased insulin sensitivity and beta-cell function are evident in premenarachal peripubertal female FDR's of PCOS without clinical or biochemical evidence of PCOS. These data suggest that having a first-degree relative with PCOS may be an independent risk factor for the development of type 2 diabetes in childhood. The implication is that FDR's of PCOS should potentially be screened more aggressively for pre-diabetic risk factors, including obesity, hypertriglyceridemia, and a pro-inflammatory state and should be considered an at-risk group in terms of efforts to prevent the development of other risk factors. Finally, the detection of impaired glucose homeostasis prior to the onset of hyperandrogenism is in agreement with the hypothesis that hyperinsulinism is a cause, rather than the result, of PCOS.

PCOS is likely the cumulative product of a number of genetic, epigenetic, environmental factors and/or familial habits [29]. PCOS may be inherited in an autosomal dominant or X-linked dominant pattern [30-32]. Genome-wide genetic and linkage studies have found associations with PCOS for many genes including fibrillin-3, PPAR-γ

Table 2 Biochemical characteristics in FDR-PCOS and Control Daughters (Cd) groups

	FDR-PCOS Group (n = 18)	Cd Group (n = 21)
DHEA-S	63 (65)	99.5 (71)
AIRg	80 (54)	97 (43)
QUICKI	0.32 (0.03) *	0.35 (0.02)
HOMA-IR	3.45 (1.7)*	2.04 (1.6)
GDI	2.6 (0.46) *	2.98 (0.27)

Data are presented as the mean ± SD. *P value < 0.05.

and IL-6, though replication has proven elusive [33-36] and development of the characteristic syndrome may occur in the absence of known mutation. In complex, heterogeneous conditions with variable presentation such as PCOS, studies of first-degree relatives of affected females may help to separate the biochemical contributions from genetic and habitual influence.

Hyperandrogenism is the consistent finding in prior studies of the adult relatives of PCOS women [22,37-39] but the data on hyperandrogenism in peripubertal FDR is scant. One study observed higher androgen levels in the later stages of puberty (Tanner 4 and 5) in PCOS-FDR subjects compared to control daughters [40], likely an expression of the normal maturation of the hypothalamic-pituitary gonadal axis.

Many have proposed that hyperinsulinism is the fundamental pathophysiological event leading to ovarian and/or adrenal production of excessive androgen [41]. Hyperandrogenism is the primary feature in the emergence of PCOS [22,42]. In our study, significant differences in the androgen precursor DHEA-S between the two groups were not detected.

Conversely, beta-cell function was impaired not only in affected PCOS probands but also in their first-degree relatives, regardless of whether PCOS or other metabolic abnormalities were yet manifest. Prior reports of insulin resistance and glucose insensitivity in first-degree relatives utilized manipulation of the less informative oral glucose tolerance test. A recent study demonstrated hyperinsulinemia and increased ovarian volumes present in PCOS daughters even prior to the onset of puberty, the hyperinsulinemia persisting throughout pubertal development. Other biochemical abnormalities of PCOS emerge only in later puberty [40], suggesting that metabolic disturbances are fundamental to establishment of permanent states of androgen excess.

Frequently-sampled IVGTT is a well-validated method of estimating insulin sensitivity and considered superior to OGTT-derived measures of insulin dynamics [43-45] as it allows determination of the glucose disposal index (GDI), a highly sensitive reflection of the capacity of pancreatic islets to compensate for lower insulin sensitivity [46]. We utilized IVGTT to assess both glucose tolerance and insulin resistance as well as the acute insulin response and glucose disposition indices that better define the beta-cell function.

Our data provides evidence of early development of insulin resistance in the peripubertal first-degree female relatives of women with PCOS. All three measures, QUICKI, HOMA-IR and GDI, demonstrated lower insulin sensitivity among PCOS first-degree relatives versus weight, Tanner, age-matched controls without family history of PCOS, diabetes mellitus and hypertension. Perturbed beta-cell dysfunction and the resulting inadequate compensation for

deteriorating insulin sensitivity has been demonstrated in the daughters of PCOS-affected women prior to puberty and independently of body weight. Our findings suggest that peripubertal insulin resistance (IR) even prior to biochemical or clinically apparent androgen excess may also be an early hallmark of risk for PCOS in the genetically vulnerable peri-adolescent population as well. This emphasizes the necessity of early and ongoing biochemical monitoring of relatives of women with PCOS, affording the opportunity for both earlier diagnosis and therapeutic intervention to prevent the long-term morbidity inherent in this disorder.

Abbreviations
PCOS: Polycystic ovarian syndrome; AIR: Acute insulin response; GDI: Glucose disposal index; QUICKI: Quantitative insulin sensitivity check index; HOMA: Homeostatic model assessment; BMI: Body mass index; IVGTT: IV glucose tolerance test; OGTT: Oral glucose tolerance test; DHEAS: Dehydroepiandrosterone sulfate.

Competing interests
NR, AK, RP, SS, SB, AB, SM, RM, J-PB, MIH, MR, ST and DG have no competing interests.

Authors' contributions
DG participated in the planning and execution of the protocols performed on study subjects, as well as the preparation of the manuscript. NR, AK, RP, SS, SB, AB, SM, RM, J-PB, MIH, MR, ST participated in the execution of the protocols performed on study subjects, as well as the preparation of the manuscript. All authors read and approved the final manuscript.

Acknowledgments
We acknowledge the Reduce Obesity and Diabetes (ROAD) project under aegis of Academy for Medical Development and Collaboration (AMDeC). We would like to gratefully acknowledge the invaluable participation of all the students, teachers, and school administrators, as well as the NYC Board of Health and Department of Education. Funding was provided through AMDeC (Academy for Medical Development and Collaboration) and NIH grant # 1 UL1 RR024156-01. The study was supported by funding from K23 HD40325 "Insulin Resistance in Adolescents at High Risk for Polycystic Ovary Syndrome" (PI: David Geller) and M01-RR000425 (Cedars-Sinai General Clinical Research Center Grant from the NCRR).

Author details
[1]Division of Pediatric Endocrinology at Infants and Children's Hospital of Brooklyn at Maimonides & SUNY Downstate Medical Center, 1068 48th St, Brooklyn, NY 11219, USA. [2]Department of Pediatrics, Division of Pediatric Endocrinology, Vanderbilt University School of Medicine, Monroe Carell Jr. Children's Hospital at Vanderbilt, 11134A Doctors' Office Tower, 2200 Children's Way, Nashville, TN 37232-9170, USA. [3]Department of Medicine, and Physiology and Biophysics, Division of Endocrinology, University of Sherbrooke, 3001, 12e Avenue Nord, Sherbrooke, QC J1H 5N4, Canada. [4]Departments of Pediatrics, Endocrinologa Infantil, Instituto de Investigaciones Materno Infantil (IDIMI), Universidad de Chile, Clinica Las Condes Santiago, Chile. [5]Department of Pediatrics, Division of Pediatric Endocrinology, Children's Hospital of New York-Presbyterian, 622 West 168th Street, PH-5E-522, New York, NY 10032, USA. [6]Department of Pediatrics, Division of Pediatric Endocrinology, Cedars-Sinai Medical Center, David Geffen- University of California, Los Angeles School of Medicine, 8700 Beverly Blvd. Room 4220 North Tower, Los Angeles, CA 90048, USA.

References
1. Asuncion M, et al: A prospective study of the prevalence of the polycystic ovary syndrome in unselected Caucasian women from Spain. J Clin Endocrinol Metabol 2000, 85(7):2434–2438.

2. Diamanti-Kandarakis E, *et al*: A survey of the polycystic ovary syndrome in the Greek island of Lesbos: hormonal and metabolic profile. *J Clin Endocrinol Metabol* 1999, **84**(11):4006–4011.

3. Azziz R, *et al*: The prevalence and features of the polycystic ovary syndrome in an unselected population. *J Clin Endocrinol Metabol* 2004, **89**(6):2745–2749.

4. Franks S, Stark J, Hardy K: Follicle dynamics and anovulation in polycystic ovary syndrome. *Hum Reprod Update* 2008, **14**(4):367–378.

5. Gilling-Smith C, *et al*: Hypersecretion of androstenedione by isolated thecal cells from polycystic ovaries. *J Clin Endocrinol Metabol* 1994, **79**(4):1158–1165.

6. Ibanez L, Potau N, Carrascosa A: Insulin resistance, premature adrenarche, and a risk of the Polycystic Ovary Syndrome (PCOS). *Trends Endocrinol Metab* 1998, **9**(2):72–77.

7. Ehrmann DA, *et al*: *Insulin secretory defects in polycystic ovary syndrome. Relationship to insulin sensitivity and family history of non-insulin-dependent diabetes mellitus. J Clin Invest* 1995, **96**(1):520–527.

8. Holte J: Disturbances in insulin secretion and sensitivity in women with the polycystic ovary syndrome. *Baillieres Clin Endocrinol Metab* 1996, **10**(2):221–247.

9. Dunaif A: Insulin resistance and the polycystic ovary syndrome: mechanism and implications for pathogenesis. *Endocr Rev* 1997, **18**(6):774–800.

10. Dunaif A, *et al*: Profound peripheral insulin resistance, independent of obesity, in polycystic ovary syndrome. *Diabetes* 1989, **38**(9):1165–1174.

11. Ehrmann DA, *et al*: Prevalence of impaired glucose tolerance and diabetes in women with polycystic ovary syndrome. *Diabetes Care* 1999, **22**(1):141–146.

12. Legro RS, *et al*: Prevalence and predictors of risk for type 2 diabetes mellitus and impaired glucose tolerance in polycystic ovary syndrome: a prospective, controlled study in 254 affected women. *J Clin Endocrinol Metabol* 1999, **84**(1):165–169.

13. Dahlgren E, *et al*: *Polycystic ovary syndrome and risk for myocardial infarction. Evaluated from a risk factor model based on a prospective population study of women. Acta Obstet Gynecol Scand* 1992, **71**(8):599–604.

14. Hull MG: Epidemiology of infertility and polycystic ovarian disease: endocrinological and demographic studies. *Gynecol Endocrinol* 1987, **1**(3):235–245.

15. Sagle M, *et al*: Recurrent early miscarriage and polycystic ovaries. *BMJ* 1988, **297**(6655):1027–1028.

16. Kahsar-Miller MD, *et al*: Prevalence of polycystic ovary syndrome (PCOS) in first-degree relatives of patients with PCOS. *Fertil Steril* 2001, **75**(1):53–58.

17. Coviello AD, *et al*: High prevalence of metabolic syndrome in first-degree male relatives of women with polycystic ovary syndrome is related to high rates of obesity. *J Clin Endocrinol Metabol* 2009, **94**(11):4361–4366.

18. Moini A, Eslami B: Familial associations between polycystic ovarian syndrome and common diseases. *J Assist Reprod Genet* 2009, **26**(2–3):123–127.

19. Reis KS, *et al*: Anthropometric and metabolic evaluation of first-degree male relatives of women with polycystic ovary syndrome. *Rev Bras Ginecol Obstet* 2010, **32**(7):334–339.

20. Sam S, *et al*: Dyslipidemia and metabolic syndrome in the sisters of women with polycystic ovary syndrome. *J Clin Endocrinol Metabol* 2005, **90**(8):4797–4802.

21. Sam S, *et al*: Evidence for pancreatic beta-cell dysfunction in brothers of women with polycystic ovary syndrome. *Metab Clin Exp* 2008, **57**(1):84–89.

22. Legro RS, *et al*: Evidence for a genetic basis for hyperandrogenemia in polycystic ovary syndrome. *Proc Natl Acad Sci U S A* 1998, **95**(25):14956–14960.

23. Zawadzki JK DA: *Diagnostic criteria for polycystic ovary syndrome: towards a rational approach.* Oxford, UK: Blackwell; 1992:59–69.

24. Kuczmarski RJ, *et al*: CDC Growth Charts for the United States: methods and development. *Vital Health Stat 11* 2000, 2002(246):1–190.

25. Bergman RN, Phillips LS, Cobelli C: Physiologic evaluation of factors controlling glucose tolerance in man: measurement of insulin sensitivity and beta-cell glucose sensitivity from the response to intravenous glucose. *J Clin Invest* 1981, **68**(6):1456–1467.

26. Matthews DR, *et al*: Homeostasis model assessment: insulin resistance and beta-cell function from fasting plasma glucose and insulin concentrations in man. *Diabetologia* 1985, **28**(7):412–419.

27. Katz A, *et al*: Quantitative insulin sensitivity check index: a simple, accurate method for assessing insulin sensitivity in humans. *J Clin Endocrinol Metabol* 2000, **85**(7):2402–2410.

28. Rosenbaum M, *et al*: beta-Cell function and insulin sensitivity in early adolescence: association with body fatness and family history of type 2 diabetes mellitus. *J Clin Endocrinol Metabol* 2004, **89**(11):5469–5476.

29. Li Z, Huang H: Epigenetic abnormality: a possible mechanism underlying the fetal origin of polycystic ovary syndrome. *Medical hypotheses* 2008, **70**(3):638–642.

30. Govind A, Obhrai MS, Clayton RN: Polycystic ovaries are inherited as an autosomal dominant trait: analysis of 29 polycystic ovary syndrome and 10 control families. *J Clin Endocrinol Metabol* 1999, **84**(1):38–43.

31. Legro RS: The genetics of polycystic ovary syndrome. *Am J Med* 1995, **98**(1A):9S–16S.

32. Givens JR: Familial polycystic ovarian disease. *Endocrinol Metab Clin North Am* 1988, **17**(4):771–783.

33. Urbanek M: The genetics of the polycystic ovary syndrome. *Nat Clin Pract Endocrinol Metab* 2007, **3**(2):103–111.

34. Prodoehl MJ, *et al*: Genetic and gene expression analyses of the polycystic ovary syndrome candidate gene fibrillin-3 and other fibrillin family members in human ovaries. *Mol Hum Reprod* 2009, **15**(12):829–841.

35. Tok EC, *et al*: Evaluation of glucose metabolism and reproductive hormones in polycystic ovary syndrome on the basis of peroxisome proliferator-activated receptor (PPAR)-gamma2 Pro12Ala genotype. *Hum Reprod* 2005, **20**(6):1590–1595.

36. Escobar-Morreale HF, *et al*: Association of polymorphisms in the interleukin 6 receptor complex with obesity and hyperandrogenism. *Obes Res* 2003, **11**(8):987–996.

37. Lenarcik A, *et al*: Hormonal abnormalities in first-degree relatives of women with polycystic ovary syndrome (PCOS). *Endokrynol Pol* 2011, **62**(2):129–133.

38. Unluhizarci K, *et al*: Investigation of hypothalamo-pituitary-gonadal axis and glucose intolerance among the first-degree female relatives of women with polycystic ovary syndrome. *Fertil Steril* 2007, **87**(6):1377–1382.

39. Yildiz BO, *et al*: Glucose intolerance, insulin resistance, and hyperandrogenemia in first degree relatives of women with polycystic ovary syndrome. *J Clin Endocrinol Metabol* 2003, **88**(5):2031–2036.

40. Sir-Petermann T, *et al*: Metabolic and reproductive features before and during puberty in daughters of women with polycystic ovary syndrome. *J Clin Endocrinol Metabol* 2009, **94**(6):1923–1930.

41. Vigouroux C: What have we learned form monogenic forms of severe insulin resistance associated with PCOS/HAIRAN? *Ann Endocrinol (Paris)* 2010, **71**(3):222–224.

42. DiMartino-Nardi J: Insulin resistance in prepubertal African-American and Hispanic girls with premature adrenarche: a risk factor for polycystic ovary syndrome. *Trends Endocrinol Metab* 1998, **9**(2):78–82.

43. Ferrannini E, Mari A: Beta cell function and its relation to insulin action in humans: a critical appraisal. *Diabetologia* 2004, **47**(5):943–956.

44. Porte D Jr: *Banting lecture 1990.* Beta-cells in type II diabetes mellitus. *Diabetes* 1991, **40**(2):166–180.

45. Rosenbaum M, *et al*: School-based intervention acutely improves insulin sensitivity and decreases inflammatory markers and body fatness in junior high school students. *J Clin Endocrinol Metabol* 2007, **92**(2):504–508.

46. Bergman RN, *et al*: Accurate assessment of beta-cell function: the hyperbolic correction. *Diabetes* 2002, **51**(Suppl 1):S212–S220.

11

Children with disorders of sex development: A qualitative study of early parental experience

Halley P Crissman[1†], Lauren Warner[1†], Melissa Gardner[1], Meagan Carr[1], Aileen Schast[2], Alexandra L Quittner[3], Barry Kogan[4] and David E Sandberg[1*]

Abstract

Background: Clinical research on psychological aspects of disorders of sex development (DSD) has focused on psychosexual differentiation with relatively little attention directed toward parents' experiences of early clinical management and their influence on patient and family psychosocial adaptation.

Objectives: To characterize parental experiences in the early clinical care of children born with DSD.

Study Design: Content analysis of interviews with parents (n = 41) of 28 children, newborn to 6 years, with DSD.

Results: Four major domains emerged as salient to parents: (1) the gender assignment process, (2) decisions regarding genital surgery, (3) disclosing information about their child's DSD, and (4) interacting with healthcare providers. Findings suggested discordance between scientific and parental understandings of the determinants of "sex" and "gender." Parents' expectations regarding the benefits of genital surgery appear largely met; however, parents still had concerns about their child's future physical, social and sexual development. Two areas experienced by many parents as particularly stressful were: (1) uncertainties regarding diagnosis and optimal management, and (2) conflicts between maintaining privacy versus disclosing the condition to access social support.

Conclusions: Parents' experiences and gaps in understanding can be used to inform the clinical care of patients with DSD and their families. Improving communication between parents and providers (and between parents and their support providers) throughout the early clinical management process may be important in decreasing stress and improving outcomes for families of children with DSD.

Keywords: disorders of sex development, qualitative, content analysis, psychosocial, health-related quality of life, genital surgery, parents

Introduction

In 2005, the Lawson Wilkins Pediatric Endocrine Society (renamed the *Pediatric Endocrine Society* in 2010) and the European Society for Paediatric Endocrinology convened a consensus conference on the management of "intersex" [1]. Conference participants recommended a new diagnostic nomenclature and introduced "disorders of sex development" (DSD) as the superordinate term for "congenital conditions in which chromosomal, gonadal, or anatomic sex development is atypical" [1].

Research on the psychological development of persons with DSD has focused on understanding the influence of atypical sex hormone exposure during steroid-sensitive periods of prenatal brain development on the process of psychosexual differentiation (i.e., gender identity, gender role, and sexual orientation) [2-5]. Analysis of clinical management strategies has focused on gender assignment and the desirability and timing of genital surgery [1,6-8].

The DSD Consensus Statement [1] recognizes that these conditions can exert substantial strain on the family; however, there have been relatively few systematic studies of how early interventions and interactions between healthcare providers and the family affect the quality of life of affected persons or their parents [9,10]. One study of parents of young children (predominantly

* Correspondence: dsandber@med.umich.edu
† Contributed equally
[1]Department of Pediatrics & Communicable Diseases Division of Child Behavioral Health University of Michigan Medical School 1500 East Medical Center Drive, SPC 5318 Ann Arbor, Michigan 48109-5318 USA
Full list of author information is available at the end of the article

46, XY) with DSD found that 19% and 13%, respectively, reported clinically significant parenting stress and diminished adaptive coping capacity [11]. Interestingly, these self-report ratings were unrelated to the degree of masculinization of the child's external genitalia. Other evidence of the burden of the medical condition on the family was reflected in the observation that over 60% of these parents experienced difficulties in discussing their child's condition with relatives and friends and 68% were concerned that the DSD would result in their child being stigmatized [11].

Similar gaps in our understanding extend to parental reactions to early medical interventions [9,10]. Although early surgery may, in some cases, be necessary to allow for unobstructed urinary output without infections or to eliminate potential malignancy risk associated with dysgenetic gonads, early timing of procedures has also been justified as a strategy to relieve parental distress and reduce the likelihood of stigmatization, despite a lack of systematic evidence to support this belief [1,8,9,12,13].

Parental understanding of DSD pathophysiology and treatment options soon after the child's birth has received scant attention [13-15]. For example, parents' conceptualizations of the relationship between biological indices of sex development (i.e., karyotype, gonadal determination, sex hormone production and genital phenotype) and psychosexual differentiation remain largely unexplored. The same holds true for parents' views of the linkages between gender assignment and necessity of genital surgery, the benefits and drawbacks of disclosure of the child's DSD to extended family and friends, and parents' experiences with healthcare providers during the earliest stages of DSD ascertainment and clinical management.

Theoretical models of adjustment to congenital chronic medical conditions recognize critical parental influences on the affected person's adjustment during childhood and beyond [16-18]. Recent reports underscore the strain experienced by parents of newborns and young children born with DSD [14,19]; however, more complete information is needed regarding parents' experiences during the diagnostic and early decision-making periods associated with DSD. The goal of the present study was to identify clinically salient aspects of the parental experience regarding the diagnosis and clinical management of their children.

Methods and Participants
Design
A secondary data analysis was performed on interview transcripts from a study designed to develop health-related quality of life (HRQoL) measures for young patients with DSD and their families. The primary study was designed to evaluate the relevance, importance and clarity of preliminary quality of life items generated via open-ended interviews with parents, health care providers and advocates [20]. Items forming the provisional parent self-report HRQoL questionnaire were clustered into 10 subscales designed to capture both common and rare DSD-specific issues (*healthcare, decision-making, talking to others, role functioning/family activities, gender concerns, social functioning, general emotional functioning, medications, surgery, doctor visits, future concerns*, and *earliest experiences*). Parents completed the questionnaires in written form and then participated in cognitive interviews during which they were asked about their responses to each item using standardized prompts, including: "What did you think of when answering this question?" and "How did you decide on your rating?" [21,22]. Parents were asked to comment on any aspects of their experience that were not covered by the existing questions at the end of each subscale and at the end of the questionnaire itself. Structured interviews were conducted by clinician-researchers and experienced research staff (MG, ALQ, AS, DES, MB, and LC), trained by ALQ to conduct cognitive interviews. This research team has extensive experience in conducting these types of interviews [23,24]. Interviewers followed a structured protocol of open-ended questions and were instructed to allow parents to explore their thoughts and experiences without interruption.

Participant responses to cognitive interview questions often involved detailed descriptions of personal experiences related to the diagnosis and management of their child's DSD that went beyond responding to the standardized prompts. Interviews were audio-recorded and transcribed verbatim. Parents' responses to the items and follow-up interviews, together with demographic information and medical chart excerpts collected in the primary study, constituted the dataset for this secondary analysis.

All study procedures were approved by participating medical centers' Institutional Review Boards.

Participants
Participants were parents of children with DSD identified by systematic medical record review at four regional medical centers located in metropolitan areas along the East Coast and Midwestern United States. Stratified, random sampling was employed to create a sample representative of a wide range of DSD diagnoses, phenotypic severity, gender assignment decisions, and age (newborn to age 6 years). Because of the sampling strategy adopted, the breakdown by diagnosis does not reflect the natural incidence of DSD. Genital surgery status was not used as a selection criterion. Participants who could not communicate in English or whose child

had a documented, significant developmental delay (e.g., autism) were excluded.

Of the 134 households with an index child meeting study eligibility criteria, three were subsequently excluded based on details provided by parents: one child exhibited marked developmental delay and two parents were unable to be interviewed in English. One non-parent caregiver who contributed data to the primary study was also excluded. Of the remaining 130 index cases, recruitment continued until it was determined that successive cognitive interviews did not yield new information or new themes (i.e., saturation of content). A total of 19 of 130 eligible households (15%) refused to participate. The final sample comprised 41 parents (27 mothers and 14 fathers; Table 1) of 28 DSD-affected children (Table 2). Participants received $50 as compensation for their time.

Details regarding the child's medical history, including diagnosis and management, were excerpted from the medical record using standardized forms completed by qualified healthcare staff at participating medical centers.

Table 1 Parent participant characteristics (n = 41)

Parenting Role	n (%)
Mother	27 (65.9)
Father	14 (34.1)
Racial Identification	**n (%)**
Non-Hispanic	28 (68.3)
Hispanic	4 (9.8)
Black	3 (7.3)
Other	2 (4.9)
Declined to Respond	4 (9.8)
Education	**n (%)**
Partial High School	2 (4.9)
High School Graduate	8 (19.5)
Some College Education	11 (26.8)
College or University Graduate	9 (22.0)
Graduate or Professional Degree	7 (17.1)
Declined to Respond	4 (9.8)
Yearly Family Income	**n (%)**
< 20,000	8 (19.5)
20,000-40,000	9 (22.0)
40,000-60,000	5 (12.2)
60,000-80,000	4 (9.8)
> 80,000	11 (26.8)
Declined to Respond	4 (9.8)
Age, *years*	
Mean (SD)	34.7 (6.7)
Range	19.5-50.8
Declined to Respond, n (%)	6 (14.6)

Data Analysis

All participants shared the experience of parenting a newborn and/or young child with DSD and associated medical management; thus, a phenomenological approach was well-suited to guide the qualitative content analysis [25]. Three investigators (HPC, LW, and MC) who were not involved with the design or evaluation of the primary study's HRQoL questionnaires, independently read the cognitive interview transcripts and highlighted parent dialogue that reflected salient thoughts, beliefs, and experiences related to their child's DSD and management. This process resulted in an initial outline of emergent categories. The same investigators then independently read the transcripts a second time to supplement and restructure the outline to better reflect parents' experiences. These outlines were merged through a process of comparison and data reduction. In contrast to the HRQoL questionnaire development process, in which we sought to capture the full range of experiences including those that were rare, this analysis focused on overarching themes expressed across multiple domains of the interview transcripts.

"Member checking" was used to improve the accuracy, credibility, and validity of the investigators' coding and interpretation of the cognitive interviews [26]: a convenience sample of study participants from one site was provided a draft of the study results for comment. Participants (n = 5) were asked to comment on the accuracy and completeness with which their experiences were represented. These respondents' comments were used to refine the results.

Results

Four overarching and clinically salient domains of parental experiences rearing young DSD-affected children emerged from the content analysis: (1) sex announcement and gender assignment, (2) surgical decision-making, (3) sharing information about the child's DSD with others, and (4) interactions with healthcare providers. Parents who participated in the member-checking interviews identified these domains as accurately reflecting the major issues they experienced.

Sex Announcement and Gender Assignment

A common feature of many DSD is atypical or ambiguous external genitalia. External genitalia ambiguity can be associated with a delayed gender announcement at birth (i.e. "It's a boy!" or "It's a girl!"). Although there is a well-recognized distinction between biologic "sex" (male/female) and "gender of rearing" (boy/girl), parents and providers often conflated the two constructs, e.g., "genetically, he was a boy." [27]

Parental perspective. Most parents voiced certainty about knowing their child's sex and gender of rearing

Table 2 Participants' children's characteristics (n = 28)

	n (%)	Gender of Rearing	
		Boy	Girl
DSD Diagnosis[a]	n (%)	n (%)	n (%)
Gender			
Boy	19 (67.9)		
Girl	9 (32.1)		
Age (years)			
Mean (SD)	4.1 (1.9)		
Range	0.75-6.99		
Number of Genital Surgeries			
Mean (SD)	2.46 (1.06)		
Range	1-4		
Sex Chromosome DSD	3 (10.7)	3 (100)	0 (0)
45XO/46XY Mixed gonadal dysgenesis	1	1	0
45XO/46XisoY Mixed gonadal dysgenesis	1	1	0
45XO/46XY/47XYY Mixed gonadal dysgenesis	1	1	0
46, XX DSD	8 (28.6)	1 (12.5)	7 (87.5)
Congenital adrenal hyperplasia	7	0	7
Ovotesticular DSD	1	1	0
46, XY DSD	17 (60.7)	15 (88.2)	2 (11.8)
Aphallia	1	1	0
Complete androgen insensitivity syndrome (AIS)	1	0	1
Partial AIS (PAIS)	1	1	0
Partial gonadal dysgenesis	3	2	1
Partial AIS vs Idiopathic vs 5α-reductase-2 deficiency	4	4	0
Severe hypospadias with cryptorchidism and chordee	1	1	0
Severe hypospadias with chordee	6	6	0

[a] see reference [1] for details of DSD nomenclature.

immediately or soon after their child's birth-despite known discordance across karyotype, gonads, or genital anatomy. Parents used (1) their personal intuitions or "gut feelings," (2) the visible appearance of the child's external genitalia or imaging reports of the internal sex organs, and/or (3) genetic testing results to justify their conviction.

A number of parents expressed confidence about knowing their child's sex and gender prior to medical testing. One mother explained that she did not need testing performed on her child to know her child was a girl: "We never even doubted it." Another parent described feeling that they "didn't really have to assign" a gender, though doctors performed a laparoscopy and, in the parent's words, determined that the child "had more boy parts than girl parts" and thus, was a boy. Others cited karyotype findings as definitively determining both their child's sex and gender, erroneously assuming that sex chromosomes are the ultimate arbiters: "We had genetic testing done. So it wasn't like we had to choose and we had to worry about whether we were doing the right thing or not."

Medical chart excerpts. In contrast to parents' nearly immediate certainty about whether their children were males or females/boys or girls, a review of children's medical records revealed healthcare provider delays in gender assignment (n = 7), gender reassignment after initial birth announcement or assignment (n = 3), and cases in which karyotype did not match assigned sex or gender of rearing [n = 6, including 3 cases of sex chromosome mosaicism (e.g., 45, XO/46, XY; Table 2)].

Surgical Decision-Making

The necessity of surgery. All children (n = 28) in this study had at least one genital surgery prior to parental participation in this study, though prior surgery was not an inclusion criterion. Reflecting on early decision-making, parents recalled strong wishes to surgically "normalize" their child's sexual anatomy, i.e., external genitalia and internal reproductive structures. Many parents viewed surgery as obvious and necessary, and did not experience it as something that involved a decision-making process. One parent stated: "The minute he was born, here he had this– it has to be fixed... It was never any question whether he was gonna go through the surgery or not." Parents frequently used the term "fix" to describe how they understood various surgical interventions.

Parents expressed a profound trust in the medical team's recommendations: "We really never had to make a decision... the doctors told us what was gonna need to be done." As one parent explained: "I wanted them to do the best that they can for my son. So umm, anything they asked for or wanted to do, I was ok with it."

Anticipated benefits. Parents expressed a strong belief that surgery would (1) "fix" the appearance and function of their child's external genitalia and reproductive structures, and (2) avert expected negative psychosocial consequences associated with DSD (i.e. non-normative gender identity and/or gender role, teasing from peers, and hardship in future romantic relationships): "We felt [surgery] would be beneficial for health and social reasons like teasing in school." This sentiment was echoed by others: "In our son's case, he would have had to pee sitting down for the rest of his life and that has both social and physical aspects." Parents sought to surgically modify aspects of the DSD that they thought would be barriers to positive daily functioning: "We want him to have as normal a life as possible. So the benefits outweigh the risks." Parents perceived the medical team as reinforcing the idea that surgery would resolve the DSD: "Dr. [Urologist] was called in and, like a ray of sunshine, said 'I can fix this.'"

Post-surgery experiences. Some parents felt all early concerns related to their child's DSD were eliminated by surgery: "We don't even talk about it anymore. It's just not an issue for us anymore, you know. It's been repaired, and that's it." In general, parents did not report thinking about their children's DSD on a day-to-day basis: "It comes and goes in waves with us definitely... he has his surgery and everything and it's 'oh my gosh, it's kinda real again.' After he recovers from the surgery he's just, you know, he's our normal little boy, doing his stuff."

Most parents expressed satisfaction with the surgery and the functioning of their child's genitalia at present; however, they also noted concerns about the future: fearing negative physical, social, or emotional changes associated with puberty and adolescence, one parent stated "I'm more concerned with it as he gets older... what things are gonna look like... things are functioning perfect right now." Another parent noted "The physically hard part is... is done with, the surgeries are all done. I think now is the emotional." For most parents who continued to express concerns about their child's genital appearance or function following surgery, the worries were future-oriented.

Parental concerns that persisted after surgery included (1) gender identity: "I worry that at some point he's going to feel like he's a woman trapped in a man's body, even though his female structures were removed," (2) gender role: "She throws in the 'Mom, will you paint my nails?' and I go fall over and do it right then and there... I dropped all that I was doing and painted her fingernails because she wanted to act like a little girl," (3) peers: "I worry he's going to be in gym class and people are going to notice things... I just always worry that, you know, that that will be frustrating for him to deal with in the future," (4) romantic partners: "The surgery can only fix so much, it's not going to look exactly normal. In the future, a husband or boyfriend may not be ok with it," (5) fertility: "[I worry about] him being able to have children and be able to feel that he is adequate," and (6) sexual orientation: "He's had so many problems. Is there a possibility of, you know, homosexuality?" No parent specifically stated that they regretted consenting to their child's surgery; however, one parent questioned the necessity in hindsight: "Did she even need to have that [surgery] in the first place? Should we have just left it alone?... It seems like with doctors, it's such a, like they just want to fix it and diagnose." Figure 1 schematically summarizes parent reports of experiences during the period of diagnostic evaluation and decision-making regarding genital surgery.

Despite parents' uncertainties and apprehensions about the future, parents in our study expressed confidence in the appropriateness of their child's gender assignment-including those whose children experienced either delayed gender assignment or reassignment. However, parents tended to express greater concerns about their child's gender development in cases in which the internal genital anatomy or sex chromosomes were discordant with the child's gender of rearing. Conversely, parents of children in whom these markers of sex development were concordant, despite an atypical genital

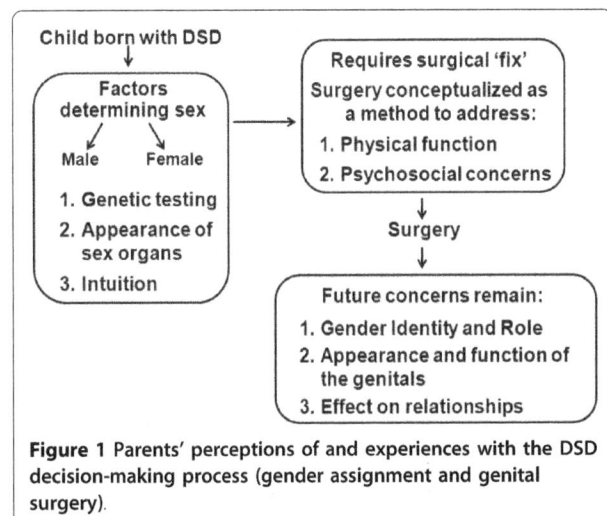

Figure 1 Parents' perceptions of and experiences with the DSD decision-making process (gender assignment and genital surgery).

phenotype (e.g., proximal hypospadias with bilateral undescended testes in child with 46, XY karyotype), expressed less concern over the child's gender development.

Sharing Information

Although parents' concerns over their child's gender development depended in part on the specific DSD, this distinction did not predict the amount of information parents shared with others about their child's condition. Instead, comfort with disclosure depended on parents' outlook regarding: (1) the likelihood of stigmatization, (2) who they believed had the right to disclose information, (3) personal comfort in talking about anatomical aspects of DSD, and (4) parents' perceived ability to accurately explain DSD to others and/or have their child's condition understood.

Concerns about talking with others. Many parents expressed the view that sharing information about their child's condition would lead to stigmatization: "I don't want people to treat her different." Parents were also concerned about rumors and gossip: "I don't want rumors to start and for it to affect him later on in life-like socially because people don't understand the condition." Most fears were not based on direct experience; however, one parent reported a negative incident with a family member: "Her father came over and said that it wasn't his child because he don't make funny babies."

Several parents noted that, because DSD was potentially stigmatizing, they wanted to preserve their child's right to make decisions about disclosure: "There's a whole stigma associated with this, and it's unfortunate, and I have kept it mostly private for [my son] because I don't know how he wants to handle it when he gets bigger." Other parents, particularly those who opted for sharing more information, felt less need to defer the decision to their child: "I'm not embarrassed about what they have. You know, it's part of life."

Several parents felt their child's condition was extremely difficult to explain, and/or not something most people would understand. Additionally, parents were concerned that their attempts to explain the condition to others would generate more questions than they wanted to answer; one parent noted: "It is kind of exhausting trying to explain." Many parents expressed discomfort in talking to others about the anatomical aspects of their child's DSD: "It's a little bit of a personal area of the body so it's... I don't know. I don't want to run around with a banner saying that my child has an issue with that part of his body."

Consequences of minimal sharing. Most parents chose to limit the amount of information shared, with whom it was shared, and who was allowed to view their child's genitals. The practice of limiting information sharing proved to be difficult and stressful for many. In some cases, parents did not share details of the DSD with anyone, including close family (e.g., child's grandparents). Nevertheless, parents reported feeling pressured to talk about their child's condition with others: "People want to know, 'What's going on?' How he is. 'Why were you at the doctor?' So you kind of have to come up with a way to talk about it," or "I had to tell somebody, 'cause it was bursting inside of me. I'm like, I've gotta get somebody else's input or something." At the same time, parents believed that keeping their children's DSD private was extremely important: "It's hard having a child with something that you can't talk to people about. That you feel like you've got to have this huge secret all the time. That in itself is stressful in that you just can't tell people how you feel... [but] I can't jeopardize it, I can't take that risk. I just can't." Parents also reported avoiding situations in which their child's genitals might be seen: "I would change [my unaffected son] into a bathing suit at a side of a pool and not think twice about it and with [my affected son], I would *never* do that" or "I was like 'Oh no, you are not changing his diaper. I don't want to talk about it.'"

Many parents decided to give others partial information about their child's DSD and its management in order to strike a balance between their desire to consult and share with others and their fear of negative consequences. One parent noted: "I guess it was a little bit easier to say, 'He had a bladder infection so we went to the doctor,' versus saying, 'Well, when he was born he had this birth defect and...'" More rarely, parents felt comfortable discussing the condition openly: "I don't think that there's really anything private... I've never thought of keeping it from anybody." Many parents reported that as time went on they became more comfortable with their child's condition and that sharing information was less pressing, particularly when their child was more independent (i.e., no longer in diapers and surgical aftercare was complete) or after genital appearance was modified. Figure 2 summarizes parents' experiences with disclosure of their child's DSD.

Interactions with Healthcare Providers

DSD education. Many parents reported that until they received their child's diagnosis, they were unaware such conditions existed: "I didn't understand it. I'd never heard of it before." Parents felt that their unfamiliarity with their child's diagnosis contributed to their stress and feelings of isolation: "[I] had never talked to anybody that had ever experienced it and I kinda felt like... I was the only one ever having to deal with this." Parents often described gaining information from the medical team as helpful in decreasing this source of stress.

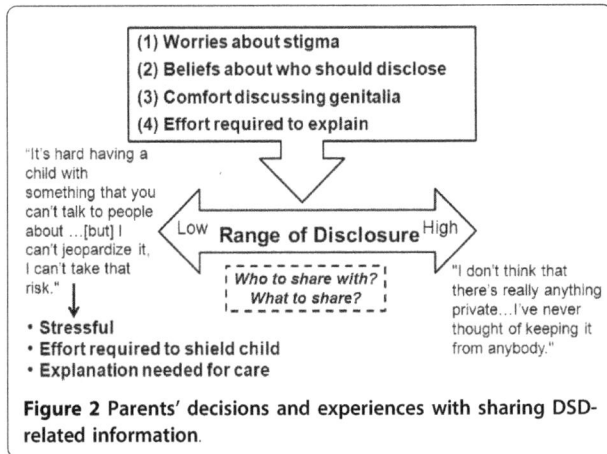

Figure 2 Parents' decisions and experiences with sharing DSD-related information.

Several parents mentioned physicians' drawings as a particularly helpful tool that enhanced their understanding.

Despite what parents believed were the providers' best efforts, some expressed frustration with the type or amount of information available to them: "The most stressful thing is just not being presented with clear-cut information." This same parent went on to explain: "[The medical staff] did give us pamphlets and they kind of explained things over and over, but you really want comprehensive information and it's hard." Still other parents noted positive experiences in obtaining information from their child's medical team, but encountered difficulties when seeking information through other sources: "The doctors don't overload you. They give you as much as you can handle, and go from there. The only problem is when you go home and you try and research this, and you get scared."

Negative experiences. Although the majority of parents described their communications with healthcare providers as supportive, a handful reported incidents described as "frustrating" or "exploitive." One parent said: "I felt like [the doctor] was looking just to look... I felt like he was just exploiting her for his own... you know—he wanted to see the surgery." While parents expressed an understanding that a hospital may also have a teaching mission, they did not feel that this justified the large number of providers interacting with them or their child or the repeated examinations of their child's genitalia: "There were so many residents and different people coming in at every time it felt like he was a show-horse and that was frustrating... you're trying to breastfeed for the first time."

Discussion

For families, the birth of a child with a DSD and the attendant uncertainty about the child's gender and future psychological and psychosexual development is believed to be extraordinarily stressful [28]. High levels of stress are likely to arise from both the unfamiliarity and perceived stigma associated with DSD and from the controversies surrounding current clinical management of these conditions. Despite parents having had access to services delivered at reputable tertiary care facilities, parents' experiences suggest a need to continue to strengthen the Consensus Statements' call for comprehensive and integrated long-term care for families affected by DSD [1]. The findings suggest, in particular, a need to improve provider-family/patient communication and to increase the availability of psychosocial support as an integral component in the delivery of care. While the parents in this study reported that early surgical interventions eased some of their immediate concerns, the findings suggest varied opportunities for enhancing education, shared decision-making, and linking families of affected children to others sharing common challenges [1].

Study participants expressed certainty about their child's sex and gender-whether announced at birth or subsequently assigned. For those parents that referenced diagnostic tests as a source of their certainty, it is unclear if such confidence stemmed from their understanding of test findings (e.g., karyotype, studies of internal reproductive anatomy), or if these results were selectively called upon to reinforce their intuitions. Several parents' reports suggested that healthcare providers framed clinical and laboratory findings to either generate or reinforce parents' beliefs that these indicators of sex development are determinative of gender identity. Until the mid-1950s, medical management of persons affected with DSD was guided by the belief that an individual's "true sex" could be revealed through examination of internal anatomy and that the person's identification as boy or girl would naturally conform to their "true sex" [28]. We now know that individual markers of biological sex can be associated with a range of gender outcomes [29-33]. Given the potential effect of this information on parental decision-making, this prompts the question to what degree and with how much detail should healthcare providers, in the promotion of the principles of shared decision-making, educate parents about the nuances of somatic sex development and their inconsistent relationship with gender identity in DSD if, by doing so, they potentially enhance cognitive and emotional conflict in the parents? Understandably, providers may fear alienating those parents who already have a strong conviction about their child's sex and gender by presenting a contrary viewpoint. However, without providing comprehensive information, providers risk breaching the ethics of informed consent for clinical interventions and the possibility that the parents will later learn about the withheld information and interpret provider's selectivity as a shortcoming or even a deception.

Delivering information that aligns with the ethics of informed consent is particularly critical when interventions are elective, non-urgent, controversial, and associated with potentially serious risks [34,35]. To enhance transparency and diminish the likelihood of decisional regret, Karkazis and colleagues recently outlined a 6-step model for shared decision-making in DSD as it pertains to genital surgery in young children [34].

Parents in our study also reported frustration over gaps in information about their child's condition. This could be due to a number of factors: (1) uncertainty about the diagnosis in the early stages which creates difficulties when discussing the condition, its course, and early management, (2) lack of educational tools that make complex medical concepts accessible to the general public, (3) parents' potentially diminished capacity to process complex medical concepts and make decisions during a time of stress, and (4) the existing gaps in medical literature surrounding DSD and DSD care. Parenting with uncertainties regarding the child's future is common in pediatric chronic illness and disease specific parent-to-parent support has been shown to be particularly useful in helping parents to cope with uncertainties and their frustrations during early decision-making; the use of support groups is additionally endorsed by the Consensus Statement [1]. Development of high quality DSD-specific educational content that adheres to the principles of health literacy [36] may also facilitate improved communication and knowledge sharing between provider and family. One exemplary sample of such content are the *Sex Development* pages of the *AboutKidsHealth* website edited by faculty and staff at the Hospital for Sick Children in Toronto [37]. Providers may also integrate HRQoL assessments into clinical care as a means of better identifying and addressing parent and child needs and concerns [29].

Parents recalled events surrounding their child's genital surgery with particular salience. Consistent with other reports, parents viewed genital surgery as a necessary and obvious "fix" for their child's DSD [9,13,38]. They justified early surgery as a means of averting negative consequences, such as stigmatization, that are associated with atypical genital appearance or function [13,39,40]. While satisfied with surgical outcomes, they continued to be concerned about the child's future experiences. Parents' worries primarily pertained to uncertainty about changes in their child's genital appearance or function associated with the onset of puberty, whether spontaneous or by hormone replacement, and the renewed risk of stigmatization or rejection by potential sexual/romantic partners and peers. These findings point out that early surgery reduces early parental concerns regarding genital appearance, but does not eliminate worries about their child's future sex development

or function. Accordingly, there is an important need to maintain contact with families in order to monitor parents' expectations and address unresolved anxiety about the child's future, even in those cases in which early surgery was considered an unqualified success.

Previous research regarding disclosure in DSD has focused on harm to affected individuals by being either uninformed or misinformed about their condition [1,6,15]. However, parents of affected individuals also appear to grapple with issues of information sharing. For the parents in the present study, withholding information from other adults was motivated by a desire to protect the child's privacy and to prevent stigmatization. However, parents varied markedly in the degree to which they disclosed details. Those who maintained fairly strict privacy experienced this approach as very stressful, whereas those who chose to share information with trusted others reported experiencing less strain. The current findings suggest that in addition to parents educating their child in a developmentally-appropriate way about their condition, they may benefit from more explicit and extensive discussions about sharing information with their usual social support system (family and friends). The extent to which such discussions between parents and providers are currently occurring is unclear. The results suggest, however, that the status quo is inadequate with respect to the counseling of parents on the challenges of information sharing and support seeking. The child's right to privacy should be balanced against the risks associated with secrecy, promoting a sense of shame, and limiting opportunities for social support. Failure to achieve this balance could contribute to unresolved parental feelings of guilt and possibly to a negative self-concept, shame or isolation for the DSD-affected person [9,41,42]. The Consensus Statement [1] identifies the timing and content of information management as warranting targeted study.

The majority of interactions between parents and their child's healthcare providers were described as positive. However, several negative interactions were noted in the context of genital examinations which parents felt were unnecessary or exploitative. There is reason to be concerned that repeated genital examinations and medical photography can have lasting and severe negative psychological consequences [43-45]. Responses to genital examinations in DSD and strategies to perform them in a way that reduces the likelihood of harm is another area in which systematic information is missing. In the interim, providers should continue to communicate openly with the patient and family, describe the purpose of the exams, ask for consent (and when appropriate, assent), and minimize patient exposure. Input from child life specialists who are trained to mitigate distress associated with medical procedures may be helpful [46].

Study Strengths and Limitations

This study presents the experiences of a relatively large sample of mothers and fathers of diagnostically diverse young children with DSD. Parent participants were identified through a systematic review of the children's medical records; only a small proportion of those contacted refused participation. An additional strength of this study was the extent of fathers' participation (35%). Frequently, studies of children with medical conditions rely exclusively on maternal reports [47,48].

All children had undergone genital surgery. It is possible that this high rate of genital surgery is related to our sampling process which identified participants via chart review at academic medical centers. This sampling approach may be suboptimal for ascertaining cases in which surgery had not been performed. The proportion of children with DSD who have not undergone surgical interventions is unknown. Accordingly, it is difficult to determine the extent to which our findings can generalize to patients and families who have elected not to have surgery performed. Research by Warne and Raza [49] encourage investigators in this area to be sensitive to variability across cultural and socioeconomic contexts.

Interviews were guided by the standardized probes to evaluate the quality of items to be incorporated into HRQoL questionnaires for parents of young children with DSD. Accordingly, although parents were asked to talk about areas of importance to them and their family that were not specifically covered in the HRQoL instrument, there may be topics of importance that did not emerge due to the interview structure. Tempering this concern is that novel questions were added to the HRQoL questionnaires based on ideas parents generated during the interviews, demonstrating that parents explored experiences beyond the confines of the cognitive interview structure. Finally, because interviews were conducted at varying intervals after some of the events being described, the potential exists for distorted recall.

Conclusions

Parents expressed a strong desire for their children's lives to be as "normal" as possible. In order to do what was best for their child with DSD, parents sought definitive information and guidance on management. Our findings suggest that parents did not always have all the information they wanted, when they wanted it, or in some cases, an accurate understanding of available information or sufficient awareness of the gaps in research on outcomes. Occasionally, parents' communication with providers was remembered and described as intentionally encouraging an oversimplified picture of DSD and factors influencing outcome or, alternatively, that parents selectively incorporated information.

Parents rationalized genital surgery as a "fix" for atypical appearance, function, and psychosocial concerns, despite a lack of empirical evidence indicating that surgery can fully address all of these challenges. Although parents reported being less concerned with the immediate implication of their child's DSD post-surgery, they remained concerned about their child's future adaptations.

The strains that parents experienced were, in some cases, ameliorated by the support of trusted family and friends. However, not all parents availed themselves of this coping strategy, viewing disclosure as too risky. This latter subgroup may be in greatest need of support from behavioral health members of the DSD interdisciplinary team [50-53].

Overall the findings suggest that families affected by DSD may benefit from enhanced adherence to the guidelines of shared decision-making, increased efforts to provide information objectively in line with the ethics of informed consent, and early and ongoing inclusion of behavioral healthcare providers in interdisciplinary teams caring for affected families.

List of Abbreviations
DSD: Disorders of Sex Development; HRQoL: Health Related Quality of Life.

Acknowledgements
We are most grateful to the parents who participated in this study. We also thank Laura Cohen and Mirranda Boshart who, in addition to some of the co-authors, conducted cognitive interviews. Thank you to Michael D. Fetters, M.D., M.P.H. for guidance with the qualitative process. We also greatly appreciate the help of Kristin Alman, Mirranda Boshart, Robert Carter, Marissa Flores, Meghan Glynn, Ross Goldberg, Mary Beth Grimley, Sharan Mullen, Talyah Sands, April Surinck, and Stephanie Stout in transcribing the cognitive interview audio-recordings, and Aimee Rolston for assistance in excerpting medical records. The project described was supported, in part, by Award Number R01HD053637 from the *Eunice Kennedy Shriver* National Institute of Child Health and Human Development granted to DES. The content is solely the responsibility of the authors and does not necessarily represent the official views of the *Eunice Kennedy Shriver* National Institute of Child Health and Human Development or the National Institutes of Health.

Author details
[1]Department of Pediatrics & Communicable Diseases Division of Child Behavioral Health University of Michigan Medical School 1500 East Medical Center Drive, SPC 5318 Ann Arbor, Michigan 48109-5318 USA. [2]Division of Urology The Children's Hospital of Philadelphia Richard D Wood Center, 3rd Floor 34th Street and Civic Center Boulevard Philadelphia, Pennsylvania 19104 USA. [3]Departments of Psychology & Pediatrics University of Miami 5665 Ponce de Leon Blvd. Coral Gables, Florida 33146-2070 USA. [4]Division of Urology Department of Surgery Albany Medical College 23 Hackett Boulevard Albany, New York 12208 USA.

Authors' contributions
HPC contributed significantly to the qualitative methods/secondary analysis research design; MG and DES supervised the design. HPC, LW, and MC executed the qualitative content analysis; MG and DES supervised the analyses. MG conducted the majority of interviews; AS and DES conducted a substantial proportion; ALQ conducted one in addition to training interviewers. LW conducted the five member-checking interviews and their analysis. HPC, LW, MG, and MC transcribed interviews. MG collected all questionnaire, demographic, and medical chart excerpt data; maintained the databases; conducted descriptive statistical analyses. MG, ALQ, BK, and DES conceived of the parent study and participated in guiding study design and

execution. AS and BK excerpted medical charts. HPC, LW, MG, and DES contributed significantly to manuscript drafts; MC contributed significantly to early drafts. All authors contributed comments throughout the writing; all read and approved the final manuscript.

Competing interests

The authors declare that they have no competing interests.

References

1. Lee PA, Houk Christopher P, Ahmed S, Faisal Hughes, Ieuan A, in collaboration with the participants in the International Consensus Conference on Intersex: **Consensus statement on management of intersex disorders.** *Pediatrics* 2006, **118**(2):e488-e500.
2. Hines M, Brook C, Conway GS: **Androgen and psychosexual development: Core gender identity, sexual orientation, and recalled childhood gender role behavior in women and men with congenital adrenal hyperplasia (CAH).** *Journal of Sex Research* 2004, **41**(1):75-81.
3. Berenbaum SA, Duck SC, Bryk K: **Behavioral effects of prenatal versus postnatal androgen excess in children with 21-hydroxylase-deficient congenital adrenal hyperplasia.** *J Clin Endo & Metab* 2000, **85**(2):727-733.
4. Collaer ML, Hines M: **Human behavioral sex differences: a role for gonadal hormones during early development?** *Psychological Bulletin* 1995, **118**(1):55-107.
5. Stout SA, Litvak M, Robbins NM, Sandberg DE: **Congenital adrenal hyperplasia: classification of studies employing psychological endpoints.** *International Journal of Pediatric Endocrinology* 2010, 11[http://www.hindawi.com/journals/ijpe/2010/191520/].
6. MacKenzie D, Huntington A, Gilmour JA: **The experiences of people with an intersex condition: a journey from silence to voice.** *Journal of Clinical Nursing* 2009, **18**(12):1775-1783.
7. de María Arana M: **A human rights investigation into the medical "normalization" of intersex people.** 2005 [http://www.sf-hrc.org/ftp/uploadedfiles/sfhumanrights/Committee_Meetings/Lesbian_Gay_Bisexual_Transgender/SFHRC%20Intersex%20Report(1).pdf], Accessed September 14, 2011.
8. Jurgensen M, Hampel E, Hiort O, Thyen U: **"Any decision is better than none" decision-making about sex of rearing for siblings with 17beta-hydroxysteroid-dehydrogenase-3 deficiency.** *Arch Sex Behav* 2006, **35**(3):359-371.
9. Frader J, Alderson P, Asch A, Aspinall C, Davis D, Dreger A, Edwards J, Feder EK, Frank A, Hedley LA, *et al*: **Health care professionals and intersex conditions.** *Archives of Pediatrics & Adolescent Medicine* 2004, **158**(5):426-428.
10. Zeiler K, Wickström A: **Why do "we" perform surgery on newborn intersexed children? The phenomenology of the parental experience of having a child with intersex anatomies.** *Feminist Theory* 2009, **10**(3):359-377.
11. Duguid A, Morrison S, Robertson A, Chalmers J, Youngson G, Ahmed SF, The Scottish Genital Anomaly Network: **The psychological impact of genital anomalies on the parents of affected children.** *Acta Pædiatrica* 2007, **96**(3):348-352.
12. Dreger AD, Sandberg DE: **Disorders of sex development.** In *Pediatric Bioethics*. Edited by: Miller G. New York, NY: Cambridge University Press; 2010:149-162.
13. Sanders C, Carter B, Goodacre L: **Parents' narratives about their experiences of their child's reconstructive genital surgeries for ambiguous genitalia.** *Journal of Clinical Nursing* 2008, **17**(23):3187-3195.
14. Fedele DA, Kirk K, Wolfe-Christensen C, Phillips TM, Mazur T, Mullins LL, Chernausek SD, Wisniewski AB: **Primary caregivers of children affected by disorders of sex development: Mental health and caregiver characteristics in the context of genital ambiguity and genitoplasty.** *International Journal of Pediatric Endocrinology* 2010, 7[http://downloads.hindawi.com/journals/ijpe/2010/690674.pdf].
15. Karkazis K: *Fixing Sex: Intersex, Medical Authority, and Lived Experience* Durham, NC: Duke University Press; 2008.
16. Wallander JL, Thompson RJ Jr, Alriksson-Schmidt A, Roberts MC: **Psychosocial adjustment of children with chronic physical conditions.** In *Handbook of Pediatric Psychology.*. Third edition. Edited by: Roberts MC. New York: Guilford Publications; 2003:141-158.
17. Mullins LL, Wolfe-Christensen C, Hoff Pai AL, Carpentier MY, Gillaspy S, Cheek J, Page M: **The relationship of parental overprotection, perceived child vulnerability, and parenting stress to uncertainty in youth with chronic illness.** *Journal of Pediatric Psychology* 2007, **32**(8):973-982.
18. Cohen MS: **Families coping with childhood chronic illness: A research review.** *Families, Systems & Health* 1999, **17**(2):149-164.
19. Kirk KD, Fedele DA, Wolfe-Christensen C, Phillips TM, Mazur T, Mullins LL, Chernausek SD, Wisniewski AB: **Parenting characteristics of female caregivers of children affected by chronic endocrine conditions: a comparison between disorders of sex development and type 1 diabetes mellitus.** *Journal of Pediatric Nursing* 2010, **26**(6):e29-e35.
20. Sandberg DE, Gardner MD, Kogan BA, Grimley MB, Cohen L, Alpern A, Quittner AL: **Assessing health-related quality of life in disorders of sex development: Phase I-item generation.** In *Hormonal and Genetic Basis of Sexual Differentiation Disorders and Hot Topics in Endocrinology: Proceedings of the 2nd World Conference, Advances in Experimental Medicine and Biology 707*. Edited by: New M, Simpson J. New York: Springer Science+Business Media; 2011:143-146.
21. Schwarz N, Sudman S: **Answering Questions: Methodology for Determining Cognitive and Communicative Processes in Survey Research.** San Francisco: Jossey-Bass Publishers; 1996.
22. Sudman S, Bradburn NM, Schwarz N: *Thinking about answers: The Application Of Cognitive Processes To Survey Methodology* San Francisco, CA, US: Jossey-Bass; 1996.
23. Modi AC, Quittner AL: **Validation of a disease-specific measure of health-related quality of life for children with cystic fibrosis.** *Journal of Pediatric Psychology* 2003, **28**(8):535-546.
24. Quittner AL, Buu A, Messer MA, Modi AC, Watrous M: **Development and validation of the Cystic Fibrosis Questionnaire (CFQ) in the United States: A health-related quality of life measure for cystic fibrosis.** *Chest* 2005, **128**(4):2347-2354.
25. Creswell JW: *Qualitative Inquiry & Research Design* Thousand Oaks, CA: Sage Publications; 2007.
26. Schwartz-Shea P: **Judging quality: Evaluative criteria and epistemic communities.** In *Interpretation and Method: Empirical Research Methods and the Interpretive Turn*. Edited by: Yanow D, Schwartz-Shea P. Armonk, NY: M.E. Sharpe; 2006:89-113.
27. Snow RC: **Sex, gender, and vulnerability.** *Global Public Health: An International Journal for Research, Policy and Practice* 2008, **3**(1 supp 1):58-74.
28. Meyer-Bahlburg HFL: **Gender assignment in intersexuality.** *Journal of Psychology & Human Sexuality* 1998, **10**(2):1-21.
29. Zucker KJ: **Intersexuality and gender identity differentiation.** *Journal of Pediatric & Adolescent Gynecology* 2002, **15**(1):3-13.
30. Bradley SJ, Zucker KJ: **Gender identity disorder and psychosexual problems in children and adolescents.** *Canadian Journal of Psychiatry-Revue Canadienne de Psychiatrie* 1990, **35**(6):477-486.
31. Meyer-Bahlburg HFL: **Gender identity outcome in female-raised 46, XY persons with penile agenesis, cloacal exstrophy of the bladder, or penile ablation.** *Archives of Sexual Behavior* 2005, **34**(4):423-438.
32. Mazur T: **Gender dysphoria and gender change in androgen insensitivity or micropenis.** *Archives of Sexual Behavior* 2005, **34**(4):411-421.
33. Cohen-Kettenis PT: **Gender change in 46, XY persons with 5α-reductase-2 deficiency and 17β-hydroxysteroid dehydrogenase-3 deficiency.** *Archives of Sexual Behavior* 2005, **34**(4):399-410.
34. Karkazis K, Tamar-Mattis A, Kon AA: **Genital surgery for disorders of sex development: implementing a shared decision-making approach.** *Journal of Pediatric Endocrinology and Metabolism* 2010, **23**(8):789-805.
35. Merz J: **Empirical analysis of the medical informed consent doctrine: search for a "standard" of disclosure.** *Risk-Issues in Health & Safety* 1991, **2**:27-76.
36. United States Department of Health and Human Services Office of Disease Prevention and Health Promotion: **Health literacy online: A guide to writing and designing easy-to-use health web sites.** 2011 [http://www.health.gov/healthliteracyonline/.], Accessed September 14, 2011.
37. AboutKidsHealth: **Sex Development.**[http://www.aboutkidshealth.ca/En/HowTheBodyWorks/SexDevelopmentAnOverview/Pages/default.aspx], Accessed September 14, 2011.

38. Daaboul J, Frader J: **Ethics and the management of the patient with intersex: a middle way.** *Journal of Pediatric Endocrinology&Metabolism* 2001, **14**(9):1575-1583.

39. Mureau MA, Slijper FM, Slob AK, Verhulst FC: **Psychosocial functioning of children, adolescents, and adults following hypospadias surgery: a comparative study.** *Journal of Pediatric Psychology* 1997, **22**(3):371-387.

40. Dayner JE, Lee PA, Houk CP: **Medical treatment of intersex: parental perspectives.** *The Journal of Urology* 2004, **172**(4, Supplement 1):1762-1765.

41. Chase C: **What is the agenda of the intersex patient advocacy movement?** *Endocrinologist* 2003, **13**(3):240-242.

42. Meyer-Bahlburg HFL: **Treatment guidelines for children with disorders of sex development.** *Neuropsychiatrie de l'Enfance et de l'Adolescence* 2008, **56**(6):345-349.

43. Money J, Lamacz M: **Genital examination and exposure experienced as nosocomial sexual abuse in childhood.** *Journal of Nervous & Mental Disease* 1987, **175**(12):713-721.

44. Creighton S, Alderson J, Brown S, Minto CL: **Medical photography: ethics, consent and the intersex patient.** *BJU International* 2002, **89**(1):67-71.

45. Phillips S, Friedman SB, Seidenberg M, Heald FP: **Teenagers' preferences regarding the presence of family members, peers, and chaperones during examination of genitalia.** *Pediatrics* 1981, **68**(5):665-669.

46. Wolfer J, Gaynard L, Goldberger J, Laidley LN, Thompson R: **An experimental evaluation of a model child life program.** *Children's Health Care* 1988, **16**(4):244-254.

47. Drotar D: **Relating parent and family functioning to the psychological adjustment of children with chronic health conditions: What have we learned? What do we need to know?** *Journal of Pediatric Psychology* 1997, **22**(2):149-165.

48. Wysocki T, Gavin L: **Paternal involvement in the management of pediatric chronic diseases: Associations with adherence, quality of life, and health status.** *Journal of Pediatric Psychology* 2006, **31**(5):501-511.

49. Warne GL, Raza J: **Disorders of sex development (DSDs), their presentation and management in different cultures.** *Rev Endocr Metab Disord* 2008, **9**(3):227-236.

50. Figueiredo MI, Fries E, Ingram KM, Figueiredo MI, Fries E, Ingram KM: **The role of disclosure patterns and unsupportive social interactions in the well-being of breast cancer patients.** *Psycho-Oncology* 2004, **13**(2):96-105.

51. Lam PK, Naar-King S, Wright K, Lam PK, Naar-King S, Wright K: **Social support and disclosure as predictors of mental health in HIV-positive youth.** *AIDS Patient Care & Stds* 2007, **21**(1):20-29.

52. Balaji AB, Claussen AH, Smith DC, Visser SN, Morales MJ, Perou R: **Social support networks and maternal mental health and well-being.** *Journal of Women's Health* 2007, **16**(10):1386-1396.

53. MacDonald J, Morley I: **Shame and non-disclosure: A study of the emotional isolation of people referred for psychotherapy.** *British Journal of Medical Psychology* 2001, **74**(1):1-21.

12

Significant gender difference in serum levels of fibroblast growth factor 21 in Danish children and adolescents

Amalie Bisgaard[1,2], Kaspar Sørensen[1,2], Trine Holm Johannsen[1,2], Jørn Wulff Helge[3], Anna-Maria Andersson[1,2] and Anders Juul[1,2]*

Abstract

Introduction: Fibroblast Growth Factor 21 (FGF21) is a novel metabolic factor with effect on glucose and lipid metabolism, and shown to be elevated in diseases related to metabolic syndrome. Due to the increasing frequency of metabolic syndrome in the pediatric population, and as FGF21 studies in children are limited, we investigated baseline serum levels of FGF21 in healthy children during an oral glucose tolerance test.

Methods: A total of 179 children and adolescents from the COPENHAGEN Puberty Study were included. An OGTT with glucose and insulin measurements, a dual energy X-ray absorptiometry (DXA) scan and a clinical examination including pubertal staging were done on all subjects. Serum levels of FGF21, adiponectin, and leptin were determined by immunoassays at baseline.

Results: The girls had significantly higher levels of FGF21 compared with boys (155 pg/mL vs. 105 pg/mL, $P = 0.04$). 38 children (21%) had levels below detection limit of assay. Baseline levels of FGF21 showed positive correlation with triglycerides, but no significant correlations were found between FGF21-concentration and body mass index (BMI), DXA-derived fat percentage, LDL- HDL- and non-HDL cholesterol, leptin or adiponectin levels, respectively. Neither was any correlation found between baseline FGF21-levels and the dynamic changes in glucose and insulin levels during the OGTT.

Conclusion: FGF21 is independent of adiposity in children, and the significant metabolic effect seems to be limited to pathological conditions associated with insulin resistance. The higher levels of triglycerides in the girls may explain the significantly higher levels of FGF21 in girls compared with boys.

Systematic review registration: The COPENHAGEN Puberty Study was registered in ClinicalTrials.gov (identifier NCT01411527), and approved by the local ethics committee (reference no. KF 01 282214 and KF 11 2006–2033).

Keywords: Fibroblast growth factor 21, Metabolic syndrome, Oral glucose tolerance test

Introduction

Metabolic syndrome in children is becoming more frequent in the pediatric population, [1,2] and pathogenetic and prognostic factors are sought for. Recently, a new protein, fibroblast growth factor 21 (FGF21), has been suggested as a factor involved in regulation of carbohydrate and lipid metabolism [3-5].

FGF21 expression is induced by an increase in free fatty acids, and is regulated by peroxisome proliferator-activated receptor-alpha (PPAR-α) in the liver [6,7] and PPAR-gamma (PPAR-γ) in white adipose tissue [8,9]. In the liver, FGF21 acts as an endocrine factor, as it increases energy production and utilization of energy during prolonged fasting [10]. In white adipose tissue FGF21 acts as an autocrine factor, as it increases glucose uptake by up-regulating glucose transporter 1 (GLUT1) in the cell membrane [5]. Glucose also stimulates FGF21 expression through carbohydrate response-element binding protein (ChREBP) in the liver [11,12]. In adipocytes, it

* Correspondence: anders.juul@regionh.dk
[1]Department of Growth and Reproduction, Rigshospitalet, Copenhagen University Hospital, section 5064 Blegdamsvej 9, DK-2100 Copenhagen, Denmark
[2]Faculty of Health and Medical Sciences, University of Copenhagen, Copenhagen, Denmark
Full list of author information is available at the end of the article

seems like PPAR-γ and ChREBP together can stimulate the expression of FGF21 [11]. Compared with insulin alone, glucose uptake into cultured adipocytes is enhanced by co-incubation with FGF21, suggesting that the effect of FGF21 is independent and additive to insulin. Accordingly, treatment with FGF21 to ob/ob mice and FGF21 transgenic mice over-expressing the human protein resulted in improved glucose clearance and insulin sensitivity during OGTT [5].

Diseases related to insulin resistance such as metabolic syndrome and type 2 diabetes mellitus have been related to increased levels of FGF21 [13-15]. In accordance, serum-concentrations of FGF21 correlated negatively with insulin sensitivity and positively with the hepatic insulin resistance index, HbA1c, fasting plasma glucose levels and two hour-plasma glucose levels after an oral glucose tolerance test in adult subjects, suggesting a relation with both hepatic and whole-body insulin resistance [13]. In children, knowledge on FGF21 and insulin resistance is limited. In a cohort study of both lean and obese children it was indicated that FGF21 levels were positively associated with free fatty acids, leptin and body mass index (BMI), respectively. This study further suggested that the increase in serum-concentrations of FGF21 in obese children was reversible with weight loss [16]. Giannini et al. confirmed this elevation of FGF21 in obese youth and in addition documented that FGF21 independent of visceral fat and insulin

sensitivity correlated with fatty liver and markers of hepatic apopotosis [17].

The aim of this study was to evaluate the fasting concentrations of serum-FGF21 in children and adolescents in relation to anthropometrical measurements, pubertal stages, concentrations of lipids, leptin and adiponectin, and concentrations of glucose and insulin during a two-hour OGTT.

Materials and methods

Participants

Subjects were recruited as part of The COPENHAGEN Puberty Study [18,19] from primary schools in the Copenhagen community. A total of 179 healthy Caucasian children (114 girls) aged 8,5-16,1 years volunteered Table 1. Sixteen children and adolescents (8 girls) were clasified as overweight (BMI > 85th percentile for age) according to the CDC reference. None of the children meet the IDF crieteria for metabolic syndrome [20]. The cohort has previously been described in details [21-23]. In brief, all participants had pubertal stages evaluated according to Tanners classification. Twenty-seven of the girls were post-menarcheal. Total body fat and lean mass was evaluated with a whole-body dual-energy X-ray absorptiometry (DXA) scan using a CDR 1000/W densitometer (Hologic Inc., Bedford MA) with software version 6.2. Aerobic fitness was evaluated by assessing maximal oxygen uptake (V_{O2}max) during a cycle ergometry test using

Table 1 General metabolic characteristics related to metabolic syndrome in a group of 179 non-obese children (65 boys, 114 girls)

	Boys	Girls	P-value
	n = 65	n = 114	
BMI (kg/m^2)	18.3 (15.0-26.21)	18.0 (13.4-30.6)	0.21
Fat percentage (%)	18.1 (7.5-29.9)	21.1 (12.3-35.0)	< 0.001
Fasting glucose (mmol/L)	4.8 (3.9-5.9)	4.9 (3.2-6.7)	0.85
2-h glucose (mmol/L)	5.1 (2.8-7.3)	4.9 (2.9-8.3)	0.69
Fasting insulin (pmol/L)	43.0 (10.0-102.0)	48.0 (8.0-168.0)	0.03
Peak glucose (mmol/L)	7.0 (4.7-11.2)	7.4 (4.7-11.2)	0.41
Triglycerides (mmol/L)	0.6 (0.4-2.4)	0.7 (0.4-2.0)	0.001
HDL (mmol/L)	1.5 (0.9-2.1)	1.5 (0.7-2.2)	0.73
LDL (mmol/L)	2.1 (0.5-3.2)	2.2 (0.8-3.8)	0.29
Total cholesterol (mmol/L)	3.6 (2.4-4.6)	3.8 (2.4-5.6)	0.003
Non-HDL cholesterol (mmol/L)	2.0 (1.1-3.2)	2.4 (0.6-3.7)	0.001
Apolipoproten A1 (mmol/L)	50.6 (38.7-64.4)	51.7 (27.1-67.6)	0.40
Apolipoproten B (mmol/L)	2.1 (1.1-3.4)	2.2 (0.7-3.7)	0.06
Leptin (ng/mL)	3476.0 (1884.0-37065.0)	6353.0 (921-49495.0)	< 0.01
Adiponectin (µg/mL)	22876.5 (977.0-57085.0)	27757.5 (9375.0-60190.0)	0.01
V_{O2}max (ml · kg^{-1} · min^{-1})	46.8 (30.3-63.2)	39.8 (25.1-51.0)	< 0.01

BMI = Body mass index; HDL = High-density lipoprotein cholesterol; LDL = Low-density lipoprotein cholesterol; Non- HDL-cholesterol = Total cholesterol minus HDL-cholesterol; VO$_2$max = Maximal oxygen uptake during a cycle ergometry test.

an electronically braked cycle ergometer (Ergomedic 839: Monark, Varberg, Sweden). V_{O2}max was measured directly using an online pulmonary gas analyzer system (Quark CPET; Cosmed, Rome, Italy).

Blood sampling

Venous fasting blood samples were drawn after 12 h of fasting from the ante-cubital vein into standard vacuum tubes and centrifuged (3000 g at 10 min) within 30 min. Plasma was immediately stored at −20°C until analysis. A standard two-hour oral glucose tolerance test with an oral glucose load of 1.75 g of glucose per kilogram body-weight (maximum 75 g glucose) was performed. Blood samples were drawn with 30 min intervals for determin-ation of glucose and insulin. The area under the curve (AUC) for plasma glucose (AUC_{glu}) and plasma insulin (AUC_{ins}), respectively, was calculated by the trapezoidal rule.

Analyses

Serum-FGF-21 concentrations were measured with a commercial enzyme-linked immunosorbent assay (Bio-Vendor Human FGF-21 ELISA, BioVendor, Brno, Czech Republic). Determination of FGF-21 was done on previ-ously unthawed biobanked serum samples. FGF21 was analyzed according to the manufacturer's instruction and measured in duplicates. According to the manufac-turer, the limit of detection was 7 pg/mL, but the lowest standard was 30 pg/mL, which then in our study was set to the limit of detection (LoD). The manufacturer re-ported the intra-assay and inter-assay coefficients of variability (CV) to be below 5%, respectively, and with no cross-reactivity with human Fibroblast Growth Factor 19 or Fibroblast Growth Factor 23. Our inter-assay CV's for the low (mean: 137.7 pg/mL) and high (mean: 536.3 pg/mL) controls were 7.0% and 5.5%, respectively.

Plasma-concentrations of adiponectin and leptin were measured using specific high-sensitive human enzyme linked immunosorbent assays. The adiponectin assay (Millipore, Human ADIPONECTIN RIA-kit, St Charles, Mi, USA) had intra-assay and inter-assay CV's of 4.9% and 5.4%, respectively. Detection limits were 1 – 200 ng/mL. The leptin assay (R&D Systems, Human Leptin Im-munoassay, Minneapolis, Mn, USA) had intra-assay and inter-assay CV's of 3.4% and 1.6%, respectively, and detection limits of 7.8 – 1000 pg/mL. Glucose, triglycer-ides, total cholesterol, high-density lipoprotein (HDL)-cholesterol, low-density lipoprotein (LDL)-cholesterol, apolipoprotein A1 and B, respectively, were all analyzed in heparin-plasma on the Modular® *ANALYTICS* SWA, Modular P-system (Roche Diagnostics GmbH, Mannheim, Germany), using the calibrator for automated systems (CFAS) and the Roche Modular® reagents for all assays [24]. Insulin was analyzed in (heparin-plasma) determined

by an electrochemiluminescence immunoassay (Elecsys in-sulin reagents kit; Roche Diagnostics GmbH, Mannheim, Germany) on the Modular® *ANALYTICS* SWA, Modular E170-system (Roche Diagnostics GmbH, Mannheim, Germany) [21]. Non-HDL-cholesterol was calculated as total cholesterol subtracted HDL-cholesterol.

Statistics

All FGF21 values below the lowest standard (30 pg/mL) were set at 15 pg/mL. Mann–Whitney U-test was used to evaluate differences in FGF21 and metabolic parame-ters between genders. Differences in median levels of FGF21 in different age groups (2-yrs intervals) and pu-bertal stages were evaluated with Kruskal-Wallis test. To account for samples below detection, sex-specific tertiles of increasing FGF21 levels were generated. Differences between several groups were evaluated with the Kruskal-Wallis test, and differences between two groups (single or combined) were evaluated by the Mann–Whitney U-test. All statistical analyses were done using the statis-tical software IBM SPSS version 19.0 for Microsoft Windows XP (Chicago, IL).

Ethics

The study was done in accordance with the ethical princi-ples of the Helsinki II declaration. The COPENHAGEN Puberty Study was registered in ClinicalTrials.gov (identi-fier NCT01411527), and approved by the local ethics committee (reference no. KF 01 282214 and KF 11 2006–2033). All children and parents gave their informed writ-ten consent.

Results

In total, 38 study participants (16 boys, 22 girls) had FGF21 levels below the lowest standard of 30 pg/mL. The serum concentrations of FGF21 in samples above this LoD ranged from 60.6 – 1715.1 pg/mL. As shown in Figure 1, the girls had significantly higher serum-levels of FGF21 (median: 155.1 pg/mL, range < LoD - 1715.1 pg/mL) compared with the boys (median: 105.1 pg/mL, range < LoD - 818.9 pg/mL, $P = 0.04$). No significant dif-ferences were found in serum FGF21 levels between age-groups and pubertal stages in boys and girls, respectively. Neither did we find any association between baseline levels of FGF21 and glucose and insulin levels during the OGTT. Due to lack of statistical significant differences in all measured parameters between the middle and highest tertiles, these two groups were combined and compared with the lowest tertile. The lowest tertile of serum FGF21 had significantly lower triglyceride (TG) levels (median: 0.61 mmol/L, range: 0.42 – 1.77 mmol/L) compared with the combined higher tertiles (median: 0.72 mmol/L, range: 0.35 – 2.38 mmol/L, $P = 0.01$).

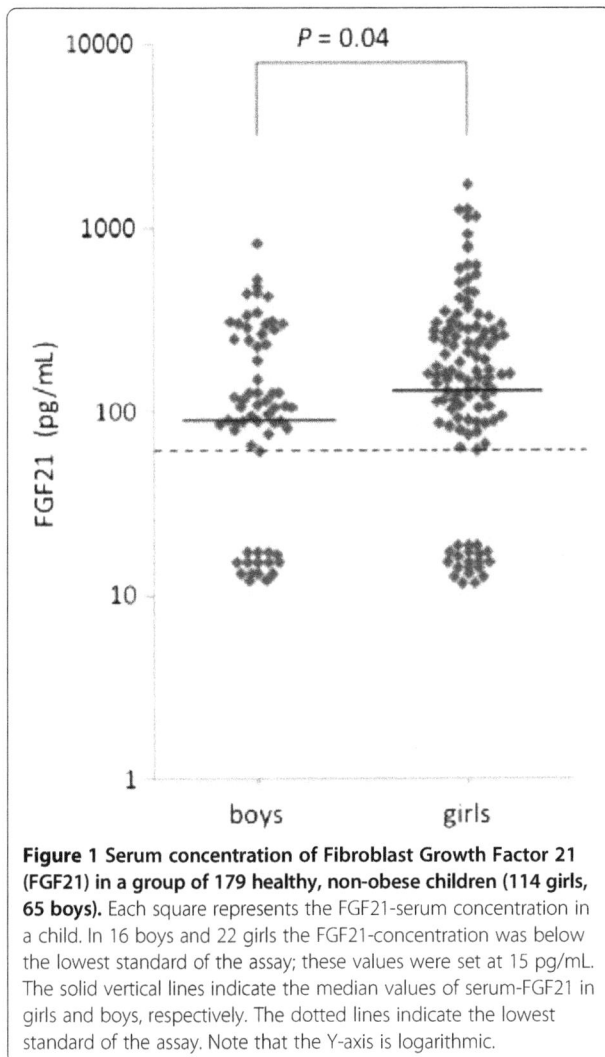

Figure 1 Serum concentration of Fibroblast Growth Factor 21 (FGF21) in a group of 179 healthy, non-obese children (114 girls, 65 boys). Each square represents the FGF21-serum concentration in a child. In 16 boys and 22 girls the FGF21-concentration was below the lowest standard of the assay; these values were set at 15 pg/mL. The solid vertical lines indicate the median values of serum-FGF21 in girls and boys, respectively. The dotted lines indicate the lowest standard of the assay. Note that the Y-axis is logarithmic.

only showed significant difference in BMI, total fat percentage, fasting insulin and leptin (p < 0.01) but no difference was found with either triglycerides, lipids, cholesterol or FGF21. These findings were consistent in a gender-specific analysis.

Discussion

In the present study, we did not find consistent evidence in favor for a regulatory function of baseline FGF21-concentrations on glucose homeostasis. This may reflect the narrow biological range in the present sample of healthy children with normal glucose tolerance. In accordance, Gälman et al. found no evidence for a relationship between FGF21 levels and metabolic parameters in healthy adult subjects, [10] indicating that significant metabolic effects of FGF21 may be limited to pathological conditions associated with glucose intolerance. In addition, as FGF21 levels were only evaluated at baseline, dynamic changes in FGF21 levels during an OGTT could not be determined in the present study. One study reported that changes of FGF21 concentrations were negatively correlated with changes of glucose levels during a standard OGTT in both healthy and insulin resistant individuals [25].

Despite the lack of association with DXA-derived total body adiposity, we found positive correlations between serum-concentrations of FGF21 and triglycerides. This is consistent with the study by Tyynismaa et al. [26] reporting that high FGF21-levels were related to higher proportions of liver fat and higher triglycerides levels rather than to total body adiposity. Due to the cross-sectional design in the present study, the cause and effect-relationship could not be determined. However, evidence suggests that FGF21 increases in response to increasing levels of lipids, which has been hypothesized as a defense mechanism against lipotoxicity [3]. Thus, FGF21 may be a marker of elevated levels of lipids even in healthy normal-weight children. In accordance with the lack of association between FGF21 and anthropometric and biochemical parameters associated with obesity, we found no correlation between FGF21 and the adipokines leptin and adiponectin [27,28].

FGF21 levels were significantly higher in girls compared with boys, which may partly be related to the higher triglyceride levels in girls. No previous studies have addressed the possible sexual differences in FGF21-concentrations in either adults or children.

A higher number of girls are represented in the present study, which might explain why a significant difference between the metabolic parameters and FGF21 levels is seen in girls only.

The strength of our study is the large unselected sample of 179 well-characterized children. However, experimental and clinical data suggest that a certain amount of

In sex-specific analyses, TG levels in girls were lower in the lowest FGF21-tertile (median: 0.70 mmol/L, range: 0.42 – 1.77 mmol/L) compared with the higher FGF21-tertiles (median: 0.82 mmol/l, range: 0.35 – 2.03 mmol/L), P = 0.03). Similar absolute differences were found for TG levels in boys between the lowest tertile (median: 0.55 mmol/L, range 0.43 – 1.41 mmol/L) and the higher tertiles of serum FGF21 (median: 0.65 mmol/L, range: 0.37 – 2.38 mmol/L), P = 0.11). In addition, LDL-cholesterol levels were lower in the lowest FGF21-tertile compared with the higher tertiles in girls only (P = 0.07).

No differences in height, weight, BMI, total body fat percentage (all p > 0.12) between the lowest FGF-21 tertile compared with the higher tertiles for girls and boys, respectively.

When the group of sixteen children and adolescents with BMI above the 85th percentile for age were compared to the large group of normal-weight children they adipose tissue should be present in order for FGF21 to exert a significant glucose lowering effect [29]. Thus, evaluation of FGF21 levels in children with obesity and glucose intolerance may shed further light on the possible regulatory actions of FGF21.

Conclusion

Fasting concentrations of FGF21 were significantly positive associated with levels of triglycerides in girls independently of adiposity and serum leptin levels. Baseline FGF21 concentrations were not associated with glucose or insulin concentrations during a two-hour OGTT. The girls showed significantly higher levels of FGF21, which may partly be explained by higher triglyceride concentrations in girls compared with boys.

Competing interests

Anders Juul is principal investigator in scientific muliticenter trial on the effects of growth hormone on growth in short SGA children. The study receives financial support from Novo Nordisk. The remaining authors have nothing to declare.

Authors' contributions

AB contributed to study design, statistical analyses, data analyses and interpretation and drafted the manuscript; KS conceived the study, contributed to study design, statistical analyses, data analyses and interpretation and made important revisions of the manuscript; THJ contributed to study design, data analyses and interpretation and made important revisions of the manuscript, JWH participated in data analyses and interpretation and made substantial revisions of the manuscript; AMA participated in data analyses and interpretation and made substantial revisions of the manuscript; AJ conceived the study, contributed to study design, data analyses and interpretation and made important revisions of the manuscript. All authors read and approved the final manuscript.

Aknowledgments

The Copenhagen Puberty Study received financial support from the Kirsten and Freddy Johansen's foundation, the Capital Region of Denmark's Research Fund for health research (R129-A3966), the Danish Research council (DFF-1331-00113) and the Danish Agency for Science, Technology and Innovation (09–067180).

Author details

[1]Department of Growth and Reproduction, Rigshospitalet, Copenhagen University Hospital, section 5064 Blegdamsvej 9, DK-2100 Copenhagen, Denmark. [2]Faculty of Health and Medical Sciences, University of Copenhagen, Copenhagen, Denmark. [3]Department of Biomedical Sciences, Xlab, Center for Healthy Aging, University of Copenhagen, Copenhagen, Denmark.

References

1. Bremer AA, Mietus-Snyder M, Lustig RH: Toward a unifying hypothesis of metabolic syndrome. *Pediatrics* 2012, 129:557–570.
2. Weiss R, Dziura J, Burgert TS, Tamborlane WV, Taksali SE, Yeckel CW, Allen K, Lopes M, Savoye M, Morrison J, Sherwin RS, Caprio S: Obesity and the metabolic syndrome in children and adolescents. *N Engl J Med* 2004, 350:2362–2374.
3. Cuevas-Ramos D, Aguilar-Salinas CA, Gomez-Perez FJ: Metabolic actions of fibroblast growth factor 21. *Curr Opin Pediatr* 2012, 24:523–529.
4. Veniant MM, Komorowski R, Chen P, Stanislaus S, Winters K, Hager T, Zhou L, Wada R, Hecht R, Xu J: Long-acting FGF21 has enhanced efficacy in diet-induced obese mice and in obese rhesus monkeys. *Endocrinology* 2012, 153:4192–4203.
5. Kharitonenkov A, Shiyanova TL, Koester A, Ford AM, Micanovic R, Galbreath EJ, Sandusky GE, Hammond LJ, Moyers JS, Owens RA, Gromada J, Brozinick JT, Hawkins ED, Wroblewski VJ, Li DS, Mehrbod F, Jaskunas SR, Shanafelt AB: FGF-21 as a novel metabolic regulator. *J Clin Invest* 2005, 115:1627–1635.
6. Inagaki T, Dutchak P, Zhao G, Ding X, Gautron L, Parameswara V, Li Y, Goetz R, Mohammadi M, Esser V, Elmquist JK, Gerard RD, Burgess SC, Hammer RE, Mangelsdorf DJ, Kliewer SA: Endocrine regulation of the fasting response by PPARalpha-mediated induction of fibroblast growth factor 21. *Cell Metab* 2007, 5:415–425.
7. Badman MK, Pissios P, Kennedy AR, Koukos G, Flier JS, Maratos-Flier E: Hepatic fibroblast growth factor 21 is regulated by PPARalpha and is a key mediator of hepatic lipid metabolism in ketotic states. *Cell Metab* 2007, 5:426–437.
8. Muise ES, Azzolina B, Kuo DW, El-Sherbeini M, Tan Y, Yuan X, Mu J, Thompson JR, Berger JP, Wong KK: Adipose fibroblast growth factor 21 is up-regulated by peroxisome proliferator-activated receptor gamma and altered metabolic states. *Mol Pharmacol* 2008, 74:403–412.
9. Dutchak PA, Katafuchi T, Bookout AL, Choi JH, Yu RT, Mangelsdorf DJ, Kliewer SA: Fibroblast growth factor-21 regulates PPARgamma activity and the antidiabetic actions of thiazolidinediones. *Cell* 2012, 148:556–567.
10. Galman C, Lundasen T, Kharitonenkov A, Bina HA, Eriksson M, Hafstrom I, Dahlin M, Amark P, Angelin B, Rudling M: The circulating metabolic regulator FGF21 is induced by prolonged fasting and PPARalpha activation in man. *Cell Metab* 2008, 8:169–174.
11. Uebanso T, Taketani Y, Yamamoto H, Amo K, Ominami H, Arai H, Takei Y, Masuda M, Tanimura A, Harada N, Yamanaka-Okumura H, Takeda E: Paradoxical regulation of human FGF21 by both fasting and feeding signals: is FGF21 a nutritional adaptation factor? *PLoS One* 2011, 6:e22976.
12. Iizuka K, Takeda J, Horikawa Y: Glucose induces FGF21 mRNA expression through ChREBP activation in rat hepatocytes. *FEBS Lett* 2009, 583:2882–2886.
13. Chavez AO, Molina-Carrion M, Abdul-Ghani MA, Folli F, Defronzo RA, Tripathy D: Circulating fibroblast growth factor-21 is elevated in impaired glucose tolerance and type 2 diabetes and correlates with muscle and hepatic insulin resistance. *Diabetes Care* 2009, 32:1542–1546.
14. Chen WW, Li L, Yang GY, Li K, Qi XY, Zhu W, Tang Y, Liu H, Boden G: Circulating FGF-21 levels in normal subjects and in newly diagnose patients with type 2 diabetes mellitus. *Exp Clin Endocrinol Diabetes* 2008, 116:65–68.
15. Cheng X, Zhu B, Jiang F, Fan H: Serum FGF-21 levels in type 2 diabetic patients. *Endocr Res* 2011, 36:142–148.
16. Reinehr T, Woelfle J, Wunsch R, Roth CL: Fibroblast growth factor 21 (FGF-21) and its relation to obesity, metabolic syndrome, and nonalcoholic fatty liver in children: a longitudinal analysis. *J Clin Endocrinol Metab* 2012, 97:2143–2150.
17. Giannini C, Feldstein A, Santoro N, Kim G, Kursawe R, Pierpont B, Caprio S: Circulating levels of FGF-21 in obese youth: associations with liver fat content and markers of liver damage. *J Clin Endocrinol Metab* 2013, 98(7):2993–3000.
18. Aksglaede L, Sorensen K, Petersen JH, Skakkebaek NE, Juul A: Recent decline in age at breast development: the Copenhagen puberty study. *Pediatrics* 2009, 123:e932–e939.
19. Sorensen K, Aksglaede L, Petersen JH, Juul A: Recent changes in pubertal timing in healthy Danish boys: associations with body mass index. *J Clin Endocrinol Metab* 2010, 95:263–270.
20. Zimmet P, Alberti KG, Kaufman F, Tajima N, Silink M, Arslanian S, Wong G, Bennett P, Shaw J, Caprio S, IDF Consensus Group: The metabolic syndrome in children and adolescents - an IDF consensus report. *Pediatr Diabetes* 2007, 8:299–306.
21. Sorensen K, Aksglaede L, Munch-Andersen T, Aachmann-Andersen NJ, Petersen JH, Hilsted L, Helge JW, Juul A: Sex hormone-binding globulin levels predict insulin sensitivity, disposition index, and cardiovascular risk during puberty. *Diabetes Care* 2009, 32:909–914.
22. Sorensen K, Mouritsen A, Mogensen SS, Aksglaede L, Juul A: Insulin sensitivity and lipid profiles in girls with central precocious puberty before and during gonadal suppression. *J Clin Endocrinol Metab* 2010, 95:3736–3744.
23. Sorensen K, Aksglaede L, Petersen JH, Andersson AM, Juul A: Serum IGF1 and insulin levels in girls with normal and precocious puberty. *Eur J Endocrinol* 2012, 166:903–910.
24. Hilsted L, Rustad P, Aksglaede L, Sorensen K, Juul A: Recommended Nordic paediatric reference intervals for 21 common biochemical properties. *Scand J Clin Lab Invest* 2012, 73:1–9.

25. Lin Z, Gong Q, Wu C, Yu J, Lu T, Pan X, Lin S, Li X: **Dynamic change of serum FGF21 levels in response to glucose challenge in human.** *J Clin Endocrinol Metab* 2012, **97**:E1224–E1228.

26. Tyynismaa H, Raivio T, Hakkarainen A, Ortega-Alonso A, Lundbom N, Kaprio J, Rissanen A, Suomalainen A, Pietiläinen KH: **Liver fat but not other adiposity measures influence circulating FGF21 levels in healthy young adult twins.** *J Clin Endocrinol Metab* 2011, **96**:E351–E355.

27. Leon-Cabrera S, Solis-Lozano L, Suarez-Alvarez K, Gonzalez-Chavez A, Bejar YL, Robles-Diaz G, Escobedo G: **Hyperleptinemia is associated with parameters of low-grade systemic inflammation and metabolic dysfunction in obese human beings.** *Front Integr Neurosci* 2013, **7**:62.

28. Mraz M, Bartlova M, Lacinova Z, Michalsky D, Kasalicky M, Haluzikova D, Matoulek M, Dostalova I, Humenanska V, Haluzik M: **Serum concentrations and tissue expression of a novel endocrine regulator fibroblast growth factor-21 in patients with type 2 diabetes and obesity.** *Clin Endocrinol (Oxf)* 2009, **71**:369–375.

29. Zhang X, Yeung DC, Karpisek M, Stejskal D, Zhou ZG, Liu F, Wong RL, Chow WS, Tso AW, Lam KS, Xu A: **Serum FGF21 levels are increased in obesity and are independently associated with the metabolic syndrome in humans.** *Diabetes* 2008, **57**:1246–1253.

13

Long-term effects of a non-intensive weight program on body mass index and metabolic abnormalities of obese children and adolescents

Rita Ann Kubicky[1,2]*, Christopher Dunne[1,2], Debika Nandi-Munshi[1] and Francesco De Luca[1,2]

Abstract

Background: Previous studies have demonstrated positive effects of short-term, intensive weight-loss programs in obese children.

Objectives: We evaluated the long-term effects of a non-intensive weight management program on the BMI, glycemic measures and lipid profiles of obese youth.

Methods: Retrospective chart review of 61 obese children followed at our Weight Management Center. During visits, dietary changes and regular physical activity were recommended. Anthropometric and laboratory parameters were evaluated.

Results: At the initial visit, the mean age was 11.1 ± 2.6 years. The follow-up period was 47.3 ± 11.1 months; the number of outpatient visits per year (OV/yr) was 2.9 ± 0.9. At the end of the follow-up, the whole group exhibited decreased BMI z-score and LDL-cholesterol when compared to the initial visit. In the subset of subjects in whom OGTT was performed, 2-hour glucose and peak insulin were decreased. Compared to children with ≤ 2 OV/year, those with > 2 OV/year (3.19 ± 0.7) exhibited a significant decrease in their BMI z-score, LDL-cholesterol, 2-hour glucose, and peak insulin.

Conclusions: Our study suggests that a periodical (~ 3 OV/yr) evaluation in a non-intensive, long-term weight management program may significantly improve the degree of obesity and cardiovascular risk factors in childhood.

Keywords: Obesity, Weight loss, Dyslipidemia, Impaired glucose tolerance, Insulin resistance

Background

It is well known that the prevalence of obesity in children has reached epidemic proportions: during the past decade, the prevalence of children with a Body Mass Index (BMI) $> 95^{th}$ percentile has tripled in all pediatric age-range groups [1]. Pediatric obesity is associated with significant medical complications during childhood [2], and it is a significant risk factor for morbidity and mortality in adulthood [2,3]. Most of the comorbidities of childhood obesity share insulin resistance as a common underlying mechanism. Such comorbidities (dyslipidemia, nonalcoholic fatty liver disease, type 2 diabetes mellitus (DM), hypertension, obstructive sleep apnea, polycystic ovary syndrome) tend to cluster in what is known as the metabolic syndrome [1,4].

Pediatric metabolic syndrome is a predictor of the metabolic syndrome and type 2 DM in adulthood [5]; in addition, obesity-associated atherosclerosis begins in childhood [6] and its rate of progression is greatly increased by lipid abnormalities. As a result, detecting and correcting obesity and its associated metabolic abnormalities in childhood may help prevent cardiovascular morbidity and mortality in adulthood.

A number of studies have demonstrated the positive effects of intensive weight-loss programs in children [7-11]. Yet, intensive programs are based on frequent interactions between children, their families, and a

* Correspondence: ritaann.kubicky@tenethealth.com
[1]Section of Endocrinology and Diabetes, St. Christopher's Hospital for Children, Department of Pediatrics, Drexel University College of Medicine, Philadelphia, PA, USA
[2]St. Christopher's Hospital for Children, Section of Endocrinology and Diabetes, 3601 A Street, Suite 3303, Philadelphia, PA 19134, USA

multi-disciplinary team of providers; thus, they are necessarily expensive and short-term. In addition, most of the beneficial effects of an intensive short-term intervention often do not persist once the program is completed [12-14].

Since little is known of the long-term impact of a non-intensive, conventional weight management program in obese children [15,16], we evaluated the effects of our Weight Management Program over a 4-year period at the Section of Endocrinology and Diabetes at St. Christopher's Hospital for Children in a subset of obese patients who maintained ongoing periodic follow-up visits. The goals of our study were: 1) to analyze the changes of BMI z-score, glycemic measures and lipid profiles at the end of the 4-year follow-up period, and 2) to correlate these changes with the frequency of the follow-up visits.

Methods

We conducted a retrospective analysis of the medical records of obese (BMI > 95th percentile for age and sex) children and adolescents evaluated between 2001 and 2008 at the Weight Management Center in the Section of Endocrinology and Diabetes at St. Christopher's Hospital for Children. All children were identified by tracking patients for whom the ICD-9 Code 783.1 was used ("abnormal weight gain"). Most of these patients were referred to us by their pediatricians for an evaluation of overweight/obesity and/or high serum insulin/abnormal lipid levels.

Inclusion criteria were the following: [1] children with a BMI > 95th percentile, [2] 1–18 years of age [3] ≥ 2 years of follow-up, and [4] fasting lipid panel, glucose and insulin obtained at the beginning and at the end of the follow-up period. Exclusion criteria included: 1) diagnosis of DM (type 1 or type 2) and 2) use of medications known to affect insulin sensitivity or glucose/lipid metabolism (metformin, insulin, growth hormone).

The Institutional Regulatory Board of Drexel University College of Medicine approved the retrospective analysis of the medical records.

At the initial visit, a physician screened the obese subjects for metabolic comorbidities, while a registered dietitian assessed their dietary habits and amount of physical activity. Generalized handouts geared towards healthy eating were provided to each subject; the dietitian reviewed each topic of the handout with the subjects and their parent/guardian. The topics included: making healthy food choices (increasing whole grains, lean meats and lower fat foods into the diet), eating three balanced meals per day using the plate method, portion control (measuring portions and learning about food labels), eliminating beverages containing more than 5 calories except for low fat milk, and making sensible snack choices. Thirty minutes of daily physical activity was recommended to all subjects with a focus on an activity that the child would enjoy.

At the subsequent visits (scheduled every 2 to 4 months), obese children and adolescents met with a pediatric nurse practitioner and the dietitian for approximately 20 minutes with each of the two providers; in order to measure implementation of the previous recommendations, during each of the follow-up visits, the child's dietary intake and physical activities were reassessed by patient history and diet and exercise recall. Patients who reported adhering to the dietary or physical activity changes were praised and encouraged to continue. If there was poor adherence to previous recommendations, or if there was need for further improvement, efforts were made by the dietitian and nurse practioner to detect barriers to change and to help determine alternative ways of engaging patients to adhere.

At each visit, body weight was measured with a balance scale, and height was measured with a wall-mounted stadiometer by a trained medical assistant. BMI was calculated as weight in kilograms divided by the height in meters squared, and expressed as a z-score by using the Centers for Disease Control and Prevention 2000 program [17]. Body weight, height and BMI were compared to the measurements/calculations of the previous visit by the nurse practitioner and dietitian in order to monitor each patient's weight loss/gain and change in the BMI as standard of care, and as an objective way to measure the likelihood that the patient was adhering to the dietary and physical activity-related recommendations.

A fasting lipid panel (total cholesterol, low-density lipoprotein [LDL] cholesterol, high-density lipoprotein [HDL] cholesterol, and triglyceride [TG] levels) was requested yearly. A 2-hour Oral Glucose Tolerance test (OGTT) was recommended to all children: impaired glucose tolerance (IGT) and DM were defined as a 2-hour glucose level of 140–199 mg/dL and ≥ 200 mg/dL, respectively [18]. Insulin resistance was estimated by using the Homeostasis Model Assessment of Insulin Resistance (HOMA-IR), calculated as fasting plasma glucose (mg/dL) x fasting insulin (µU/mL) ÷ 405 [19]. Dyslipidemia was defined as high TG (≥ 90th percentile for age and sex) and/or low HDL-cholesterol (≤ 10th percentile for age and sex) concentrations [4].

Data were analyzed with SPSS software version 17.0 for Windows (SPSS, Chicago, IL). All data were expressed as the mean plus or minus SD or range. A p-value < 0.05 was considered to be statistically significant. Differences in the mean values between groups were evaluated using a Student's t-test or analysis of variance.

Results

A total of 61 children and adolescents met our inclusion criteria. 39 children were females and 24 were prepubertal; the mean age was 11.1 ± 2.6 years (mean $\pm$ SD). With respect to their ethnicity, 25 were African American, 26 were Hispanic, 7 were Caucasian, 2 Asian and 1 identified himself as other. The duration of the follow-up period was 47.3 ± 11.1 months while the number of outpatient visits per year (OV/yr) was 2.9 ± 0.9.

At the end of the follow-up, children exhibited a significant decrease in their BMI z-score (p = 0.03) and LDL-cholesterol (p = 0.022) (Table 1). In the subset of children in whom OGTT was performed both at the beginning and at the end of the follow-up period (n = 42), there was a significant decrease in both the 2-hour glucose (p = 0.004) and peak insulin (p = 0.043) (Table 1).

All children with an initially normal OGTT (n = 37) maintained a normal OGTT by the end of the follow-up period, with the exception of 1 child who developed IGT (2-hr glucose, 141 mg/dL); his HOMA-IR increased and BMI z-score decreased. 5 children were found with IGT on their initial OGTT; their BMI z-score and HOMA-IR were similar to those of children with normal OGTT. In 4 children with IGT, the OGTT normalized by the end of the follow-up, while the 5th child developed DM. Of the 4 children with normalized OGTT, 1 child experienced increased BMI z-score and HOMA-IR, 1 child decreased BMI z-score and increased HOMA-IR, and 2 children increased BMI z-score and decreased HOMA-IR. The child who became diabetic had decreased BMI z-score and HOMA-IR by the end of the follow-up period.

When children were grouped according to changes in BMI z-score [increased vs. same/decreased BMI z-score (0.2 ± 0.15 vs. -0.32 ± 0.3, p < 0.001)], those with the same or decreased BMI z-score exhibited decreased fasting insulin (136.7 ± 98.6 vs. 153.5 ± 91 pmol/L, last vs. initial visit, p < 0.001) and LDL-cholesterol (2.4 ± 0.5 vs. 2.7 ± 0.9 mmol/L, last vs. initial visit, p = 0.02).

Among the 60 subjects for whom a fasting lipid panel was obtained at the initial visit, 25 children had dyslipidemia: 5 with low HDL and high TG, 11 with isolated low HDL and 9 with isolated high TG; when compared to those with normal lipid levels, children with abnormal levels had similar BMI z-scores (Table 2). At the end of the follow-up period, lipid levels normalized in 15 children and remained abnormal in 10 children: the 15 children with normalized lipid levels exhibited a significantly decreased BMI z-score (Table 3), unlike those with persistently abnormal lipid profile.

5 children with normal HDL and TG at baseline developed dyslipidemia at the end of the follow-up period: 1 child developed both elevated TG and low HDL, 3 children had low HDL and 1 developed high TG. These 5 children did not experience any significant change of the mean BMI-z-score or HOMA-IR at the end of the follow-up period (Table 3).

When children were divided in two groups according to their mean number of OV per year (≤ 2 vs. >2; 1.53 ± 0.5 vs. 3.19 ± 0.7, p < 0.001), there were no differences at the initial visit for any of the metabolic variables analyzed or for BMI z-score (Table 4). At the end of the follow-up, children with > 2 OV/yr exhibited a significant decrease in their LDL-cholesterol (Table 4) and BMI z-score (Table 4), while children with ≤ 2 OV/yr did not. In the group of children who underwent OGTT, those with > 2 OV/yr experienced a significant decrease of both the 2-hour glucose (n = 33), (Table 4, p = 0.0001) and peak insulin (n = 32), (Table 4, p = 0.0036), while children with ≤ 2 OV/yr did not (n = 8 and 6, respectively).

Discussion

In our multi-ethnic population sample, a non-intensive ($\sim$ 3 visits per year) weight management program that reinforced healthy dietary modifications and regular daily activity over a 4-year period resulted in a statistically

Table 1 Anthropometric and metabolic characteristics of the population sample

	Initial Visit	Last Visit	p-value
BMI z-score	2.49 ± 0.4	2.33 ± 0.4	**0.03**
Fasting glucose (mmol/L)[a]	4.8 ± 0.5	4.6 ± 0.5	0.08
Fasting insulin (pmol/L)[b]	145.1 ± 90.3	135.4 ± 100.7	0.56
HOMA-IR	4.5 ± 3	4.1 ± 2.9	0.38
HDL-cholesterol (mmol/L)[c]	1.2 ± 0.3	1.2 ± 0.3	0.61
LDL-cholesterol (mmol/L)[c]	2.9 ± 0.9	2.5 ± 0.6	**0.022**
Triglycerides (mmol/L)[d]	2.8 ± 1.8	2.3 ± 0.9	0.057
2-hour glucose (mmol/L)[a]	2.9 ± 0.6	2.5 ± 0.7	**0.004**
Peak insulin (pmol/L)[b]	1445.9 ± 869.5	1070.9 ± 748.7	**0.043**

Results are expressed as mean $\pm$ SD. p-values < 0.05 are in bold.
[a]To convert to mg/dL divide by 0.0555.
[b]To convert to μIU/mL divide by 6.945.
[c]To convert to mg/dL divide by 0.0259.
[d]To convert to mg/dL divide by 0.0113.

Table 2 Comparison of BMI z-score and metabolic parameters according to the presence of dyslipidemia at the initial visit

	Dyslipidemia (n=25)	Normal Lipids (n=35)	p-value
BMI z-score	2.42 ± 0.4	2.51 ± 0.4	0.42
HDL-cholesterol (mmol/L)[a]	1.0 ± 0.2	1.3 ± 0.2	**< 0.001**
Triglycerides (mmol/L)[b]	1.6 ± 1.0	0.9 ± 0.3	**< 0.001**
HOMA-IR	4 ± 1.8	4.6 ± 3.1	0.45

Results are expressed as mean $\pm$ SD. p-values < 0.05 are in bold.
[a]To convert to mg/dL divide by 0.0259.
[b]To convert to mg/dL divide by 0.0113.

Table 3 Changes of BMI z-score and metabolic parameters at the last visit according to changes of lipid levels

	Abnormal HDL & TG ↓ Abnormal HDL & TG (n=10)		Abnormal HDL & TG ↓ Normal HDL & TG (n=15)		Normal HDL & TG ↓ Abnormal HDL & TG (n=5)		Normal HDL & TG ↓ Normal HDL & TG (n=30)	
	Initial Visit	Last Visit	Initial Visit	Last Visit	Initial Visit	Last Visit	Initial Visit	Last Visit
BMI z-score	2.36 ± 0.4	2.32 ± 0.5	2.49 ± 0.4	2.19 ± 0.3*	2.47 ± 0.5	2.47 ± 0.5	2.52 ± 0.4	2.37 ± 0.4
HDL-cholesterol (mmol/L)[a]	0.9 ± 0.1	0.9 ± 0.1	1.1 ± 0.3	1.1 ± 0.2	1.2 ± 0.1	1 ± 0.1*	1.3 ± 0.2	1.3 ± 0.3
Triglycerides (mmol/L)[b]	1.9 ± 1.4	1.3 ± 32	1.6 ± 0.7	1 ± 0.3*	1 ± 0.3	1.3 ± 0.4	0.9 ± 0.3	0.9 ± 0.3
HOMA-IR	4.2 ± 1.9	5.3 ± 3.3	4.7 ± 3.4	3.7 ± 2	4 ± 2.4	3.3 ± 2.4	4.7 ± 3.2	3.9 ± 3.2

Results are expressed as mean ± SD. *p-value < 0.05, last vs. initial visit.
[a]To convert to mg/dL divide by 0.0259.
[b]To convert to mg/dL divide by 0.0113.

significant reduction of BMI z-score and LDL-cholesterol, and improvement of glucose tolerance.

Extensive evidence previously published supports the effectiveness of intensive weight-loss programs in children. In a study conducted by Wilfley et al., 204 overweight children were enrolled to determine the short-term and long-term efficacy of weight-loss and weight maintenance programs [7]. After 5 months of intensive weekly meetings focused on weight-loss treatment with a multi-disciplinary team, almost 90% of children exhibited a decreased BMI z-score. At the end of the weight-loss intervention, the 2 active maintenance groups experienced a mean change in BMI z-score of − 0.22 from baseline to 2-year follow-up versus the control group. Such BMI z-score reduction is similar to the one shown in our study by the end of the 4-year follow-up (−0.16); however, Wilfley et al. did not evaluate the impact of weight loss on metabolic parameters. Savoye et al. studied a population of 209 obese children to evaluate the effects of a 12-month weight management program on adiposity and metabolic parameters [8]. The program included exercise, nutrition, and behavior modification: intervention occurred biweekly the first 6 months and bimonthly thereafter. At the end of study, the weight-management group experienced a significant decrease of BMI and HOMA-IR compared to the control group; conversely, no difference was found relative to changes in fasting glucose, HDL-cholesterol, LDL-cholesterol, or blood pressure. Reinehr et al. studied changes in weight status and cardiovascular disease (CVD) risk factors in 203 obese children who attended a 1-year outpatient intervention program; enrolled subjects were then evaluated 1 year after the end of the intervention [20]. The program included weekly meetings with an exercise physiologist as well as once to twice monthly with a dietitian and a psychologist. Children who experienced a reduction of BMI SDS (72% of the group) at the end of the 12-month intervention maintained this reduction 1 year later. In addition, children with reduced BMI SDS (but not those without)

showed improved HDL-cholesterol, LDL-cholesterol, blood pressure, and HOMA-IR.

Although the positive effects of all these studies were sustained for a relatively long period of time, the high costs associated with the frequent utilization of a team of dietitians, social workers, and exercise physiologists render this format not widely applicable. In contrast, our findings suggest that weight management programs based on less frequent encounters with a smaller team (pediatric nurse practitioner and a registered dietitian) may result in a similarly effective and lasting reduction of obesity and obesity-associated metabolic abnormalities.

The importance of preventing or reducing the severity of overweight in childhood is supported by a number of studies demonstrating the link between pediatric obesity and morbidity and mortality in adulthood. Three previous studies have identified an association between overweight in children and adolescents with increased rates of death due to coronary heart disease [21,22] and with death from all causes [22,23]. In a large cohort of American-Indian subjects followed since childhood [3], the rate of premature death (before 55 years of age) from endogenous causes among children in the highest quartile of BMI was more than double than that in children in the lowest quartile. Of note, the association between BMI and premature death was attenuated but remained significant after adjustment for glucose level, cholesterol level, and blood pressure: thus, some of the effects of overweight on the risk of premature death may not depend on abnormal glucose and lipid metabolism, or on hypertension.

In our cohort of 61 children, 5 were found with IGT at baseline; in 4 of these children, the OGTT normalized by the end of the 4-year follow-up period, while one child became diabetic. In a similar study, Weiss et al. identified 33 children with IGT in a population sample of 117 obese children [24]. By the end of a 2-year period, 15 of those with IGT reverted to normal glucose tolerance while 8 developed Type 2 DM. When compared to those who reverted to normal glucose tolerance, subjects

Table 4 Changes of BMI z-score and metabolic parameters according to the frequency of clinic visits

	≤ 2 Outpatient visits (n=13)		p-value	>2 Outpatient visits (n=48)		p-value
	Initial Visit	Last Visit		Initial Visit	Last Visit	
Age (years)	10.9 ± 1.64			11.2 ± 2.9		0.71
Sex (male/female)	5/8			17/31		0.84
BMI z-score	2.44 ± 0.4	2.37 ± 0.4	0.66	2.5 ± 0.4	2.32 ± 0.4	**0.03**
Fasting glucose (mmol/L)[a]	4.8 ± 0.32	4.5 ± 0.4	0.09	4.8 ± 0.6	4.7 ± 0.5	0.21
Fasting insulin (pmol/L)[b]	151.4 ± 59.0	150.01 ± 95.8	0.97	143.8 ± 97.2	131.3 ± 102.1	0.54
HOMA-IR	4.7 ± 1.8	4.4 ± 2.9	0.8	4.5 ± 3.2	4 ± 2.9	0.4
HDL-cholesterol (mmol/L)[c]	1.2 ± 0.2	1.1 ± 0.3	0.25	1.2 ± 0.3	1.2 ± 0.3	0.98
LDL-cholesterol (mmol/L)[c]	106.2 ± 84.4	97.9 ± 12.3	0.16	111.3 ± 36.7	96.4 ± 23.5	**0.022**
Triglycerides (mmol/L)[d]	1.6 ± 1	1.2 ± 0.4	0.20	1.1 ± 0.7	1 ± 0.4	0.13
2-hour glucose (mmol/L)[a]	(n=8) 5.8 ± 1.2	5.3 ± 1.3	0.44	(n=34) 6.3 ± 1.2	5.2 ± 1.0	**0.0001**
Peak insulin (pmol/L)[a]	(n=6) 1486.9 ± 1039.0	1474.4 ± 1206.3	0.98	(n=32) 1472.3 ± 817.4	952.9 ± 563.2	**0.0036**

Results are expressed as mean ± SD. p-values < 0.05 are in bold.
[a]To convert to mg/dL divide by 0.0555.
[b]To convert to µIU/mL divide by 6.945.
[c]To convert to mg/dL divide by 0.0259.
[d]To convert to mg/dL divide by 0.0113.

who developed DM were significantly more obese at baseline and increased their BMI during the follow-up period; in our study, the relationship between OGTT results and initial BMI z-score and/or change in BMI z-score overtime is less clear. While the association between IGT and risk to develop DM has not been well defined in children, it has been clearly demonstrated in adults [25,26]; in addition, IGT in adults appears to be linked to an increased risk for cardiovascular disease and mortality [27,28].

In the present study, 25 of the 60 subjects had dyslipidemia at the initial visit: by the end of the 4-year follow-up period, in 15 of these 25 subjects the abnormal lipid levels normalized: unlike those with persistently abnormal lipid panel, the 15 children with normalized lipid levels exhibited a significantly decreased BMI z-score during the 4-year follow-up period. Previous cross-sectional studies have shown a high prevalence of low HDL-cholesterol and elevated TG in obese children [29,30]. A longitudinal study conducted in the United Kingdom in more than 5,000 children showed that 1 SD greater BMI at age 9–12 years was associated with high TG and low HDL-cholesterol at age 15–16 years [31]; in the same study, changing from overweight/obese at age 9–12 to normal weight at age 15–16 was associated with better cardiovascular risk profiles than remaining overweight/obese from childhood through adolescence. Data from 4 prospective cohorts have demonstrated that cardiovascular risk factors in childhood (including high TG) significantly predict subclinical atherosclerosis as early as 9 years of age [32], thus justifying sustained efforts to correct obesity and lipid abnormalities in children.

There are some limitations of our study, such as the lack of a control group and the relatively small sample size. However, the fact that our results are consistent with those of studies including a larger number of subjects and a control group supports the validity of our findings. In addition, there may have been a selection bias regarding the subjects included in the retrospective analysis, since only a small number of children initially evaluated at our Weight Management Center were eventually followed for 2 or more years. We can speculate that the effects of the program were less significant for those subjects followed for less than 2 years. Those subjects having a longer duration of follow-up may have experienced weight loss early in the program, greater adherence to the lifestyle changes, or more family involvement. Our results demonstrate that a non-intensive weight management program offers potential medical benefits to children and adolescents who are sufficiently motivated to continue their follow-up visits.

The long duration of our retrospective study, and the non-intensive approach of our intervention, has rendered unfeasible the concomitant evaluation of a control, completely untreated, group of obese children. To circumvent such limitation, we have used two historical control groups followed longitudinally by Reinehr et al. [33] and by D'Hondt et al. [34]. In the former study, 100 overweight children [BMI-SDS 1.92 (1.27-2.75)] with a mean age of 9 years (6–15 years) were periodically evaluated during a 2-year period without any intervention. This control group did not experience any significant change in their BMI-SDS. In the latter study by D'Hondt et al., at baseline 50 overweight children (8 of which were obese) had a mean age of 11.6 ± 0.8 years and a baseline BMI z-score range of 1.55 ± 0.39 (1.00; 2.64). 2 years later, even these children's BMI z-scores remained unchanged. These finding suggests that the significant reduction of BMI-SDS observed in our study likely depends on the lifestyle modifications reinforced by our team, rather than simply reflecting a physiological change in adiposity.

In conclusion, our study suggests that a non-intensive, long-term weight management program may significantly improve the degree of obesity and some cardiovascular risk factors in childhood. In addition, this non-intensive treatment (a small team approach) is more likely to be reimbursed by 3rd party payors making it more financially sustainable. Prospective studies with a larger population sample and comparison to a control group are warranted to confirm these findings.

Abbreviations
BMI: Body Mass Index; OV/yr: Outpatient visits per year; DM: Diabetes Mellitus; HDL: High-density lipoprotein; LDL: Low-density lipoprotein; TG: Triglycerides; OGTT: Oral Glucose Tolerance Test; IGT: Impaired glucose tolerance; HOMA-IR: Homeostasis Model Assessment of Insulin Resistance; CVD: Cardiovascular disease.

Competing interests
The authors disclose no potential, perceived, or real conflict of interest.

Authors' contributions
DN and CD initiated data collection; CD continued data collection and started literature search. RAK continued data collection and completed literature search with FDL. CD, RAK and FDL analyzed data. RAK and FDL as well as CD wrote the paper. All authors had final approval of the submitted version.

References
1. McCrindle BW, Urbina EM, Dennison BA, Jacobson MS, Steinberger J, Rocchini AP, et al: Drug Therapy of High-Risk Lipid Abnormalities in Children and Adolescents: A Scientific Statement From the American Heart Association Atherosclerosis, Hypertension, and Obesity in Youth Committee, Council of Cardiovascular Disease in the Young, With the Council on Cardiovascular Nursing. Circulation 2007, 115:1948–1967.
2. Weiss R, Kaufman FR: Metabolic Complications of Childhood Obesity. Diabetes Care 2008, 31(Suppl 2):S310–S316.
3. Franks PW, Hanson RL, Knowler W, Sievers M, Bennett PH, Looker HC: Childhood Obesity, Other Cardiovascular Risk Factors, and Premature Death. N Engl J Med 2010, 3624(6):85–493.
4. Cook S, Auinger P, Huang TTK: Growth Curves for Cardio-Metabolic Risk Factors in Children and Adolescents. J Pediatr 2009, 155(3):S6.e15-26. doi:10.1016/j.jpeds.2009.04.05.
5. Morrison JA, Friedman LA, Wang P, Glueck CJ: Metabolic Syndrome in Childhood Predicts Adult Metabolic Syndrome and Type 2 Diabetes Mellitus 25 to 30 Years Later. J Pediatr 2008, 152:201–206.
6. Morrison J, et al: Metabolic Syndrome in Childhood Predicts Adult Cardiovascular Disease 25 years Later: The Princeton Lipid Research Clinics Follow-up Study. Pediatrics 2007, 120:340–345.
7. Wilfley DE, Stein RI, Saelens BE, Mockus DS, Matt GE, Hayden-Wade HA, et al: Efficacy of Maintenance Treatment Approaches for Childhood Overweight: A Randomized Controlled Trial. JAMA 2007, 298(14):1661–1672.
8. Savoye M, Berry D, Dziura J, Shaw M, Serrecchia J, Barbetta G, et al: Anthroprometric and Psychosocial Changes in Obese Adolescents Enrolled in a Weight Management Program. J Am Diet Assoc 2005, 105(3):364–369.
9. Berry D, Savoye M, Melkus G, Grey M: An Intervention for multiethnic obese parents and overweight children. Appl Nurs Res 2007, 20:63–71.
10. Savoye M, Shaw M, Dziura J, Tamborlane W, Rose P, Guandalini C, et al: Effects of a Weight Management Program on Body Composition and Metabolic Parameters in Overweight Children: A Randomized Controlled

11. Gately PJ, Cooke CB, Barth JH, Bewick BM, Radley D, Hill AJ: Children's Residential Weight-Loss Programs Can Work: A Prospective Cohort Study of Short-Term Outcomes for Overweight and Obese Children. Pediatrics 2005, 116:73–77.
12. Goldfield GS, Raynor HA: Epstein LH Treatment of pediatric obesity. In Handbook of Obesity Treatment. Edited by Wadden TA, Stunkard AJ. New York: Guildford Press; 2002:532–555.
13. Weiss EC, Galuska DA, Kettel Khan L, Gillespis C, Serdula MK: Weight regain in U.S. adults who experienced substantial weight loss, 1999–2002. Am J Prev Med 2007, 33:34–40.
14. Dansinger ML, Tatsioni A, Wong JB, Chung M, Balk EM: Meta-analysis: The effect of dietary counseling for weight loss. Ann Intern Med 2007, 147:41–50.
15. Jeffery RW, Hinkle LK, Carr RE, Anderson DA, Lemmon CR, Engler LB, et al: Long-Term Maintenance of Weight Loss: Current Status. Health Psychol 1997, 19:5–16.
16. Perri MG, Nezu AM, Patti ET, McCann KL: Effect of length of treatment on weight loss. J Consult Clin Psychol 1989, 57:450–452.
17. Kuczmarski RJ, Ogden CL, Grummer-Strawn HM, Flegal KM, Guo SS, We R, et al: CDC growth charts: United States. Advance data from vital and health statistics, no. 314. Hyattsville(MD): National Center for Health Statistics; 2000.
18. Expert Committee on the Diagnosis and Classification of Diabetes Mellitus: Report of the Expert Committee on the Diagnosis and Classification of Diabetes Mellitus. Diabetes Care 1997, 20:1183–1197.
19. Matthews DR, Hosker JP, Rudenski AS, Naylor BA, Treacher DF, Turner RC: Homeostasis Model assessment: insulin resistance and [beta]-cell function from fasting plasma glucose and insulin concentration in man. Diabetologia 1985, 28:412–419.
20. Reinehr T, de Sousa G, Toschke AM, Andler W: Long-term follow-up of cardiovascular disease risk factors in children after an obesity intervention. Am J Clin Nutr 2003, 84:490–496.
21. Must A, Jacques PF, Dallal GE, Bajema CJ, Dietz WH: Long-term morbidity and mortality of overweight adolescents: a follow-up of the Harvard Growth Study of 1922 to 1935. N Engl J Med 1992, 327:1350–1355.
22. DiPietro L, Mossberg HO, Stunkard AJ: A 40-year history of overweight children in Stockholm: life-time overweight, morbidity, and mortality. Int J Obes Relat Metab Disord 1994, 18:585–590.
23. Gunnell DJ, Frankel SJ, Nanchahal K, Peters TJ, Davey Smith G: Childhood obesity and adult cardiovascular mortality: a 57-y follow-up study based on the Boyd Orr cohort. Am J Clin Nutr 1998, 67:1111–1118.
24. Weiss R, Taksali SE, Tamborlane WV, Burgert TS, Savoye M, Caprio S: Predictors of Changes in Glucose Tolerance Status in Obese Youth. Diabetes Care 2005, 28(4):902–909.
25. Lee ET, Welty TK, Cowan LD, Wang W, Rhoades DA, Devereux R, et al: Incidence of Diabetes in American Indians of Three Geographic Areas: The Strong Heart Study. Diabetes Care 2002, 25:49–54.
26. Gerstein HC, Santaguida P, Raina P, Morrison KM, Balion C, Hunt D, et al: Annual incidence and relative risk of diabetes in people with various categories of dysglycemia: a systematic overview and meta-analysis of prospective studies. Diabetes Res Clin Pract 2007, 78(3):305–312.
27. Barr EL, Zimmet PZ, Welborn TA, Jolley D, Magliano DJ, Dunstan DW, et al: Risk of cardiovascular and all-cause mortality in individuals with diabetes mellitus, impaired fasting glucose, and impaired glucose tolerance: the Australian Diabetes, Obesity, and Lifestyle Study (AusDiab). Circulation 2007, 116(2):151–157.
28. Sourij H, Saely CH, Schmid F, Zweiker R, Marte T, Wascher TC, et al: Post-challenge hyperglycaemia is strongly associated with future macrovascular events and total mortality in angiographied coronary patients. Eur Heart J 2010, 31(13):1583–1590.
29. Pinhas-Hamiel O, Lerner-Geva L, Copperman NM, Jacobson MS: Lipid and Insulin Levels in Obese Children: Changes with Age and Puberty. Obesity 2007, 15:2825–2831.
30. Raitakari OT, Juonala M, Kähönen M, Taittonen L, Laitinen T, Mäki-Torkko N, et al: Cardiovascular risk factors in childhood and carotid artery intima-media thickness in adulthood: the Cardiovascular Risk in Young Finns Study. JAMA 2003, 290(17):2277–2283.
31. Lawlor DA, Benfield L, Logue J, Tilling K, Howe LD, Fraser A, et al: Association between general and central adiposity in childhood, and change in these, with cardiovascular risk factors in adolescence: prospective cohort study. BMJ 2010, 341:c6224.

Trial. JAMA 2007, 297(24):2697–2704.

32. Juonala M, Magnussen CG, Venn A, Dwyer T, Burns TL, Davis PH, et al: **Influence of age on associations between childhood risk factors and carotid intima-media thickness in adulthood: the Cardiovascular Risk in Young Finns Study, the Childhood Determinants of Adult Health Study, the Bogalusa Heart Study, and the Muscatine Study for the International Childhood Cardiovascular Cohort (i3C) Consortium.** *Circulation* 2010, **122**(24):2514–2520.

33. Reinehr T, Kersting M, Alexy U, Andler W: **Long-Term Follow-Up of Overwight Children: After Training, After a Single Consultation, and Without Treatment.** *J Pediatr Gastroenterol Nutr* 2003, **37**:72–74.

34. D'Hondt E, Deforche B, Gentier I, De Bourdeaudhuij I, Vaeyens R, Philippaerts, Lenoir M: **A longitudinal analysis of grow motor coordination in overweight and obese children versus normal-weight peers.** *Int J Obes* 2012. doi:10.1038/ijo.2012.55.

14

Prediction of post-treatment hypothyroidism using changes in thyroid volume after radioactive iodine therapy in adolescent patients with Graves' disease

Nobuhiro Nakatake*, Shuji Fukata and Junichi Tajiri

Abstract

Background: The goal of iodine-131 therapy for pediatric Graves' disease is to induce hypothyroidism. However, changes in post-treatment thyroid volume have not been investigated in pediatric and/or adolescent patients.

Objective: The aim of this retrospective study was to examine whether changes in thyroid volume predict post-treatment hypothyroidism in adolescent Graves' disease patients.

Patients and Methods: We used ultrasonography to examine changes in thyroid volume, and also assessed thyroid functions, at 0, 1, 3, 5, 8 and 12 months after iodine-131 treatment in 49 adolescents ranging in age from 12 to 19 years retrospectively. Based on thyroid function outcome at 12 months, patients were divided into two groups: 29 patients with overt hypothyroidism requiring levothyroxine replacement and 20 without overt hypothyroidism. We compared changes in post-radioiodine thyroid volume between the two groups.

Results: About 90% of patients whose thyroid volume at 3 months after iodine-131 administration was less than 50% of the original volume were hypothyroid by one year after treatment (positive predictive value 88%, sensitivity 75.9%, specificity 85.0%).

Conclusions: We believe ultrasonographic measurement of thyroid volume at 3 months after iodine-131 to be clinically useful for predicting post-treatment hypothyroidism in adolescent Graves' disease patients.

Introduction

Graves' disease (GD) is the most common cause of hyperthyroidism in children, adolescents and adults [1-3]. Treatments available for GD include anti-thyroid medications (methimazole or propylthiouracil), surgery and radioactive iodine (RAI) [4,5]. There is ongoing debate worldwide regarding the most suitable therapy for GD in pediatric patients. Although anti-thyroid medications are commonly used as first-line therapy for pediatric GD, long-term remission occurs in only 20% to 30% of pubertal cases and 15% of pre-pubertal cases treated pharmacologically [3,6-8]. Consequently, either surgery or RAI is needed to achieve a long-term cure in most pediatric GD patients.

RAI therapy is generally considered to be safe, inexpensive and effective, with relatively few side effects [8-10]. Radioiodine was introduced for the treatment of GD more than 50 years ago [11], and at present is the most commonly used treatment for adult GD in the North America [12]. In 107 young GD patients who had been treated with RAI before age 20 years, no increased risk of adverse events was reported [13]. In some facilities, RAI is becoming the first-line therapy for GD in children and adolescents [14,15].

The goal of iodine-131 therapy for pediatric GD is to induce hypothyroidism [16,17]. When children are treated with 330 µCi/g of iodine-131, hypothyroidism is achieved in nearly 95% of patients [18]. Higher dose ablative therapy (13.8 to 15.6 mCi) is effective in nearly all children with GD [19]. The use of high dose iodine-131 will destroy most thyroid tissue, thereby decreasing the risk of

* Correspondence: nakatake@j-tajiri.or.jp
Tajiri Thyroid Clinic, Kumamoto 862-0950, Japan

RAI-induced thyroid tumors, and is thus preferable especially in children [20]. The long-term risks of thyroid cancer appear to be lower when the thyroid gland is largely ablated than when residual thyroid tissue remains [21,22]. Changes in post-RAI thyroid volume have been investigated in adult GD patients [10,23-26], but not in pediatric and/or adolescent patients [3].

The objective of this retrospective study was to investigate changes in post-radioiodine thyroid volume in adolescent GD patients (< 20 years old) and also to examine whether these changes predict post-treatment hypothyroidism.

Patients and Methods

The medical records of all adolescent patients (< 20 years old) at Tajiri Thyroid Clinic who received a single RAI treatment for GD during the decade from January 2000 to January 2010 were examined retrospectively. The present study was approved by the Institutional Review Board of our clinic.

GD was diagnosed based on elevated free thyroxine and suppressed thyrotropin concentrations, elevated TSH receptor antibodies (TRAb), and diffuse, elevated uptake of radioiodine or technetium-99 m within the thyroid. Thyrotropin, free thyroxine and TSH receptor antibody were measured by electrochemiluminescence immunoassay (Cobas e601; Roche Diagnostics, Tokyo, Japan).

The iodine-131-absorbed radiation dose was calculated from RAIU and thyroid weight, using the formula: dose (μCi/g) = oral iodine-131 dose (mCi) × estimated 24 h RAIU (%) × 10/thyroid weight (g). Twenty-four hour RAI uptake was estimated using 4-hour uptake of iodine-123 [27] or 20-minute uptake of technetium-99 m [28]. Thyroid volume was estimated by ultrasound (SSA-350A; Toshiba Inc. Ltd., Tokyo, Japan) as previously reported [29]. Thyroid function (free thyroxine and thyrotropin) and ultrasonographic thyroid volume were determined at 1, 3, 5, 8 and 12 months after RAI therapy. When free thyroxine values dropped below 0.8 ng/dL and/or thyrotropin levels rose above 20 μIU/mL, replacement therapy with levothyroxine was initiated.

Statistical analyses were performed using Student's t test and the chi-squared test. Values are shown as means ± standard deviation (SD). A P-value of less than 0.05 was considered to indicate a statistically significant difference.

Results

There were 10 males and 39 females ranging in age from 12 to 19 years (mean ± SD, 16.4 ± 1.8 years old). All 49 patients were initially treated with anti-thyroid medications for 1 to 108 months (80% with methimazole, 20% with propylthiouracil). RAI therapy was performed due to lack of remission after 14 to 108 months (39%) of

medical treatment, the development of a presumed toxic reaction to anti-thyroid drugs (44%; rash, arthralgia, hepatitis, neutropenia), or a desire for definitive therapy (17%). Anti-thyroid drugs were discontinued 3 to 5 days before RAI treatment. After administration of iodine-131, patients were treated with anti-thyroid drugs with or without propranolol to control symptoms of hyperthyroidism until hyperthyroxinemia abated.

The mean RAI dose for our 49 patients was 184 ± 84 μCi/g (range 44 - 393 μCi/g) and mean thyroid volume decreased significantly from 34.5 ml to 8.3 ml during the one year period after RAI (P < 0.00001). Based on thyroid functions at one year after RAI, patients were divided into two groups: 29 (59.2%) with overt hypothyroidism (hypothyroid patients) requiring levothyroxine replacement therapy (mean time until hypothyroidism: 4 ± 1.5 months, range 1 - 8 months) and 20 (40.8%) without hypothyroidism (non-hypothyroid patients) taking no medication at one year after RAI. The 20 non-hypothyroid patients consisted of 8 euthyroid and 12 hyperthyroid patients. Euthyroid patients included two who experienced transient hypothyroidism at 3 months after I-131 but had recovered without intervention at 1 year and one with subclinical hypothyroidism (TSH 6.53 μIU/ml (normal range: 0.20 - 3.30 μIU/ml)) at 1 year. Hyperthyroidism was subclinical in 8 patients and mild in 4 with serum free T4 levels of 1.93 - 2.03 ng/dl (normal range: 0.90 - 1.80 ng/dl). None of the hyperthyroid patients took anti-thyroid drugs at one year after RAI because all were asymptomatic. There were no statistically significant differences between euthyroid and hyperthyroid patients with respect to pre- and post-treatment thyroid volumes, or in percent volume reductions at 1, 3, 5, 8 and 12 months. The characteristics of adolescent GD patients who received RAI therapy, divided into hypothyroid and non-hypothyroid groups, are summarized in Table 1. There were no significant differences between the two groups in gender (P = 0.20), age (P = 0.18), pre-treatment thyroid volume (P = 0.30) or pre-treatment TRAb values measured by cosmic TRAb coated-tube kit (P = 0.45). The two groups differed only in the RAI dose administered (P = 0.048).

We compared changes in post-RAI administration thyroid volume during the one year period after treatment between hypothyroid and non-hypothyroid patients. As shown in Figure 1, post-treatment thyroid volume was significantly smaller in hypothyroid than in non-hypothyroid patients, especially after 8 months (8.2 ml vs. 13.1 ml at 8 months; P = 0.003, 6.3 ml vs. 10.9 ml at 12 months; P = 0.0005). The mean percent reduction in thyroid volume was significantly greater in hypothyroid than in non-hypothyroid patients at all measurement time points (P < 0.005) (Figure 2). We examined whether changes in thyroid volume predict post-treatment hypothyroidism at one year. The optimal

Table 1 Characteristics of Adolescent GD Patients Receiving Iodine-131 Therapy

	Hypothyroid (n = 29)	Non-hypothyroid (n = 20)	P-value
Gender, female/male	20/9	19/1	NS (0.06)
Age (yr)	16.1 ± 1.9	16.8 ± 1.6	NS (0.18)
Pre-treatment thyroid volume (ml)	36.3 ± 17.5	31.9 ± 11.6	NS (0.30)
Pre-treatment TRAb (%)	60.2 ± 27.8 (n = 22)	53.5 ± 29.1	NS (0.45)
I-131 dose (μCi/g)	202.7 ± 88.6	156.3 ± 71.2	0.048

NS: not significant. All values are means ± SD.

cut-off point for predicting post-treatment hypothyroidism is considered to be a 50% reduction, as compared to the original volume of the thyroid gland, at 3 months after iodine-131 administration (Table 2). The sensitivity, specificity, positive predictive value, negative predictive value, positive likelihood ratio, and negative likelihood ratio were 75.9%, 85.0%, 88.0%, 70.8%, 5.1 and 0.3, respectively.

We also examined the relationship between iodine-131 doses and post-RAI administration thyroid volume at 3 months in all 49 patients. Three iodine-131 doses (mean ± SD) were compared: 120 ± 32 μCi/g (n = 25, range 44 - 171 μCi/g), 200 ± 20 μCi/g (n = 11, range 174 - 224 μCi/g) and 300 ± 62 μCi/g (n = 13, range 225 - 393 μCi/g). When doses of 120 μCi/g, 200 μCi/g and 300 μCi/g were used, post-RAI administration thyroid volumes at 3 months were less than 50% of the pre-treatment thyroid volume in 36% (9/25), 55% (6/11) and 85% (11/13) of patients, respectively. We also found that doses of 120 μCi/g, 200 μCi/g and 300 μCi/g resulted in hypothyroidism at 1 year after RAI in 48% (12/25), 55% (6/11) and 85% (11/13) of the patients, respectively.

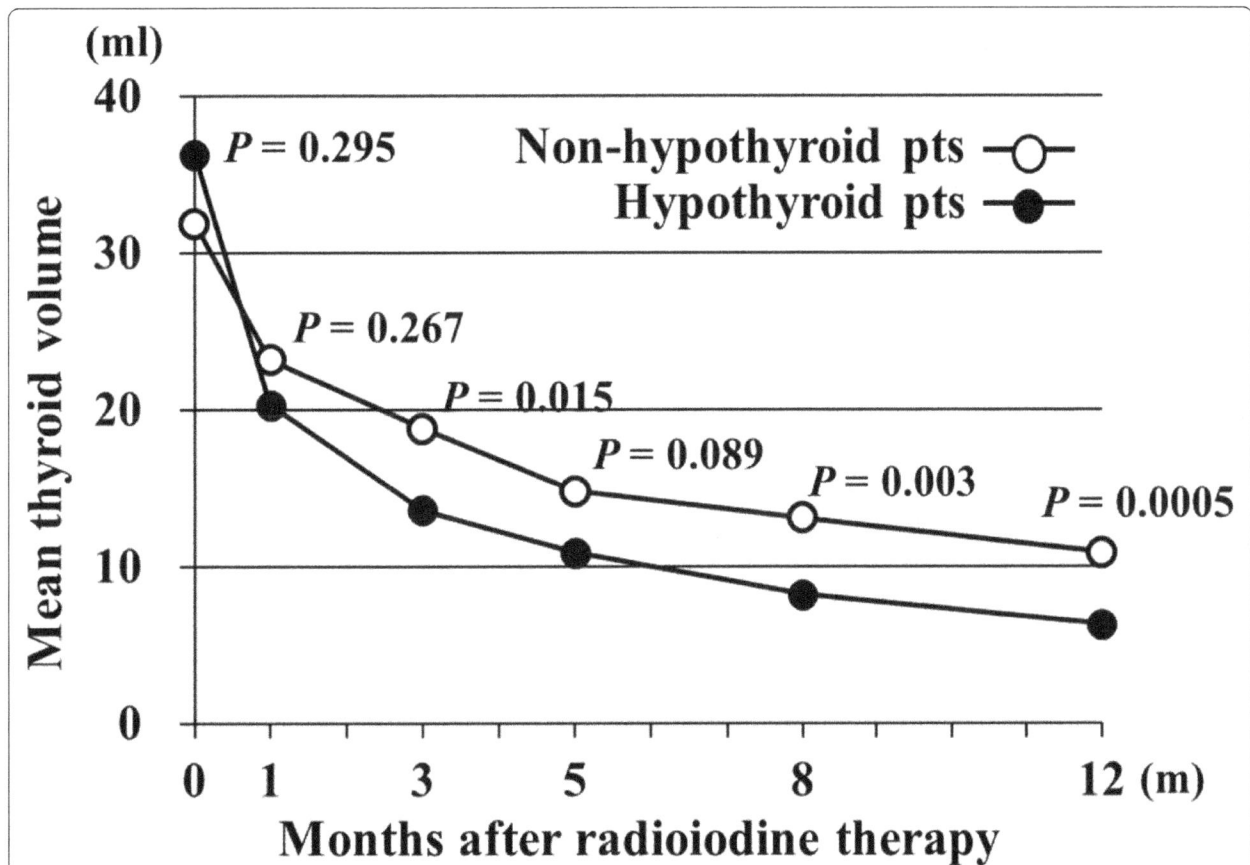

Figure 1 Changes in thyroid volume during the one year period after iodine-131 therapy in hypothyroid and non-hypothyroid patients. Mean thyroid volumes in hypothyroid vs. non-hypothyroid patients were 36.3 ml vs. 31.9 ml at 0 months (m), 20.3 ml vs. 23.2 ml at 1 m, 13.6 ml vs. 18.8 ml at 3 m, 10.9 ml vs. 14.8 ml at 5 m, 8.2 ml vs. 13.1 ml at 8 m, and 6.3 ml vs. 10.9 ml at 12 m after iodine-131 therapy.

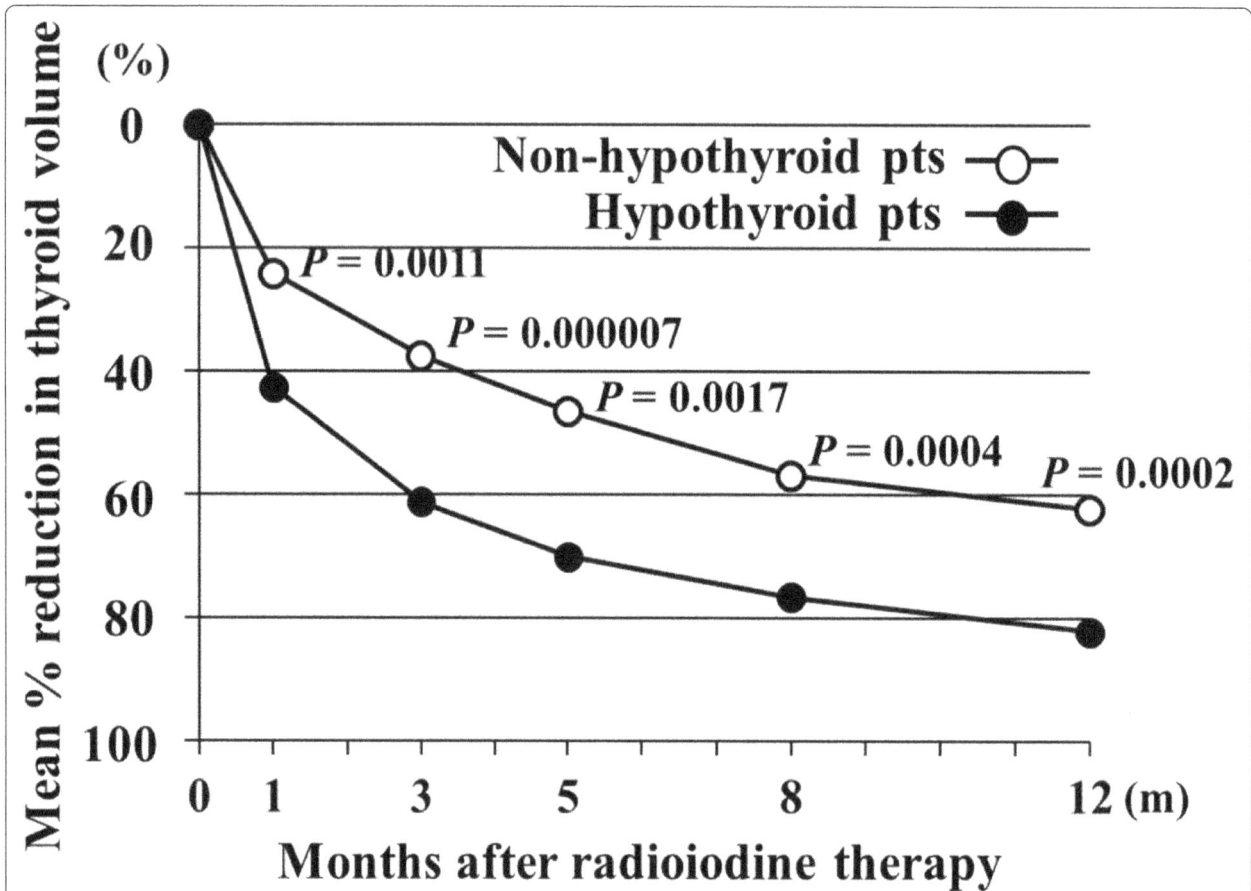

Figure 2 Percent reductions in thyroid volume during the one year period after iodine-131 therapy in hypothyroid and non-hypothyroid patients. Mean percent reductions in thyroid volume in hypothyroid vs. non-hypothyroid patients were 42.6% vs. 24.2% at 1 month (m), 61.2% vs. 37.6% at 3 m, 70.1% vs. 46.5% at 5 m, 76.6% vs. 56.9% at 8 m, and 82.2% vs. 62.4% at 12 m after iodine-131 therapy.

Discussion

This retrospective study showed mean post-treatment thyroid volume to be significantly decreased, from 34.5 ml to 8.3 ml (P < 0.00001), at one year after RAI in 49 adolescent GD patients (age range: 12 - 19 years), as has been demonstrated in adult GD patients (10,23-26).

The goal of iodine-131 therapy for pediatric GD is to ablate the thyroid gland, in order to decrease the risk of RAI-induced thyroid tumors [18]. However, changes in post- RAI administration thyroid volume have not been investigated in pediatric and/or adolescent patients [3]. We found thyroid volume at one year after RAI administration

Table 2 Sensitivity and Specificity of Percent Reductions in Thyroid Volume at Each Measurement Time Point after Iodine-131 Therapy

	Month(s) after iodine-131 therapy				
	1	3	5	8	12
% reduction*	Sens Spec	Sens Spec	Sens Spec	Sens Spec	Sens Spec
30%	75.9 55.0				
40%	55.2 80.0	79.3 60.0			
50%	41.4 95.0	75.9 85.0	92.6 53.3		
60%		55.2 90.0	73.3 74.1	96.2 57.9	
70%			51.9 93.3	73.1 78.9	85.2 60.0
80%				46.2 94.7	74.1 85.0
90%					18.5 100.0

*% reduction: cut-off point for percent reduction in thyroid volume

Sens: sensitivity for predicting hypothyroidism at one year after iodine-131 therapy using %reduction

Spec: specificity for predicting hypothyroidism at one year after iodine-131 therapy using %reduction for adolescent Graves' hyperthyroidism to be significantly smaller in hypothyroid than in non-hypothyroid patients (mean 6.3 ml vs. 10.9 ml; P < 0.001). As the post- RAI administration thyroid volume is smaller in hypothyroid patients, apparently conferring a lower risk of thyroid neoplasm development, this underscores the need for hypothyroidism to be a goal of therapy when using iodine-131 to treat GD in children [18].

A correlation between changes in thyroid volume and thyroid function outcome in adult patients with GD has been described (10,23-25). However, these studies did not investigate the relationship between the degree of thyroid volume reduction and thyroid function outcome. Chiovato et al reported that the degree of thyroid volume reduction after RAI administration was the best predictor of early (within 1 year) thyroid function outcome in adult Graves' hyperthyroidism [26]. In fact, we found that about 90% of our patients had become hypothyroid at one year when thyroid volume was less than 50% of the original volume at 3 months after iodine-131 administration (positive predictive value 88%, sensitivity 75.9%, specificity 85.0%).

We also found that 85% of patients treated with a dose of 300 µCi/g (range: 225 - 393 µCi/g) showed remarkable thyroid gland shrinkage (< 50% of the original thyroid gland volume at 3 months) and 85% were hypothyroid at one year. These data indicate that doses of approximately 300 µCi/g are needed to insure ablation of thyroid tissue. Our findings are thus consistent with those reported by Rivkees et al [18].

High thyroid-stimulating antibody levels before iodine-131 seem to be associated with a relative resistance to therapy (24, 26). On the other hand, TRAb levels did not show any predictive value for iodine-131 therapeutic outcome [25]. In our present study, pre-treatment TRAb values were not correlated with iodine-131 therapeutic outcome.

In conclusion, thyroid volume progressively diminished for one year after iodine-131 administration for adolescent GD. Decreases were more significant in hypothyroid than in non-hypothyroid patients. We also demonstrated that approximately 90% of patients became hypothyroid within one year when thyroid volume was less than 50% of the original volume at 3 months after RAI therapy. We believe ultrasonographic thyroid volume measurement at 3 months after iodine-131 administration to be clinically useful for predicting post-treatment hypothyroidism.

Authors' contributions

All authors contributed to the development and writing of this manuscript and each has many years of clinical experience in the care of individuals with Graves' disease. All authors read and approved the final manuscript.

Competing interests

The authors declare that they have no competing interests.

References

1. Saxena KM, Crawford JD, Talbot NB: Childhood thyrotoxicosis: a longer term perspective. *Br Med J* 1964, **2**:1153-1158.
2. Brent GA: Clinical practice. Graves' disease. *N Engl J Med* 2008, **358**:2594-2605.
3. Rivkees SA, Sklar C, Freemark M: Clinical review 99: the management of Graves' disease in children, with special emphasis on radioiodine treatment. *J Clin Endocrinol Metab* 1998, **83**:3767-3775.
4. Franklyn JA: The management of hyperthyroidism. *N Engl J Med* 1994, **330**:1731-1738.
5. Levy WJ, Schumacher P, Gupta M: Treatment of childhood Graves' disease. A review with emphasis on radioiodine treatment. *Cleve Clin J Med* 1988, **55**:373-382.
6. Hamburger JI: Management of hyperthyroidism in children and adolescents. *J Clin Endocrinol Metab* 1985, **60**:1019-1024.
7. Lazar L, Kalter-Leibovici O, Pertzelan A, Weintrob N, Josefsberg Z, Phillip M: Thyrotoxicosis in prepubertal children compared with pubertal and postpubertal patients. *J Clin Endocrinol Metab* 2000, **85**:3678-3682.
8. Shulman DI, Muhar I, Jorgensen EV, Diamond FB, Bercu BB, Root AW: Autoimmune hyperthyroidism in prepubertal children and adolescents: comparison of clinical and biochemical features at diagnosis and responses to medical therapy. *Thyroid* 1997, **7**:755-760.
9. Spencer RP, Kayani N, Karimeddini MK: Radioiodine therapy of hyperthyroidism: socioeconomic considerations. *J Nucl Med* 1985, **26**:663-665.
10. Nygaard B, Hegedüs L, Gervil M, Hjalgrim H, Hansen BM, Søe-Jensen P, Hansen JM: Influence of compensated radioiodine therapy on thyroid volume and incidence of hypothyroidism in Graves' disease. *J Intern Med* 1995, **238**:491-497.
11. Chapman EM: History of the discovery and early use of radioactive iodine. *JAMA* 1983, **250**:2042-2044.
12. Ma C, Kuang A, Xie J, Liu GJ: Radioiodine treatment for pediatric Graves' disease (Review). *The Cochrane Library* 2009, , **3**: 1-31.
13. Read CH Jr, Tansey MJ, Menda Y: A thirty-six year retrospective analysis of the efficacy and safety of radioactive iodine in treating young Graves' patients. *J Clin Endocrinol Metab* 2004, **89**:4229-4233.
14. Foley TP Jr, Charron M: Radioiodine treatment of juvenile Graves' disease. *Exp Clin Endocrinol Diabetes* 1997, **4(Suppl 105)**:61-65.
15. Chao M, Jiawei X, Guoming W, Jianbin L, Wanxia L, Driedger A, Shuyao Z, Qin Z: Radioiodine treatment for pediatric hyperthyroid Grave's disease. *Eur J Pediatr* 2009, **168**:1165-1169.
16. Rivkees SA: Pediatric Graves' Disease: Controversies in Management. *Horm Res Paediatr* 2010, **74**:305-311.
17. Bahn Chair RS, Burch HB, Cooper DS, Garber JR, Greenlee MC, Klein I, Laurberg P, McDougall IR, Montori VM, Rivkees SA, Ross DS, Sosa JA, Stan MN: Hyperthyroidism and Other Causes of Thyrotoxicosis: Management Guidelines of the American Thyroid Association and American Association of Clinical Endocrinologists. *Thyroid* 2011, **21**:593-646.
18. Rivkees SA, Cornelius EA: Influence of iodine-131 dose on the outcome of hyperthyroidism in children. *Pediatrics* 2003, **111**:745-749.
19. Nebesio TD, Siddiqui AR, Pescovitz OH, Eugster EA: Time course to hypothyroidism after fixed-dose radioablation therapy of Graves' disease in children. *J Pediatr* 2002, **141**:99-103.
20. Rivkees SA, Dinauer C: Controversy in clinical endocrinology. An optimal treatment for pediatric Graves' disease is radioiodine. *J Clin Endocrinol Metab* 2007, **92**:797-800.
21. Ron E, Doody MM, Becker DV, Brill AB, Curtis RE, Goldman MB, Harris BS, Hoffman DA, McConahey WM, Maxon HR, Preston-Martin S, Warshauer ME, Wong FL, Boice JD Jr: Cancer mortality following treatment for adult hyperthyroidism. Cooperative Thyrotoxicosis Therapy Follow-up Study Group. *JAMA* 1998, **280**:347-355.
22. Dobyns BM, Sheline GE, Workman JB, Tompkins EA, McConahey WM, Becker DV: Malignant and benign neoplasms of the thyroid in patients treated for hyperthyroidism: a report of the Cooperative Thyrotoxicosis Therapy Follow-up Study. *J Clin Endocrinol Metab* 1974, **38**:976-998.
23. Peters H, Fischer C, Bogner U, Reiners C, Schleusener H: Reduction in thyroid volume after radioiodine therapy of Graves' hyperthyroidism: results of a prospective, randomized, multicentre study. *Eur J Clin Invest* 1996, **26**:59-63.

24. Murakami Y, Takamatsu J, Sakane S, Kuma K, Ohsawa N: **Changes in thyroid volume in response to radioactive iodine for Graves' hyperthyroidism correlated with activity of thyroid-stimulating antibody and treatment outcome.** *J Clin Endocrinol Metab* 1996, **81**:3257-3260.

25. Gómez-Arnaiz N, Andía E, Gumà A, Abós R, Soler J, Gómez JM: **Ultrasonographic thyroid volume as a reliable prognostic index of radioiodine-131 treatment outcome in Graves' disease hyperthyroidism.** *Horm Metab Res* 2003, **35**:492-497.

26. Chiovato L, Fiore E, Vitti P, Rocchi R, Rago T, Dokic D, Latrofa F, Mammoli C, Lippi F, Ceccarelli C, Pinchera A: **Outcome of thyroid function in Graves' patients treated with radioiodine: Role of thyroid-stimulating and thyrotropin-blocking antibodies and of radioiodine-induced thyroid damage.** *J Clin Endocrinol Metab* 1998, **83**:40-46.

27. Vemulakonda US, Atkins FB, Zissman HA: **Therapy dose calculation in Graves' disease using early I-123 uptake measurements.** *Clin Nucl Med* 1996, **21**:102-105.

28. Smith JJ, Croft BY, Brookeman VA, Teates CD: **Estimation of 24-hour thyroid uptake of I-131 sodium iodide using a 5-minute uptake of technetium-99m pertechnetate.** *Clin Nucl Med* 1990, **15**:80-83.

29. Tajiri J: **Radioactive iodine therapy for goitrous Hashimoto's thyroiditis.** *J Clin Endocrinol Metab* 2006, **91**:4497-4500.

FGF23 is correlated with iron status but not with inflammation and decreases after iron supplementation: a supplementation study

Vickie Braithwaite[1*], Andrew M Prentice[2,3], Conor Doherty[2,3] and Ann Prentice[1,3]

Abstract

Background: Recent studies have described relationships between iron status and fibroblast growth factor-23 (FGF23) but the possible confounding effects of inflammation on iron status have not been considered. The aims of this study were a) to consider a relationship between FGF23 and inflammation b) to identify relationships between iron status and FGF23 whilst correcting for inflammation and c) to assess the relationship between changes in FGF23 and iron status after supplementation.

Study design and methodology: Blood samples from an iron supplementation study in children ($n=79$) were collected at baseline and after 3 months supplementation with iron sulphate. The children were from a rural Gambian population where rates of iron deficiency and infection/inflammation are high. This study identified cross-sectional and longitudinal relationships between FGF23, inflammation (C-reactive protein (CRP)) and iron status (ferritin, haemoglobin, and zinc protoporphyrin). CRP $\geq$ 5 mg/dL was used to indicate inflammation and FGF23 $\geq$ 125 RU/mL was considered elevated.

Results: FGF23 was not significantly correlated with CRP. At baseline, all markers of iron status were significantly correlated with FGF23. Ferritin was the strongest independent inverse predictor of FGF23 in subjects with and without elevated CRP (coefficient (SE)): All subjects=-0.57 (0.12), R^2=22.3%, $P\leq0.0001$; subjects with CRP < 5 mg/dL=-0.89 (0.14), R^2=38.9%, $P\leq0.0001$. FGF23 was elevated in 28% of children at baseline and 16% post supplementation ($P=0.1$). Improved iron status was associated with a decrease in FGF23 concentration in univariate (ferritin =-0.41 (0.11), R^2=14.1%, $P=0.0004$; haemoglobin=-2.22 (0.64), R^2=12.5%, $P=0.0008$; zinc protoporphyrin=1.12 (0.26), R^2=18.6%, $P\leq0.0001$) and multivariate analysis (R^2=33.1%; ferritin=-0.36 (0.10), $P=0.0007$, haemoglobin = -1.83 (0.61), $P=0.004$, zinc protoporphyrin=0.62 (0.26), $P=0.02$).

Conclusions: Iron status rather than inflammation is a negative predictor of plasma FGF23 concentration. Improvements in iron status following iron supplementation are associated with a significant decrease in FGF23 concentration.

Keywords: Fibroblast growth factor-23, Iron status, Inflammation, Africa, Iron supplementation

Background

Fibroblast growth factor-23 (FGF23) is a bone derived, phosphate regulating hormone which is often elevated in genetic hypophosphataemic disorders [1] and in chronic kidney disease [2]. Recent studies have identified relationships between FGF23 and various markers of iron status. These include an inverse correlation between FGF23 and serum iron (Fe) [3,4], haemoglobin (Hb) [5], and ferritin (Ferr) [6]. However each of these markers of iron status is affected by the acute phase response and consequently they have limited use as markers of nutritional iron status when used in isolation from markers of inflammation [7]. It is plausible that the inverse correlation between markers of iron status and FGF23 [3-6] is the result of confounding by the inflammatory response. The potential role of the inflammatory response in FGF23 pathways has not yet been considered [8].

* Correspondence: Vickie.braithwaite@mrc-hnr.cam.ac.uk
[1]MRC Human Nutrition Research, Elsie Widdowson Laboratory, Cambridge CB1 9NL, United Kingdom
Full list of author information is available at the end of the article

The aims of this study were a) to consider a relationship between FGF23 and inflammation b) to identify relationships between iron and FGF23 whilst correcting for inflammation and c) to assess the change of FGF23 after supplementation with iron. The study used data from children in a rural Gambian population where dietary calcium intakes are low, rates of iron deficiency [9] and infection are high, and where a wide range of FGF23 concentrations have been reported [5].

Methods
Subjects and study information

A subset of samples (n=79) from a cohort of children (n=821) who participated in a non-controlled iron supplementation study designed to assess the variability of response to supplementation during the malaria season were included in this study. The children in the cohort were recruited from the local community in West Kiang, The Gambia and were aged between 0.5-7.0 y. Baseline measurements and start of supplementation were conducted in August 2004 and post supplementation measurements were conducted in December 2004 [10]. Subjects were given Fe 6x/week for three months in the form of Fe sulphate tablets (Nutriset, Malaunay, France). Daily consumption of the supplement was supervised by trained fieldworkers. The dose given was dependent on age and, if present, the severity of baseline anaemia (<7 g/dL): 25 mg elemental Fe in 76 subjects and 50 mg in 3 severely anaemic subjects. A blood sample and anthropometric data were collected at both time-points. All samples from subjects aged between 4.8–6.0 y with sufficient residual EDTA-plasma stored from samples at the beginning and end of supplementation (n=79, 47 female/32 male) were included in this study and analysed for plasma FGF23. The mean (SD) time from measurements at baseline to post supplementation was 118 (2) days.

Ethical statement

Ethical approval from The Gambian Government/MRC Laboratories Joint Ethics Committee for the original iron supplementation trial (n=821) and the subset study (n=79) was obtained. Written informed consent from the parents of the children involved were obtained for both the original iron supplementation trial and for any further analyses performed on stored samples.

Anthropometry

Weight was measured (kg) using a calibrated electronic scale (model HD-314, Tanita B.V., Hoofddorp, The Netherlands). Height was measured (cm) using a portable stadiometer (Leicester Height Measure, Seca GmbH & Co., Hamburg, Germany). Body mass index (BMI) was calculated (kg/m^2).

Fasting blood samples

In the original study an overnight fasting, venous blood sample had been collected into lithium-heparin (LiHep) and EDTA coated tubes. Fresh blood had been used to measure Hb by haemoglobinometer (Medonic CA, 530 Oden 16 Parameter System) and zinc protoporphyrin (ZnPP) by haematofluorimeter (Aviv Biomedical Lakewood, NJ). The remainder of the blood had been separated by centrifugation at 4°C and frozen at −70°C, and had been later transported frozen on dry ice to MRC Human Nutrition Research (HNR), Cambridge, UK where it had been stored at −80°C until analysis. Ferr and CRP had been measured in LiHep by Immunoassay (Abbot Laboratories, IL, USA and Dade Dimension®, respectively) [10]. For the purpose of this study, the residual, frozen EDTA samples were analysed for FGF23 using a 2nd generation C-terminal, two-site enzyme-linked immunosorbent assay (Immutopics Inc., Ca, USA). Assay accuracy and precision were monitored using kit controls supplied by the manufacturer.

Statistical analysis

All statistical analyses were performed using DataDesk 6.1 (Data Description Inc., NY, USA) with the exception of two-tailed Chi-square tests (without Yates' correction) which were performed using GraphPad QuickCalcs (GraphPad Software, Inc., CA, USA). Normally distributed data are presented as mean (1SD), positively skewed distributions of data are presented as geometric mean (−1SD, +1SD) obtained from the antilog of mean (−1SD, +1SD) of the logged values. Variables with positively skewed distributions were transformed to natural logarithms before further statistical analysis. Paired t-tests were used to assess the significance of change in anthropometric and biochemical variables from baseline and after supplementation.

A regression model was used with $\log_e$ FGF23 as the independent variable. Age was not significantly correlated with any of the biochemical variables and was therefore not adjusted for in the regression model. CRP $\geq$ 5 mg/dL was used to indicate the presence of inflammation [11] and an upper-limit of $\geq$ 125 RU/mL, as defined by the manufacturers, was used for FGF23. Subjects were defined as being anaemic according to WHO guidelines: Hb $\leq$ 11.0 g/dL for < 4.99 y, and $\leq$ 11.5 g/dL for 5–12 y [7,11]. Subjects with Ferr < 15 ng/mL were considered low [11]. Selectors for CRP < 5 and $\geq$ 5 mg/dL were used in regression analysis. Relative change (Δ) in variables (X) over time was calculated by: $\Delta X = \log_e X_{post} - \log_e X_{pre}$. Univariate analyses were conducted to determine the relationships between ΔFGF23 as the dependent variable, with Δ in Ferr, Hb and ZnPP in turn. Multivariate analysis was conducted to determine the relationship between ΔFGF23 as the dependent variable, and Δ in the three markers of iron status markers together and results are described as coefficient (SE).

Results

At baseline the mean age of the subjects was 5.5 (0.3) y, 28% had elevated FGF23, 87% were anaemic, 24% had low Ferr, and 13% had a CRP $\geq$ 5 mg/dL. After supplementation, the prevalence of elevated FGF23 was 16% (P=0.1), the prevalence of anaemia had decreased to 62% (P=0.0005), there were no subjects with low Ferr ($P\leq$0.0001) and the frequency of subjects with CRP $\geq$ 5 mg/dL did not significantly change (P=1.0).

After supplementation both Hb and Ferr had significantly increased from baseline (Hb (g/dL) from 10.3 (1.3) to 11.3 (1.0) $P\leq$0.0001; Ferr (ng/mL) from 26.6 (12.3, 57.6) to 46.9 (28.6, 76.9) $P\leq$0.0001). ZnPP (μmol/ mol haem) significantly decreased by the end of supplementation (from 61.9 (32.4, 118.3) to 24.7 (15.8, 38.5), $P\leq$0.0001). Mean FGF23 concentration had not significantly changed from baseline to after supplementation (from 96.0 (38.4, 240.4) to 82.8 (47.1, 145.7) RU/mL, P=0.1) (Table 1); although there was a wide range of changes observed (mean (−1SD, +1SD) change in FGF23 = 16.2 (4.6, 56.9) RU/mL).

There was no correlation between FGF23 and CRP at baseline (coefficient (SE)=-0.01 (0.11), R^2=-1.3%, P=0.9) or at the end of supplementation (0.11 (0.07), R^2=1.8%, P=0.1).

At baseline, FGF23 was significantly correlated with all markers of iron status. Ferr was the strongest, independent predictor of FGF23 in $\log_e$-$\log_e$ models (−0.57 (0.12), R^2=22.3%, $P\leq$0.0001). When excluding subjects with CRP $\geq$ 5 mg/dL, the relationship between FGF23 and

Ferr strengthened (−0.89 (0.14), R^2=38.9%, $P\leq$0.0001) (Figure 1).

The ΔFGF23 was significantly negatively correlated with Δ in markers of iron status in univariate (Ferr = - 0.41 (0.11), R^2=14.1%, P = 0.0004, Hb=−2.22 (0.64), R^2=12.5%, P = 0.0008 and ZnPP = 1.12 (0.26), R^2 = 18.6%, $P \leq$ 0.0001) analysis. In multivariate analysis, Δ in all three markers of iron status predicted R^2 = 33.1% of the variation of ΔFGF23 (Ferr = - 0.36 (0.10), P = 0.0007, Hb = −1.83 (0.61), P = 0.004, ZnPP = 0.62 (0.26), P = 0.02).

Discussion

This study has shown the existence of elevated FGF23, both before and at the end of iron supplementation (28% and 16% respectively) in apparently healthy, although generally undernourished children. This rate is in keeping with previous prevalence findings in Gambian children of similar age [5].

In this study, we have used a combination of iron status markers coupled with CRP, an acute phase marker [11], to provide further evidence of an inverse relationship between FGF23 and iron status.

In keeping with previous reports [9], ~90% of children in this study were anaemic at baseline. Overall Hb concentration increased after supplementation, although ~60% of children were still defined as anaemic [11]. Furthermore, after supplementation the concentration of the other markers of iron status, namely Ferr and ZnPP, changed sufficiently to indicate that the cohort had improved iron status.

Although CRP was not a significant predictor of FGF23, the association between FGF23 and Ferr was further strengthened when children with a raised CRP were removed from the regression model (R^2=38.9%, $P\leq$0.0001). All of the iron status markers were independently correlated with FGF23 at baseline and Ferr was the strongest predictor of FGF23 concentration (R^2=22.3%, $P\leq$0.0001). In addition the decrease in FGF23 concentration was significantly correlated with the improvement of all of iron status markers (both in univariate and multivariate analyses) during the period of iron supplementation. A point to note is that due to the wide range of FGF23 concentrations within subjects the decrease in mean FGF23 concentrations after supplementation compared with baseline was not statistically significant (P=0.1).

Although a causal relationship cannot be established, this study shows that FGF23 concentration decreased when iron status improved. This differs from a previous report which described an increase in FGF23 concentration in response of intravenous iron therapy in patients with iron deficiency anaemia and normal baseline FGF23 concentrations [12] but is in keeping with the observation that poor iron status was associated with

Table 1 Anthropometric and biochemical variables at baseline and after iron supplementation

Dependent Variable	Baseline $n= 79$	After supplementation $n= 79$	Paired t-test P-Value
Age (y)	5.48 (0.32)	5.81 (0.32)	-
Sex (F/M)	47/32	47/32	-
Height (cm)	105.6 (6.8)	107.7 (6.5)	$\leq$0.0001
Weight (kg)	15.6 (2.2)	16.3 (2.2)	$\leq$0.0001
BMI (kg/m^2)	13.9 (1.2)	14.0 (1.2)	0.2
ZnPP (μmol/ mol haem)*	61.9 (32.4, 118.3)	24.7 (15.8, 38.5)	$\leq$0.0001
Hb (g/dL)	10.3 (1.3)	11.3 (1.0)	$\leq$0.0001
Ferr (ng/mL)*	26.6 (12.3, 57.6)	46.9 (28.6, 76.9)	$\leq$0.0001
FGF23 (RU/mL)*	96.0 (38.4, 240.4)	82.8 (47.1, 145.7)	0.1
CRP (mg/dL)*	2.45 (1.00, 6.01)	1.99 (0.83, 4.78)	0.1

Data shown as mean (SD) or geometric mean (−1SD, +1SD) for skewed variables (*).

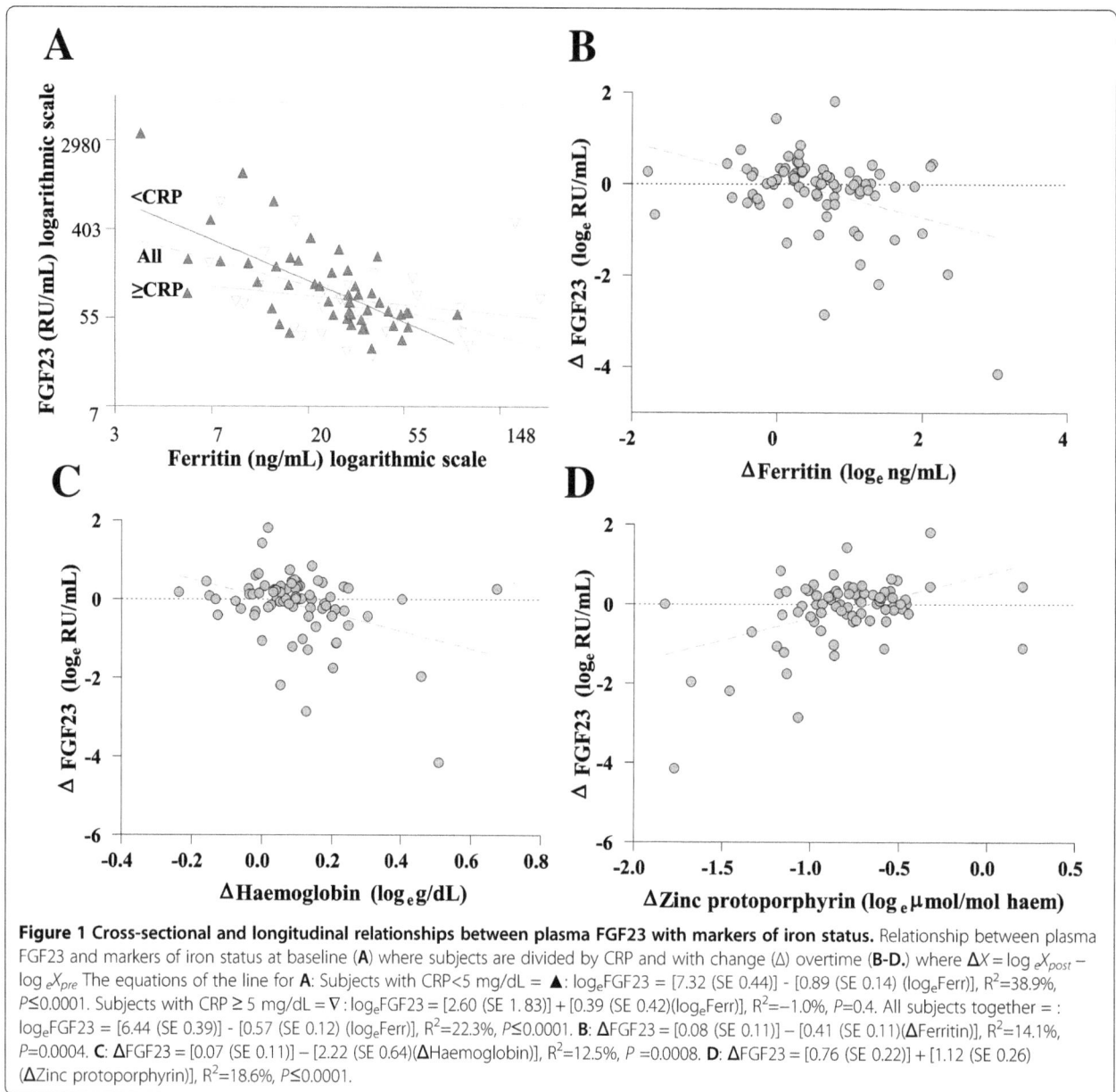

Figure 1 Cross-sectional and longitudinal relationships between plasma FGF23 with markers of iron status. Relationship between plasma FGF23 and markers of iron status at baseline (**A**) where subjects are divided by CRP and with change (Δ) overtime (**B-D.**) where $\Delta X = \log_e X_{post} - \log_e X_{pre}$ The equations of the line for **A**: Subjects with CRP<5 mg/dL = ▲: $\log_e FGF23 = [7.32 \text{ (SE 0.44)}] - [0.89 \text{ (SE 0.14)} (\log_e Ferr)]$, $R^2 = 38.9\%$, $P \leq 0.0001$. Subjects with CRP ≥ 5 mg/dL = ∇: $\log_e FGF23 = [2.60 \text{ (SE 1.83)}] + [0.39 \text{ (SE 0.42)}(\log_e Ferr)]$, $R^2 = -1.0\%$, $P = 0.4$. All subjects together = : $\log_e FGF23 = [6.44 \text{ (SE 0.39)}] - [0.57 \text{ (SE 0.12)} (\log_e Ferr)]$, $R^2 = 22.3\%$, $P \leq 0.0001$. **B**: $\Delta FGF23 = [0.08 \text{ (SE 0.11)}] - [0.41 \text{ (SE 0.11)}(\Delta Ferritin)]$, $R^2 = 14.1\%$, $P = 0.0004$. **C**: $\Delta FGF23 = [0.07 \text{ (SE 0.11)}] - [2.22 \text{ (SE 0.64)}(\Delta Haemoglobin)]$, $R^2 = 12.5\%$, $P = 0.0008$. **D**: $\Delta FGF23 = [0.76 \text{ (SE 0.22)}] + [1.12 \text{ (SE 0.26)} (\Delta Zinc protoporphyrin)]$, $R^2 = 18.6\%$, $P \leq 0.0001$.

higher C-FGF23 in Gambian children [5] and in British adults [6]. It has been suggested that low iron may result in an increased rate of proteolytic cleavage of the intact and biologically active hormone to inactive C- and N-terminal fragments. However, recent western-blotting analysis of plasma from Gambian children has not provided any evidence in support of this [13].

In light of this, the more plausible scenario is that iron is involved in the expression and/or secretion of FGF23 rather than having effects on the degradation pathway. This scenario could be further substantiated through the use of the intact FGF23 assay. Unfortunately, the intact FGF23 assay was not available for use in this study.

A limitation of this study is that there was no control group as all subjects were iron supplemented as part of the original study. Therefore, changes seen in FGF23 may not be attributable to the supplementation. Another limitation of this study is that only one marker of inflammation was measured and CRP is a marker of acute rather than chronic inflammation.

Conclusion

In conclusion this study has demonstrated that FGF23 concentration is not correlated with inflammation but is negatively correlated with markers of iron status. Furthermore an improvement in iron status, associated with

FGF23 is correlated with iron status but not with inflammation and decreases after iron...

111

iron supplementation in a population with endemic iron deficiency, is associated with a decrease in plasma FGF23.

Abbreviations

FGF23: Fibroblast growth factor-23; CRP: C-reactive protein; SE: Standard error; Hb: Haemoglobin; Ferr: Ferritin; EDTA: Ethylenediaminetetraacetic acid; Fe: Iron; BMI: Body mass index; ZnPP: Zinc protoporphyrin; MRC HNR: Medical Research Council Human Nutrition Research; LiHep: Lithium-heparin; SD: Standard deviation.

Competing interests

The authors have no competing interests to declare.

Authors' contributions

Study design: VB, AMP, CD, AP. Data analysis: VB, AMP, AP. Data interpretation: VB, AMP, AP. Drafting manuscript: VB, CD, AMP, AP. AP takes responsibility for the integrity of the data analysis. All authors read and approved the final manuscript.

Acknowledgments

The work was performed at MRC HNR, Cambridge, UK and MRC Keneba. The work was funded by Medical Research Council UK programme numbers U105960371, U123261351 and MC-A760-5QX00. We should like to thank the study participants; the clinical scientific, field staff and research assistants at MRC Keneba; the scientists and lab staff at MRC HNR, especially Miss Veronica Bell.

Author details

[1]MRC Human Nutrition Research, Elsie Widdowson Laboratory, Cambridge CB1 9NL, United Kingdom. [2]MRC International Nutrition Group, London School of Hygiene and Tropical Medicine, London WC1E 7HT, UK. [3]MRC Keneba, Keneba, West Kiang, The Gambia.

References

1. Yu X, White KE: **FGF23 and disorders of phosphate homeostasis.** *Cytokine Growth Factor Rev* 2005, **16**:221–232.
2. Harald J: **Phosphate and FGF23.** *Kidney Int* 2011, **79**:s24–s27.
3. Imel EA, Peacock M, Gray AK, Padgett LR, Hui SL, Econs MJ: **Iron modifies plasma FGF23 differently in autosomal dominant hypophosphatemic rickets and healthy humans.** *J Clin Endocrinol Metab* 2011, **96**(11):3541–3549.
4. Farrow EG, Yu X, Summers LJ, Davis SI, Fleet JC, Allen MR, Robling AG, Stayrook KR, Jideonwo V, Magers MJ, Garringer HJ, Vidal R, Chan RJ, Goodwin CB, Hui SL, Peacock M, White KE: **Iron deficiency drives an autosomal dominant hypophosphatemic rickets (adhr) phenotype in fibroblast growth factor-23 (FGF23) knock-in mice.** *Proc Natl Acad Sci USA* 2011, **108**:E1146–E1155.
5. Braithwaite V, Jarjou LMA, Goldberg GR, Prentice A: **Iron status and fibroblast growth factor-23 in gambian children.** *Bone* 2012, **50**:1351–1356.
6. Durham BH, Joseph F, Bailey LM, Fraser WD: **The association of circulating ferritin with serum concentrations of fibroblast growth factor-23 measured by three commercial assays.** *Ann Clin Biochem* 2007, **44**:463–466.
7. The Scientific Advisory Committee on Nutrition: *Iron and health United Kingdom.* London: The Stationary Office; 2010.
8. Prentice A, Braithwaite V, Schoenmakers I, Pettifor JM: **Serum iron, FGF23 and the acute phase response, Letter to the editor.** *JCEM* 2011, http://jcem.endojournals.org/content/96/11/3541/reply#jcem_el_90005.
9. Republic of the Gambia: *Nationwide survey on the prevalence of vitamin A and iron deficiency in women and children in the Gambia.* Banjul (The Gambia): The National Nutrition Agency (NaNA) and the Medical Research Council The Gambia; 2001.
10. Doherty CP, Cox SE, Fulford AJ, Austin S, Hilmers DC, Abrams SA, Prentice AM: **Iron incorporation and post-malaria anaemia.** *PLoS One* 2008, **3**:1–5.
11. World Health Organization, Centers for Disease Control and Prevention: *Assessing the iron status of populations.* Geneva: World Health Organization Department of Nutrition for Health and Development; 2007.
12. Schouten BJ, Hunt PJ, Livesey JH, Frampton CM, Soule SG: **FGF23 elevation and hypophosphatemia after intravenous iron polymaltose: a prospective study.** *J Clin Endocrinol Metab* 2009, **94**:2332–2337.
13. Braithwaite V, Bruggraber SF, Prentice A: **Intact fibroblast growth factor-23 and fragments in plasma from gambian children.** *Osteoporos Int* 2012, doi:10.1007/s00198-012-2029-3.

16

Differences in adjustment by child developmental stage among caregivers of children with disorders of sex development

Stephanie E Hullmann[1]*, David A Fedele[1], Cortney Wolfe-Christensen[2], Larry L Mullins[1] and Amy B Wisniewski[3]

Abstract

Background: The current study sought to compare levels of overprotection and parenting stress reported by caregivers of children with disorders of sex development at four different developmental stages.

Methods: Caregivers ($N = 59$) of children with disorders of sex development were recruited from specialty clinics and were asked to complete the Parent Protection Scale and Parenting Stress Index/Short Form as measures of overprotective behaviors and parenting stress, respectively.

Results: Analyses of covariance (ANCOVAs) were conducted to examine differences between caregiver report of overprotection and parenting stress. Results revealed that caregivers of infants and toddlers exhibited more overprotective behaviors than caregivers of children in the other age groups. Further, caregivers of adolescents experienced significantly more parenting stress than caregivers of school-age children, and this effect was driven by personal distress and problematic parent-child interactions, rather than having a difficult child.

Conclusions: These results suggest that caregivers of children with disorders of sex development may have different psychosocial needs based upon their child's developmental stage and based upon the disorder-related challenges that are most salient at that developmental stage.

Keywords: disorder of sex development, parenting stress, overprotection

Introduction

Disorders of sex development, or DSD, are a group of congenital medical conditions in which affected individuals experience discordance between their genetic, gonadal, and/or phenotypic sex [1]. Caring for a child with a chronic medical condition can be a significant stressor for parents such that they may experience guilt and uncertainty regarding their child's disease, treatment, and long-term prognosis [2]. Parents of children with DSD must make many decisions regarding the social, emotional, medical, and surgical management of their child's illness throughout the child's life, and these choices often vary depending on the age and developmental level of their child. For example, decisions about sex of rearing are typically made by caregivers of infants

and young toddlers [1], whereas judgments about whether or not to pursue gonadectomy or genital surgery for their child may persist into adolescence [1,3,4]. Throughout the child's life, caregivers must also make decisions regarding how much and with whom to share information regarding the child's diagnosis (e.g., family members, childcare workers, teachers, and their child). Furthermore, as children mature into puberty, caregivers may be faced with choices regarding hormone therapy to support development of their child's secondary sexual characteristics.

Child development is often conceptualized as a multifaceted process that occurs in four relatively distinct stages based largely upon physical and mental development and degree of independence from caregivers. These stages include infancy and toddlerhood, preschool age, school age, and adolescence [5]. During the first three years of life (i.e., infancy and toddlerhood), children experience rapid physical development, and it is during this time

* Correspondence: stephanie.hullmann@okstate.edu
[1]Department of Psychology, Oklahoma State University, Stillwater, Oklahoma, 74078, USA
Full list of author information is available at the end of the article

that gender identity is established [6,7]. Though children continue to grow during the preschool- and school-age stages, their rate of growth slows. During adolescence, individuals, once again, undergo drastic physical changes when the hypothalamic-pituitary-gonadal (HPG) axis is reactivated, and they experience puberty [5]. Adolescence is also a time when children ostensibly learn to exert their independence from their family and further develop their autonomy [5] by developing close peer relationships and beginning to enter into romantic and sexual relationships. The major role of the HPG axis during pre- and peri-natal development in boys, and in adolescence for both boys and girls, combined with the development of gender and sexuality at these ages, may make the challenge of caring for a child with a DSD particularly salient to parents at these developmental stages.

Parental overprotection and parenting stress are both *parenting capacity variables* [8] that involve discrete aspects of a caregiver's psychosocial adjustment. Both of these constructs have been conceptualized as measures of adjustment within the parent-child relationship [9,10]. Parental overprotection describes overt behaviors on the part of the parent to protect their child. Importantly, these behaviors are considered excessive for the child's current developmental level [11]. On the other hand, parenting stress is a measure of the parent's stress regarding their role as a parent and their relationship with their child [12]. Both of these caregiver adjustment variables are related to adjustment outcomes of children with chronic illnesses. Specifically, parental overprotection has been shown to be related to poorer quality of life and higher rates of behavior problems in children with chronic illnesses [13-15]. Similarly, higher levels of parenting stress are related to poorer emotional, behavioral, and social adjustment and worse physical health in children with chronic illnesses [16-18]. Notably, age differences have been observed in both rates of overprotective behaviors and parenting stress such that caregivers of younger children are more overprotective and experience more parenting stress than caregivers of older children [11,12]. To date, few studies have examined these parenting capacity variables in caregivers of children with DSD. Notably, recent research with this population suggests that caregivers of children with DSD experience similar levels of these parenting capacity variables as caregivers of children with Type 1 diabetes mellitus [19]. Additionally, parenting stress and overprotection are related to medical factors such as genitoplasty and age at genitoplasty in children with DSD [20].

To date, no studies have examined the differential effect of the child's developmental stage on adjustment in caregivers of children with DSD. It stands to reason that, given the specific needs of children with DSD at each developmental stage, caregiver adjustment would change as the child's needs change and as the child's illness characteristics become more or less salient to the family. Specifically, we hypothesized that caregivers of infants and toddlers and caregivers of adolescents would exhibit the most overprotective behaviors and experience greater parenting stress than caregivers of children at other developmental stages.

Methods

Participants

Participants for the current examination included 59 caregivers (66.1% female) of children (69.5% girls) between the ages of .5 and 17.83 years (M = 5.54, SD = 4.75). Children in the current study had been diagnosed with 46,XX DSD due to 21-hydroxylase deficiency or transposition of the SRY gene reared female (n = 37) or 46,XY DSD due to androgen biosynthetic defects, androgen insensitivity or unknown causes reared male or female (n = 22). At birth, each child was assigned a Prader score describing the appearance of their external genitalia prior to medical and/or surgical intervention. Prader scores for females in the sample ranged from 1 to 5 (M = 2.78, SD = 1.10), and the scores ranged from 2 to 5 (M = 3.50, SD = .79) for males.

The caregivers in the sample were 19 to 47 years old (M = 34.24, SD = 7.16), and the majority of caregivers reported being married (63.8%). Additionally, 22.8% of the respondents reported an annual household income less than $20,000, 14% reported an income between $20,000 and $40,000, 24.6% reported an income between $40,000 and $60,000, and 38.6% reported an income over $60,000. With regard to race and ethnicity, the majority of participants self-identified as Caucasian (74.1%), 10.3% self-identified as African American, 5.2% as Native American, 5.2% as Hispanic, 3.4% as Asian American, and 1.7% as "other".

Measures

The caregiver participants completed the following questionnaires as part of a larger study of psychosocial adjustment in caregivers of children with DSD. As such, part of this dataset was utilized in our earlier research [19,20].

Demographic Questionnaire

Parent participants completed a demographic questionnaire to provide information regarding their age, race, and marital status, their child's age, and their household income.

Parent Protection Scale

Parental overprotection was assessed using the Parent Protection Scale (PPS) [11]. The PPS, a 25-item, self-report measure, examines several dimensions of overprotective parenting behaviors. Caregivers are asked to rate the extent to which each statement is descriptive of their behavior with their child on a four-point scale ranging from *never* to *always*. A higher total score indicates a higher level of protective parenting behaviors. A score one standard deviation above the sample mean indicates clinically significant levels of overprotection [21]. Normative studies examining the PPS have demonstrated adequate internal reliability (.73) and moderate test-retest reliability (.86) [11]. The PPS has been utilized to measure protective parenting behaviors in a several different pediatric populations [17,22]. The internal reliability coefficient for the current sample was adequate (.71).

Parenting Stress Index/Short Form

The amount of stress present in the caregiver-child relationship was assessed using the Parenting Stress Index/ Short Form (PSI/SF) [12]. The PSI/SF is a 36-item instrument that asks caregivers to rate the extent to which each statement is descriptive of their relationship with their child on a five-point scale ranging from *strongly agree* to *strongly disagree*. The PSI/SF yields a total parenting stress score as well as three subscale scores (i.e., stress attributable to the caregiver's personal distress, distress related to the child, and relational distress between the caregiver and child). Higher scores on all scales indicate higher levels of parenting stress. A total score of 90 or greater indicates clinically significant parenting stress. The PSI/SF is highly correlated with the full-length PSI instrument ($r = .94$), and the two-week test-retest reliability of the PSI with the PSI/SF is also very high (.95) [12]. The validity of the PSI and PSI/SF has been established in a range of populations, including parents of children with chronic illnesses [17,22-24]. The internal consistency for the current sample was excellent (.95).

Procedure

Caregivers were invited to participate in the current study if they had a child who had been diagnosed with some type of 46,XX or 46,XY DSD. The study was IRB approved and all aspects of the projects were conducted in compliance with the APA ethical guidelines for research. For inclusion in the study, caregivers must have been at least 18 years old, able to provide informed consent, and able to read English at an 8th grade reading level. All caregivers of these children were invited to participate; however, only data from one caregiver participant per child was used for the current study. For those families in which multiple caregivers participated ($n = 33$), one caregiver was randomly selected to be included in the analyses. Caregivers were recruited from their DSD specialty clinic at the University of Oklahoma Children's Hospital, Johns Hopkins Hospital, and the Women's and Children's Hospital of Buffalo. Additionally, caregivers of children with DSD receiving treatment at other hospitals who contacted the senior author regarding participation were included in the study.

All caregivers provided informed consent, and the study questionnaires were subsequently mailed to them for completion. Upon receipt of the study questionnaires, all caregivers were compensated with a $25 gift card to thank them for their participation. Three caregivers, one whose child has an XX, DSD and two whose children have an XY, DSD, declined participation, yielding a consent and completion rate of 97% for all caregivers approached to participate.

Overview of Analyses

To determine whether levels of parental overprotection and parenting stress differed by a child's developmental level, an analysis of covariance (ANCOVA) was conducted, controlling for child and caregiver sex. Developmental level was divided into four categories based upon previously published guidelines [5]: 1) infants and toddlers (0 - 2 year-olds, $n = 20$), 2) preschool-age children (3 - 6 year-olds, $n = 21$), 3) school-age children (7 - 11 year-olds, $n = 10$), and 4) adolescents (12 - 18 year-olds, $n = 8$). Planned post-hoc comparisons using a Bonferroni alpha adjustment were conducted in order to examine pairwise differences among the marginal means while controlling for Type I error. The assumptions of homogeneity of regression slopes and variances were tenable for all analyses. Partial η^2 was used for an effect size estimate because it estimates the factor of interest while controlling for covariates.

Results

Preliminary Analyses

The sample was first examined to determine the percentage of caregivers meeting criteria for clinically significant levels of parenting stress and overprotective behaviors. In accordance with the authors' recommendations, a cutoff score of 90 on the PSI/SF [12] and 41 on the PPS (i.e., one standard deviation above the sample mean) [21] were utilized to identify clinically significant reports of parenting stress and overprotection, respectively. Please see Table 1 for clinical cutoff information by developmental level.

Caregiver Overprotection

Analyses demonstrated a significant main effect for developmental level, $F(3,50) = 11.94$, $p <, 001$, $\eta_p^2 = .42$. Planned post-hoc comparisons revealed that, on average, caregivers of infants and toddlers ($M = 40.64$, $SEM = 1.61$, 95% CI [37.42, 43.87]) evidenced significantly higher levels of parental overprotection than caregivers of preschool-age children ($M = 32.00$, $SEM = 1.44$, 95% CI [29.11, 34.89], $p = .001$), school-age children ($M = 27.14$, $SEM = 2.10$, 95% CI [22.93, 31.35], $p < .001$), or adolescents ($M = 27.46$, $SEM = 2.37$, 95% CI [22.71, 32.21], $p < .001$). There were no other significant

Table 1 Clinical Cut-off Percentages by Developmental Level

Variable	Overall M(SD)	Ages 0-2	Ages 3-6	Ages 7-11	Ages 12-18
Parental Overprotection	33.12(8.29)	58.80%	4.80%	0.00%	0.00%
Parenting Stress	72.68(21.69)	15.00%	23.80%	0.00%	37.5%

Note. Clinical cut-offs were ≥ 41 for Parental Overprotection and ≥ 90 for Parenting Stress.

differences in parental overprotection between any of the other developmental levels (see Figure 1).

Caregiver Stress

Results revealed a significant main effect for developmental level, $F(3,53) = 3.30$, $p = .027$, $\eta_p^2 = .16$. Planned post-hoc comparisons showed that, on average, caregivers of adolescents ($M = 89.89$, $SEM = 7.34$, 95% CI [75.17, 104.61]) reported significantly higher levels of stress than caregivers of school-age children ($M = 60.89$, $SEM = 6.50$, 95% CI [47.85, 73.93], $p = .028$]. There were no other significant differences in parenting stress between any of the other developmental levels (see Figure 2).

Exploratory Analyses

Exploratory analyses sought to examine the subscales of the PSI/SF by the developmental levels. For the personal distress subscale, results revealed a significant main effect for developmental level, $F(3,59) = 3.31$, $p = .036$, $\eta_p^2 = .148$. Planned post-hoc comparisons showed that, on average, caregivers of adolescents ($M = 33.105$, $SEM = 2.714$, 95% CI [27.662, 38.548]) reported significantly higher levels of personal distress than caregivers of

infants and toddlers ($M = 26.348$, $SEM = 1.696$, 95% CI [22.947, 29.749], $p = .041$) and caregivers of school-age children ($M = 22.207$, $SEM = 2.404$, 95% CI [17.385, 27.028], $p = .004$). There were no other significant differences in caregiver personal distress between any of the other developmental levels. For the caregiver-child dysfunctional interaction subscale, results revealed a significant main effect for developmental level, $F(3,59) = 3.291$, $p = .028$, $\eta_p^2 = .157$. Planned post-hoc comparisons revealed that, on average, caregivers of adolescents ($M = 26.50$, $SEM = 2.63$, 95% CI [21.23, 31.77]) reported significantly higher levels of caregiver-child dysfunctional interactions than caregivers of infants and toddlers ($M = 18.40$, $SEM = 1.64$, 95% CI [15.11, 21.69], $p = .012$), caregivers of preschool-age children ($M = 19.13$, $SEM = 1.60$, 95% CI [15.91, 22.34], $p = .021$), and caregivers of school-age children ($M = 15.94$, $SEM = 2.33$, 95% CI [11.27, 20.61], $p = .004$). There were no other significant differences in caregiver-child dysfunctional interaction between any of the other developmental levels. For the difficult child subscale, the main effect for developmental level was found to be nonsignficant, $p > .05$.

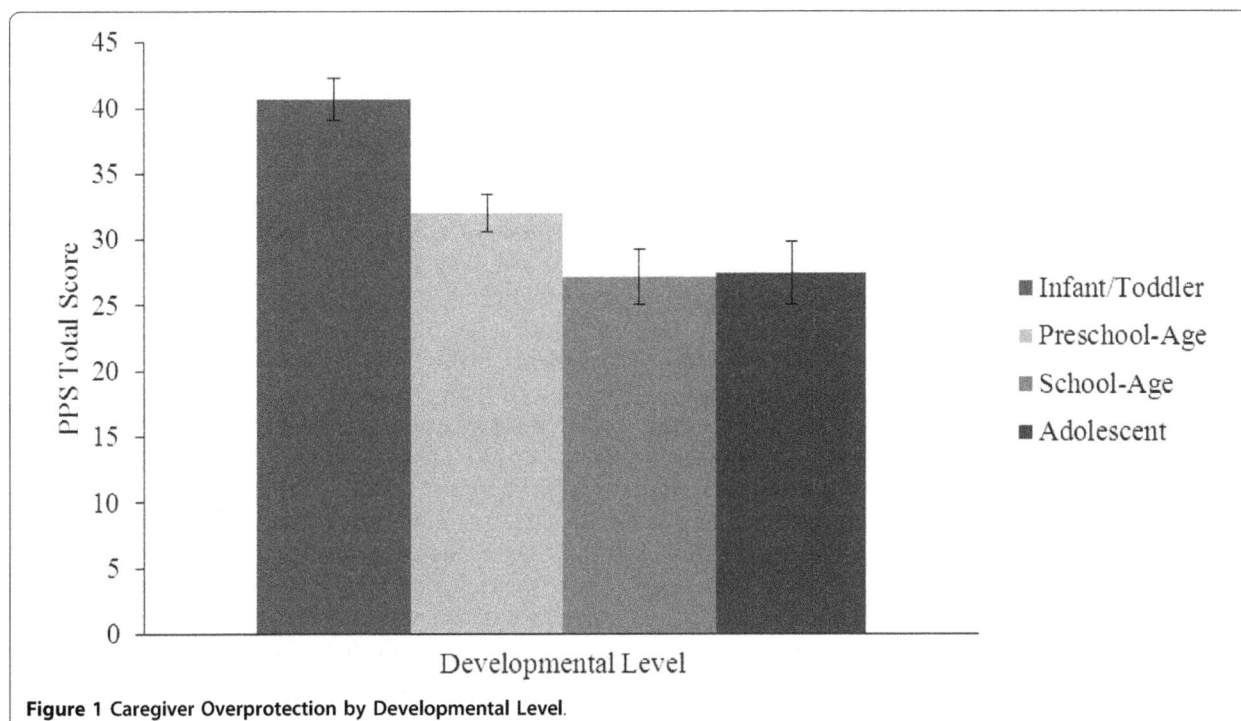

Figure 1 Caregiver Overprotection by Developmental Level.

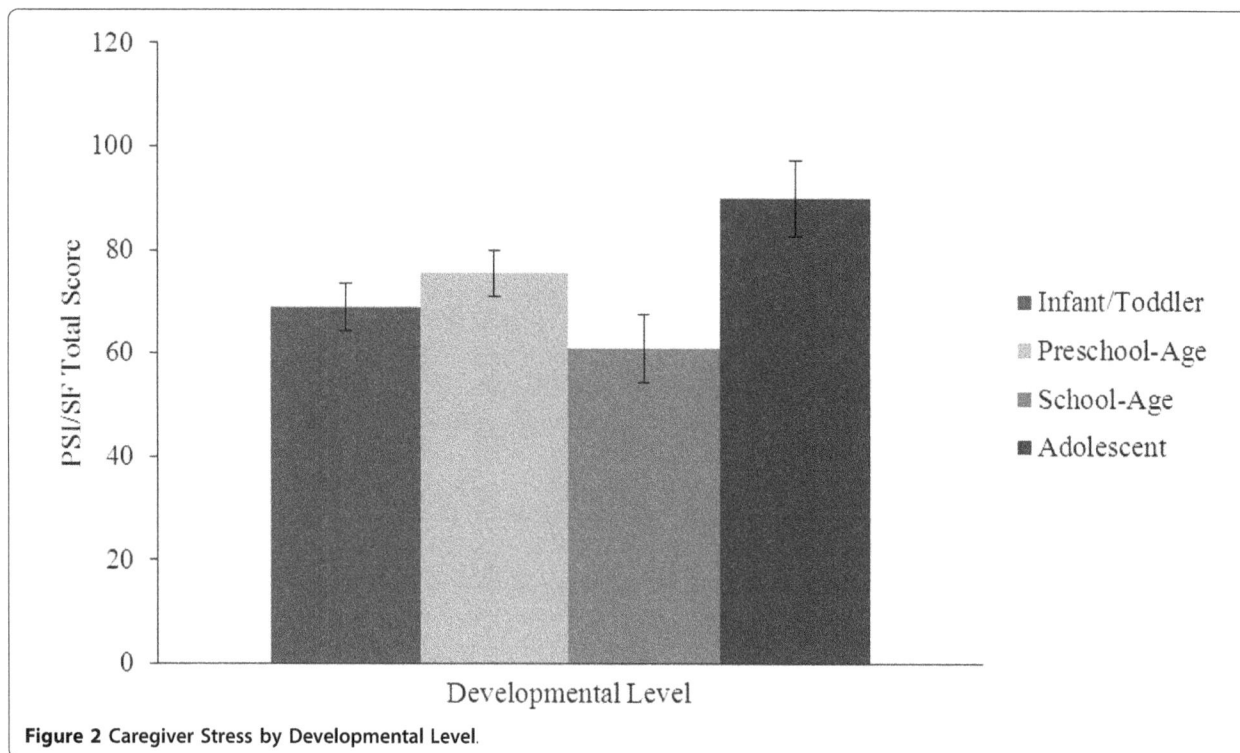

Figure 2 Caregiver Stress by Developmental Level.

Discussion

The current study sought to examine differences in levels of parental overprotection and parenting stress in caregivers of children with DSD across four developmental stages. Specifically, it was hypothesized that caregivers of infants and toddlers and caregivers of adolescents would exhibit the greatest rates of overprotective behaviors and parenting stress. The results partially supported this hypothesis in that caregivers of infants and toddlers were found to exhibit significantly more overprotective behaviors than caregivers of children in the other age groups. Caregivers of adolescents were not found to exhibit higher rates of overprotective behavior than the other groups. These results are consistent with the extant literature on parental overprotection, which states that caregivers of younger children exhibit more overprotective behavior than caregivers of older children [11]. In other words, developmental theory suggests that as children mature, they are expected to become more independent and autonomous [25]. As children grow more autonomous, caregivers may also have more opportunities to observe their child's resiliency, perhaps reducing the perceived benefits of their protective behavior. In this regard, caregivers of children with DSD do not differ from caregivers of children with other chronic illnesses in their ratings of parental overprotection.

Although speculative, it is possible that parental overprotection impacts decisions regarding their child's early medical care in a manner that is specific to DSD. For example, surgery to "normalize" ambiguous genitalia may be chosen for young children with DSD, in part, because this is when some surgeons recommend such procedures [4] but also because caregivers believe that early surgery will spare their child from future problems. In other words, caregivers may see surgery as a way to protect their child and to exert control over their child's long-term medical prognosis and psychosocial adjustment. This speculation is testable and should be studied further.

The results regarding parenting stress also partially supported our hypothesis. Caregivers of adolescents experienced significantly higher rates of parenting stress than those of school-age children, but caregivers of infants and toddlers did not experience more stress than the other groups. Upon examination of the parenting stress subscales, caregivers of adolescents were found to experience higher rates of personal distress and distress related to their interaction with their child than the other groups, but no differences were observed between the groups on the difficult child subscale. These results suggest that much of the stress caregivers of adolescents with DSD are experiencing is not due to their child exhibiting particularly challenging behaviors, but it is due to their own personal distress (e.g., *I feel trapped by my responsibilities as parent*) and challenging interactions with their child (e.g., *Most times I feel that my child does not like me and does not want to be close to me*).

These results argue against the notion that caregivers are reacting negatively to their child's gender or sexuality. Rather, their stress may originate from personal maladjustment (e.g., depressive symptoms) and perhaps their own perceived difficulties in parenting their child. Again, we can speculate about DSD-specific scenarios that may increase caregiver distress in this way. For example, caregivers of older children may be faced with educating their child about their medical history, fertility, and long-term prognosis, and perhaps, they feel unprepared to do so. Challenging caregiver-child interactions may also be a result of negative feelings experienced by caregivers and fear of disclosing information to adolescents regarding their illness. There may be tension in their interactions because the adolescents sense that their caregivers are withholding information. By comparing parenting stress levels among caregivers who have educated their child prior to adolescence with caregivers who have not done so, this possibility could be tested. Another important study would be to compare caregivers who take advantage of DSD support groups to those who do not in order to determine if such activities increase their confidence in speaking candidly with and caring for an adolescent with a DSD.

Certainly, the current study has a number of limitations, including its cross-sectional design, exclusive use of self-report methodology, and relatively small sample size. Further, the study examined caregivers of children with several different medical conditions which fall under the umbrella of DSD. In addition, the lack of a control group precludes any conclusions that can be drawn concerning the uniqueness of this finding to caregivers of children with a DSD, though the extant literature would suggest that the finding regarding parenting stress in adolescents is unique [12]. Notwithstanding these limitations, this study is the first to address possible differences in caregiver adjustment to DSD as a function of developmental level of the child.

Overall, the current results suggest that caregivers of children with DSD experience different parenting challenges across their child's development. Understanding the unique challenges faced by caregivers of children with DSD relative to their child's developmental stage in the context of gender development will help to inform the development of optimal resources and support services for these caregivers and their families. In regard to clinical implications, when children are very young, caregivers may benefit from education regarding their child's diagnosis and developmentally appropriate expectations of their child. They may also benefit from support groups and mental health services targeted at normalizing their experience to decrease their need to shelter and protect their children. When children reach adolescence, caregivers may benefit from interventions targeted at their

own distress as a parent, but perhaps more importantly, interventions designed to enhance communication between adolescents with DSD and their caregivers are warranted. This will help to resolve dysfunctional interactions between caregivers and adolescents and facilitate open communication regarding the child's diagnosis, fertility, and long-term prognosis.

Acknowledgements
This research was supported by the Study Network of Pediatric Endocrinologists (SNoPE) of the Lawson Wilkins Pediatric Endocrine Society, the Presbyterian Health Foundation (PHF) of Oklahoma, and Sigma Theta Tau International Honor Society of Nursing. The authors wish to thank the caregivers who participated in this study.

Author details
[1]Department of Psychology, Oklahoma State University, Stillwater, Oklahoma, 74078, USA. [2]Department of Pediatric Urology, Children's Hospital of Michigan, Detroit, Michigan, 48201, USA. [3]Department of Urology, University of Oklahoma Health Sciences Center, Oklahoma City, Oklahoma, 73104, USA.

Authors' contributions
SH conceived of the study, performed statistical analyses, and drafted the manuscript. DF performed statistical analyses and drafted the manuscript. CW collected the data and revised the manuscript. LM participated in the design and coordination of the study and revised the manuscript. AW participated in the design and coordination of the study and drafted the manuscript. All authors read and approved the final manuscript.

Competing interests
The authors declare that they have no competing interests.

References
1. Hughes IA, Houk C, Ahmed SF: Consensus statement on management of intersex disorders. *Arch Dis Child* 2006, **91**:554-563.
2. van Dongen-Melman JE, Pruyn JF, de Groot A, Koot HM, Hahlen K, Verhulst FC: Late psychosocial consequences for parents of children who survived cancer. *J Pediatr Psychol* 1995, **20**:567-586.
3. Speiser PW, Azziz R, Baskin LS: A summary of the Endocrine Society clinical practice guidelines on congenital adrenal hyperplasia due to steroid 21-hydroxylase deficiency. *Intl J Pediatr Endocrinol* 2010.
4. Vidal I, Brindusa Gorduza D, Haraux E: Surgical options in disorders of sex development (DSD) with ambiguous genitalia. *Best Pract Res Cl En* 2010, **24**:311-324.
5. Bogin B: *Patterns of human growth.* 2 edition. Cambridge: Cambridge University Press; 1999.
6. Money J, Ehrhardt AA: Gender identity differentiation. *Man and woman, boy and girl* Baltimore, MD: The Johns Hopkins Press; 1972, 146-175.
7. Green R: Gender identity disorders. In *Kaplan & Sadock's Comprehensive Textbook of Psychiatry. Volume 1..* 8 edition. Edited by: Sadock BJ, Sadock VA. Philadelphia, PA: Lippincott Williams 2005:1979-1990.
8. National Institutes of Health (NIH) 2006 PA-06-97: *Parenting capacities and health outcomes in youths and adolescents (R21)* [http://grants.nih.gov/grants/guide/pa-files/PA-06-097.html].
9. Sameroff AJ, Emde RN: Relationship disturbances in early childhood: a developmental approach. New York, NY: Basic Books, Inc; 1992.
10. Deater-Deckard K: *Parenting stress* New Haven: Yale University Press; 2004.
11. Thomasgard M, Metz WP, Edelbrock C, Shonkoff JP: Parent-child relationship disorders. Part I. Parental overprotection and the development of the Parent Protection Scale. *J Dev Behav Pediatr* 1995, **16**:244-250.
12. Abidin RR: *Parenting Stress Index* Odessa, FL: Psychological Assessment Resources; 1990.
13. Hullmann SE, Wolfe-Christensen C, Meyer WH, McNall-Knapp RY, Mullins LL: **The relationship between parental overprotection and health-related**

quality of life in pediatric cancer: the mediating role of perceived child vulnerability. *Qual Life Res* 2010, **19**:1373-1380.

14. Cappelli M, McGrath PJ, MacDonald NE: **Parental care and overprotection of children with cystic fibrosis.** *Br J Med Psychol* 1989, **62**:281-289.

15. Holmbeck GN, Johnson SZ, Wills KE, McKernon W, Rose B, Erklin S, Kemper T: **Observed and perceived parental overprotection in relation to psychosocial adjustment in preadolescents with a physical disability: the mediational role of behavioral autonomy.** *J Consult Clin Psych* 2002, **70**:96-110.

16. Colletti CJM, Wolfe-Christensen C, Carpentier MY, Page MC, McNall-Knapp RY, Meyer WH, Chaney JM, Mullins LL: **The relationship of parental overprotection, perceived vulnerability, and parenting stress to behavioral, emotional, and social adjustment in children with cancer.** *Pediatr Blood Cancer* 2008, **51**:269-274.

17. Mullins LL, Fuemmeler BF, Hoff A, Chaney JM, Van Pelt J, Ewing CA: **The relationship of parental overprotection and perceived child vulnerability to depressive symptomatology in children with type 1 diabetes mellitus: the moderating influence of parenting stress.** *Child Health Care* 2004, **33**:21-34.

18. Patterson JM, Budd J, Goetz D, Warwick WJ: **Family correlates of 10-year pulmonary health trends in cystic fibrosis.** *J Pediatr* 1993, **91**:383-389.

19. Kirk K, Fedele DA, Wolfe-Christensen C, Phillips TM, Mazur T, Mullins LL, Chernausek SD, Wisniewski AB: **Parenting characteristics of female caregivers of children affected by chronic endocrine conditions: a comparison between disorders of sex development and type 1 diabetes mellitus.** *J Pediatr Nurs* .

20. Fedele DA, Kirk K, Wolfe-Christensen C, Phillips TM, Mazur T, Mullins LL, Chernausek SD, Wisniewski AB: **Primary caregivers of children affected by disorders of sex development (DSD): mental health and caregiver characteristics in the context of genital ambiguity and genitoplasty.** *Int J Pediatr Endocrinol* 2010.

21. Thomasgard M, Metz WP: **Parental overprotection and its relation to perceived child vulnerability.** *Am J Orthopsychiatry* 1997, **67**:330-335.

22. Hullmann SE, Wolfe-Christensen C, Ryan J, Fedele DA, Rambo PL, Chaney JM, Mullins LL: **Parental overprotection, perceived child vulnerability, and parenting stress: a cross-illness comparison.** *J Clin Psychol Med S* 2010, **17**:357-365.

23. Carson DK, Schauer RW: **Mothers of children with asthma: perceptions of parenting stress and the mother-child relationship.** *Psychol Rep* 1992, **71**:1139-1148.

24. Wysocki T, Huxtable K, Linscheid TR, Wayne W: **Adjustment to diabetes mellitus in preschoolers and their mothers.** *Diabetes Care* 1989, **12**:524-529.

25. Williams PG, Holmbeck GN, Neff-Greenley R: **Adolescent health psychology.** *J Consult Clin Psych* 2002, **70**:828-842.

17

Proteomic analysis allows for early detection of potential markers of metabolic impairment in very young obese children

Gabriel Á Martos-Moreno[1,2,3], Lucila Sackmann-Sala[1,4,5], Vicente Barrios[2,3], Darlene E Berrymann[1], Shigeru Okada[1,6], Jesús Argente[2,3]* and John J Kopchick[1,5,6]*

Abstract

Background: Early diagnosis of initial metabolic derangements in young obese children could influence their management; however, this impairment is frequently not overt, but subtle and undetectable by routinely used clinical assays. Our aim was to evaluate the ability of serum proteomic analysis to detect these incipient metabolic alterations in comparison to standard clinical methods and to identify new candidate biomarkers.

Methods: A cross-sectional study of fasting serum samples from twenty-two prepubertal, Caucasian obese (**OB**; 9.22 ± 1.93 years; 3.43 ± 1.08 BMI-SDS) and twenty-one lean controls (**C**; 8.50 ± 1.98 years; -0.48 ± 0.81 BMI-SDS) and a prospective study of fasting serum samples from twenty prepubertal, Caucasian obese children (11 insulin resistant [**IR**]) before (4.77 ± 1.30 BMI-SDS) and after weight reduction (2.57 ± 1.29 BMI-SDS) by conservative treatment in a reference hospital (**Pros-OB**) was performed. Proteomic analysis (two-dimension-eletrophoresis + mass spectrometry analysis) of serum and comparative evaluation of the sensitivity of routinely used assays in the clinics to detect the observed differences in protein expression level, as well as their relationship with anthropometric features, insulin resistance indexes, lipid profile and adipokine levels were carried out.

Results: Study of the intensity data from proteomic analysis showed a decrease of several isoforms of apolipoprotein-A1, apo-J/clusterin, vitamin D binding protein, transthyretin in **OB** *vs.* **C**, with some changes in these proteins being enhanced by **IR** and partially reversed after weight loss. Expression of low molecular weight isoforms of haptoglobin was increased in **OB**, enhanced in **IR** and again decreased after weight loss, being positively correlated with serum interleukin-6 and NAMPT/visfatin levels. After statistical correction for multiple comparisons, significance remained for a single isoform of low MW haptoglobin (OB vs. C and IR vs. non-IR) and Apo A1 (IR vs. non-IR). Assays routinely used in the clinical setting (ELISA/kinetic nephelometry), only partially confirmed the changes observed by proteomic analysis (ApoA1 and haptoglobin).

Conclusion: Proteomic analysis can allow for the identification of potential new candidate biomarkers as a complement to routinely used assays to detect initial changes in serum markers of inflammation and lipid metabolism impairment in young obese children.

Keywords: Proteomic, Two dimension electrophoresis, Childhood obesity, Insulin resistance

* Correspondence: argentefen@terra.com; kopchick@ohio.edu
[2]Hospital Infantil Universitario Niño Jesús, Department of Endocrinology, Instituto de Investigación la Princesa, Universidad Autónoma de Madrid, Department of Pediatrics, Av. Menéndez Pelayo, 65, E-28009 Madrid, Spain
[1]Edison Biotechnology Institute, Ohio University, Konneker Research Laboratories, 1 Water Tower Drive, The Ridges, 45701 Athens, Ohio, USA
Full list of author information is available at the end of the article

Background

Early-onset obesity is a definite risk factor for adult obesity, its associated comorbidities and reduced life expectancy [1,2]. Most of the metabolic comorbidities overtly observed in obese adults are usually subtle or even undetectable in most young (prepubertal) obese children when the currently available biomarkers, including the growing number of adipokines, are used. Adipokines play a preeminent role in carbohydrate metabolism, the derangement of which is the most important metabolic comorbidity of obesity, which can ultimately lead to type 2 diabetes mellitus ([T2DM] [3,4]). Impaired adipokine synthesis and secretion, which can be detected even in young obese children, contributes to the generation of insulin resistance (IR) in a dual fashion. Obesity induces changes in serum levels of insulin sensitizing adipokines [4-7] and also generates a generalized proinflammatory environment by increasing the circulating levels of resistin, interleukin 6 (IL-6) and tumoral necrosis factor alpha (TNF-α) [6,8]. However, these changes in circulating adipokines related with carbohydrate metabolism have not been shown to be of value for the detection of early stages of homeostatic derangement in young obese children. Hence, there is a lack of sensitive markers for the initial stages of carbohydrate metabolism impairment in childhood obesity. A similar situation is observed with regard to the obesity related impairment of lipid metabolism, mainly represented by the decrease in high density lipoprotein (HDL) levels in this age range and definitely influenced by the existence of IR.

Consequently, analysis of the serum proteome of young children in different weight-related conditions (normal, excess and later reduction), with or without IR, could be useful for the detection of new more sensitive diagnostic biomarkers. An advantageous tool for the study of the circulating proteome in serum under different conditions is the use of two dimension electrophoresis (2DE). This technique allows for the isolation and identification of proteins in a given sample and has previously been applied to human serum samples for different purposes, with a limited amount (below 0.5 ml) of serum needed to identify up to 300 protein spots [9-12]. Therefore, the aims of this study were: 1) To investigate the influence of obesity and weight loss on the serum proteomic profile of young prepubertal obese children. 2) To evaluate the differences in the serum proteome between young obese children according to the presence or lack of estimated IR and 3) To identify new candidate biomarkers of early metabolic impairment in young obese children.

Subjects and methods

Subjects

Three groups of children were enrolled for this study: obese patients (**OB**), controls (**C**) and a second cohort of prospectively followed obese patients (**Pros-OB**).

Obese patients (OB)

This group was made up of twenty-two prepubertal (Tanner stage I) obese (BMI > +2 SDS according to Spanish standards [13]) Caucasian children (13 males / 9 females). Their mean age at recruitment was 9.22 ± 1.93 years (range 5.53-12.89) and their mean BMI 3.43 ± 1.08 SDS. Samples from these patients were obtained exclusively at the time of enrollment in the study.

Control group (C)

This group was made up of twenty-one prepubertal (Tanner stage I) lean (BMI between -1.5 and + 1.5 SDS according to Spanish standards [13]) Caucasian children (16 boys/ 4 girls). Their mean age at recruitment was 8.50 ± 1.98 years (range 5.64-11.95) and their mean BMI -0.48 ± 0.81 SDS. These children were referred to our department but found to be healthy, with no pathological auxological, clinical or analytical findings. Samples from controls were obtained exclusively at the time of enrollment in the study.

Prospectively followed obese patients (Pros-OB)

A subgroup of a larger cohort of obese patients that were prospectively followed for 18 months in an intensive program of behavioural modification [6] was used in these studies. It was made up of twenty children, all of whom had achieved extensive BMI reduction (over 2 SDS regarding their BMI at enrollment) during the first 12 months of follow-up. All of them were prepubertal (Tanner stage I), obese (BMI > +2 SDS according to Spanish [13]) and Caucasian (16 boys/ 4 girls). Their mean age at recruitment was 8.64 ± 1.56 years (range 5.44-11.70) and serum samples were obtained at two different time-points: at diagnosis (**D**, mean BMI 4.77 ± 1.30 SDS) and after reducing their BMI by over 2 SDS (weight loss [**WL**], mean BMI 2.57 ± 1.29 SDS). These patients underwent an oral glucose tolerance test at D (OGTT, 1.75g/kg, maximum 75g) to estimate their degree of IR. Body composition analyses were performed by DXA (Hologic QDR4500W) at time-points D and WL, confirming that the observed weight loss was due exclusively to body fat mass reduction, without bone density or lean mass impairment [6]. Blood samples were obtained at both time-points (D and WL).

All samples were obtained after overnight fasting. Those samples from children in groups OB and C were centrifuged and serum stored at −80°C until preparation for proteomic analysis. The samples from the patients in the Pros-OB, both at D and at WL, underwent a lyophylization process for better preservation after collection and were reconstituted immediately before preparation for proteomic analysis.

All patients and controls and their parents or guardians gave informed consent as required by the local ethics committee, which had previously approved the study. The study was also approved by the Ohio University Institutional Review Board.

Biochemical measurements

Serum lipid profile (triglycerides, total cholesterol, HDL, LDL and VLDL), glucose, insulin, total (T) and high molecular weight (HMW) adiponectin, resistin, IL-6, TNF-α, NAMPT/visfatin and vaspin levels were measured in separated aliquots of each sample by using commercial assays as previously reported [6,7]. The findings in proteomic analysis were contrasted with validated commercial assays by ELISA [Apolipoprotein-A1 (Apo-A1; Assaypro[R]), haptoglobin (Assaypro[R]), apo-J/clusterin (BioVendor[R]), alpha-1B-acid glycoprotein (α-1-BAGP; Assaypro[R]), alpha-1-antitrypsin (α1-AT; Assaypro[R]); vitamin D binding protein (vD-BP; R&D Systems[R]); retinol binding protein 4 (RBP4; R&D Systems[R])] or kinetic nephelometry [transthyretin (Immage. Beckman[R]).

HOMA index was calculated as glucose [mmol/l] × insulin [μUI/ml]/22.5 and S_A as HMW-(μg/ml)/(T)-adiponectin(μg/ml). IR was estimated in patients in the **Pros-OB** at **D** according to the patient's insulin secretion rate in the OGTT and classified at baseline as insulin resistant (**IR**, n = 11) if they met any of the following criteria: basal insulin > 15 μU/ml, peak insulin > 150 μU/ml or insulin at 120 minutes > 75 μU/ml or as not IR (**non-IR**, n = 9) if they did not [14].

Sample preparation for proteomic analysis

The serum samples were thawed or reconstituted (according to their preservation process). Fifty milliliters of each selected serum sample were albumin and Ig-G-depleted using an albumin and IgG Depletion kit (ProteoPrep® Blue Albumin Depletion Kit, Sigma-Aldrich, St. Louis, MO) and diluted in sample buffer containing 7 M urea, 2 M thiourea, 1% w/v SB 3–10, 3% w/v CHAPS, 0.25% v/v Bio-Lyte 3/10 ampholytes (Bio-Rad Laboratories Inc., Hercules, CA), and 1.5% v/v protease inhibitor cocktail (Sigma, St. Louis, MO). Disulfide bonds were reduced by addition of tributylphosphine and sulfhydryl groups were alkylated with iodoacetamide.

Two-dimensional gel electrophoresis (2DE) + mass spectrometry (MS)

All of the 2DE, image processing and analysis, mass spectrometry (MS) and tandem MS (MS-MS) analysis procedures (MALDI-TOF) have been detailed previously for human samples [9-12,15]. Identities obtained after MS and MS-MS analysis were verified using the MS and MS/MS data obtained to search online databases with the software Mascot (www.matrixscience.com) [9-12,15].

Sets of comparison

Due to the different sample processing and preservation procedures undergone by the samples from the patients in the Pros-OB group (lyophylization), regarding the OB and C groups (exclusively freezing), the obese patients from these groups were not pooled for analysis at baseline. The following sets of comparison were established in order to achieve the proposed objectives avoiding any possible bias derived from differences in the process of sample preservation:

1) Influence of obesity on serum proteomic profile: OB (n = 22) *vs.* C (n = 21).
2) Differences in the serum proteome due to insulin resistance: Pros-OB group at baseline (B): IR (n = 11) *vs.* non-IR (n = 9).
3) Effect of extensive weight reduction on serum proteomic profile: Pros-OB: Paired comparison between time-points D and WL (n = 20 at each time-point).

Statistical analysis

All 2DE intensity data were log-transformed. Variables fitting a normal distribution (p > 0.05 in a Shapiro–Wilk test) were compared between pairs of groups using a Student-t test for independent samples (OB *vs.* C; IR *vs.* non-IR) or a paired t-test for repeated samples (D *vs.* WL). The remaining variables were analyzed using the nonparametric Mann & Whitney U test (OB *vs.* C; IR *vs.* non-IR) or Wilcoxon test (D *vs.* WL). Correlation analysis was performed by using Pearson's r or Spearman's rho for parametric and non parametric variables, respectively. A value of $p < 0.05$ was chosen as the level of significance. These tests were performed using the software Statistical Package for Social Sciences (SPSS v. 14.0. MapInfo Corporation, Troy, NY, USA). Due to the high number of variables considered for every comparison set, statistical correction for multiple comparisons was performed by using the false discovery rate (FDR) test after initial comparisons (PRISM v. 6.0. GraphPad Software, Inc., La Jolla, CA, USA).

Results

Influence of obesity on the serum proteomic profile

The study of the serum proteomic profile in OB (n = 22) and C (n = 21) allowed for the analysis of 231 protein spots. The comparison of the protein spot intensities revealed that 17 of them showed differences between groups (p < 0.05). Among these, 6 proteins were overexpressed in OB compared to C, whereas the expression of the remaining 11 protein spots was decreased in OB (Table 1, Figure 1).

Among the observed changes, the down-regulation of several isoforms of Apo A1 (#2201, #3201, #3202; #6203;

Table 1 Protein spot displaying intensity differences (p < 0.05) between obese children (OB) and controls (C) before FDR analysis

Spot	Spot intensity in OB Significance level	MS Score/ Cut-off	MS Matched fragments	MS Sequence coverage (%)	MS -MS Score/ Cut-off	MS-MS Matched (Significant) fragments	MS-MS Sequence coverage (%)	Identification
1809	Upregulated, p < 0.05	68/66	15	26	45/40	2 (1)	6	Alpha 1B acid glycoprotein
2201	Downregulated, p < 0.01	115/66	12	50	98/41	9 (6)	40	Apolipoprotein A1
2203	Downregulated, p < 0.05	44/66	3	–	102/41	3(3)	6	Clusterin (Apolipoprotein J)
2301	Downregulated, p < 0.05	56/66	7	–	95/41	5(4)	23	Clusterin (Apolipoprotein J)
2306	Upregulated, p < 0.05	75/66	7	30	71/41	6(2)	17	Haptoglobin
3201	Downregulated, p < 0.05	137/66	16	59	81/41	8(4)	33	Apolipoprotein A1
3202	Downregulated, p < 0.01	71/66	8	34	81/41	6(4)	25	Apolipoprotein A1
3307	Upregulated, p < 0.05	91/66	7	36	61/58	3(1)	6	Haptoglobin
4401	Downregulated, p < 0.05	68/66	6	83	95/59	2(2)	28	Transthyretin chain A
5603	Downregulated, p < 0.05	71/66	6	11	79/59	3(1)	6	Haptoglobin
5604	Downregulated, p < 0.01	82/66	11	49	84/58	2(1)	4	Haptoglobin
6203	Downregulated, p < 0.05	127/66	17	65	76/58	6(3)	29	Apolipoprotein A1
7102	Upregulated, p < 0.01	55/66	8	–	64/56	2(1)	13	Haptoglobin (alpha2)
7201	Downregulated, p < 0.01	106/66	16	66	76/59	3(2)	13	Apolipoprotein A1
7503	Downregulated, p < 0.05	53/66	5	–	64/58	2(2)	7	Vitamin D binding protein
8102	**Upregulated, p < 0.01**	**68/66**	**5**	**20**	**70/57**	**3(1)**	**8**	**Haptoglobin (alpha2)**
9101	Upregulated, p < 0.05	49/66	3	–	105/55	1(1)	4	Haptoglobin (alpha2)

Protein spots displaying significant intensity differences between obese children (**OB**) and controls (**C**) prior to the false discovery rate (FDR) analysis. The spot in bold (8102) remained significantly different after FDR analysis. The second column shows the direction of the change observed in **OB** vs. **C**. *Abbreviations: MS* Mass spectrometry; *MS-MS* Tandem mass spectrometry.

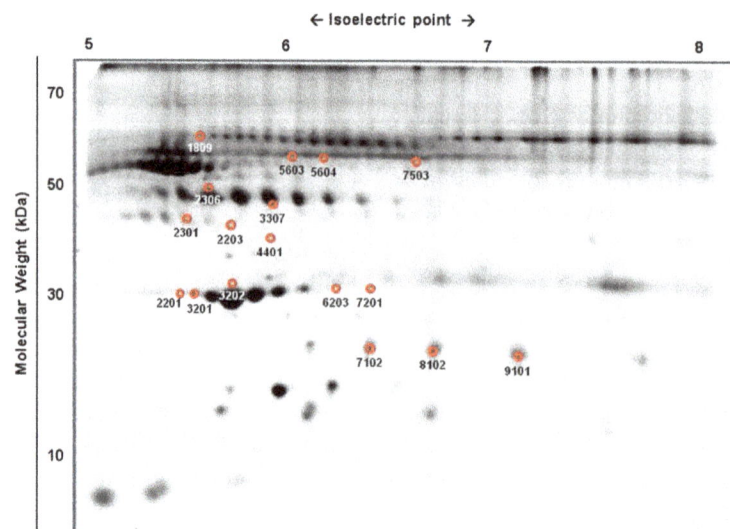

Figure 1 Proteomic profile comparison of OB vs. C. Protein identification of spots displaying differences (p < 0.05) between obese (OB) and control (C) children before FDR analysis. For spot identification, please see Table 1.

#7201), clusterin/Apo J (#2203; #2301), vD-BP (#7503) and transthyretin (#4401) was remarkable. OB patients showed a decreased expression of the highest molecular weight (MW) isoforms of haptoglobin (#5603, #5604), whereas those isoforms with a medium (#2306; #3307) or low MW (#7102; #8102; #9101) were up-regulated, as was α-1-BAGP (#1809).

After FDR analysis, only differences between groups in spot #8102 (low MW haptoglobin) remained significant ($p < 0.001$).

When analyzed by ELISA, lower serum levels of Apo-A1 (120.7 ± 56.9 vs. 236.3 ± 91.7 mg/dl, $p < 0.001$) in OB were observed, as was HDL cholesterol (46.22 ± 10.64 vs. 62.87 ± 12.53 mg/dl, $p < 0.001$). Similarly, ELISA was successful in discriminating the increase in α-1-BAGP (179.3 ± 78.2 vs. 125.8 ± 49.1; $p < 0.01$) and total haptoglobin (162.5 ± 103.5 vs. 85.84 ± 60.63 mg/dl) in OB vs. C.

In contrast, ELISA assays did not detect differences between OB and C in serum clusterin/Apo J (61.07 ± 9.75 vs. 57.29 ± 12.81 mcg/ml) or vD-BP levels (223.1 ± 62.5 vs. 236.2 ± 71.2 mcg/ml). No differences between groups were found after transthyretin quantification by kinetic nephelometry (22.72 ± 6.23 vs. 22.71 ± 4.91 mcg/ml), nor in its substrate (RBP4) serum levels by ELISA (750.3 ± 206.8 vs. 794.9 ± 173.2 mcg/ml).

To explore the eventual effect of excess BMI on the expression of these protein spots, correlation studies were performed in the whole study group (22 OB + 21 C: n = 43) between the relative intensity of spots showing differences between groups prior to the FDR analysis and the BMI-SDS of the patients. As expected, significant negative correlations were found between BMI-SDS and several isoforms of Apo-A1, clusterin/Apo J , vD-BP and haptoglobin isoforms with high MW, whereas positive correlation coefficients were observed exclusively with those haptoglobin isoforms with a lower MW, including spot #8102 (Table 2).

Effect of insulin resistance on serum proteomic profile

Comparison of the serum proteomic profile between IR (n = 11) and non-IR (n = 9) obese children (the Pros-OB group at diagnosis) allowed for the analysis of 237 protein spots, with 12 of them showing differences between groups ($p < 0.05$). Among these, 5 proteins were overexpressed in IR compared to non-IR obese children, whereas the expression of the remaining 7 protein spots was decreased in IR (Table 3, Figure 2).

Among the observed changes, it was remarkable that the presence of IR in obese children induced a further down-regulation of isoforms of Apo-A1 (#3101; #4101; #4103) and clusterin/Apo J (#3301; #4402). In contrast, no significant differences between the IR and non-IR groups were found in serum levels of clusterin/Apo J (54.67 ± 14.70 vs. 56.87 ± 14.80 mg/dl), Apo-A1 ($235.4 \pm$

Table 2 Correlation between BMI-SDS and protein spot intensity

Protein	Correlation	Protein	Correlation
#2201 (ApoA1)	r = -0.41; $p < 0.01$	#5604 (Haptoglobin)	r = -0.42; $p < 0.05$
#2203 (Clusterin)	r = -0.38; $p < 0.05$	#6203 (ApoA1)	r = -0.36; $p < 0.05$
#2301 (Clusterin)	r = -0.32; $p < 0.05$	#7102 (HP)	r = +0.36; $p < 0.05$
#3201 (ApoA1)	r = -0.32; $p < 0.05$	#7201 (ApoA1)	r = -0.35; $p < 0.05$
#3202 (ApoA1)	r = -0.43; $p < 0.05$	#8102 (HP)	r = +0.44; $p < 0.01$
#3307 (HP)	r = +0.32; $p < 0.05$	#9101 (HP)	r = +0.44; $p < 0.01$
#5603 (HP)	r = -0.35; $p < 0.05$		

Correlation coefficients (Spearman's rho) and significance levels between patient's standardized BMI (SDS) and protein spot intensity in the whole cohort of 43 prepubertal children studied, made up of 22 obese (**OB**) and 21 controls (**C**). *Abreviations: ApoA1* Apoprotein A1, *HP* Haptoglobin.

74.4 vs. 250.5 ± 79.4 mg/dl) or HDL (45.79 ± 8.82 vs. 45.89 ± 10.40 mg/dl) using standard immuno and enzymatic assays.

IR obese children also showed an increased expression of the 4 low MW isoforms of haptoglobin (#3002; #7101; #8101; #9101) and one of α1-AT (#1703), whereas the haptoglobin isoforms with the highest MWs (#4503; #5503) were down-regulated. When analyzed by ELISA, no significant differences between the IR and non-IR groups were found in serum levels of haptoglobin (202.7 ± 109.6 vs. 149.5 ± 49.5) or α1-AT (124.6 ± 60.1 vs. 115.2 ± 70.8).

After FDR analysis, differences between groups in spots #4101 (Apo A1) and #8101 (low MW haptoglobin) remained significant (both $p < 0.0001$).

To explore the relationship between the level of expression of these proteins and insulin resistance, the correlation between the relative intensity of protein spots showing differences between groups and the HOMA index of each patient in the entire study group was determined. As expected, significant negative correlations were found between HOMA and several isoforms of Apo-A1 (including spot #4101; rho -0.40 to -0.48; $p < 0.05$) and clusterin/Apo J (rho -0.45; $p < 0.05$), whereas positive correlation coefficients were observed with low MW isoforms of haptoglobin (including spot #8101; r = +0.55 to +0.61; $p < 0.01$).

Similar correlation studies were performed between these protein spot intensities at diagnosis and circulating levels of adipokines and the HMW to T adiponectin ratio (S_A index). No significant correlations were found for HMW adiponectin, T- adiponectin or S_A, or for resistin, TNF-alpha or vaspin. In contrast, a significant positive correlation was found between serum IL-6 levels and the intensity of protein spots #8101 (r = +0.53; $p < 0.05$) and

Table 3 Protein spot displaying intensity differences (p < 0.05) between insulin resistant (IR) and non-IR obese children before FDR analysis

Spot	Spot intensity in IR, Significance level	MS Score/Cut-off	MS Matched fragments	MS Sequence coverage (%)	MS -MS Score/Cut-off	MS-MS Matched fragments	MS-MS Sequence coverage (%)	Identification
1703	Upregulated, p < 0.05	111/66	15	54	100/40	6(4)	26	Alpha-1-Antitrypsin
3002	Upregulated, p < 0.05	48/66	4	–	52/38	1(1)	4	Haptoglobin
3101	Downregulated, p < 0.05	160/66	20	69	116/40	11(8)	43	Apolipoprotein A1
3301	Downregulated, p < 0.05	85/66	7	22	79/41	5(4)	23	Clusterin (Apo J)
4101	**Downregulated, p < 0.01**	**165/66**	**23**	**73**	**150/49**	**11(5)**	**43**	**Apolipoprotein A1**
4103	Downregulated, p < 0.05	161/66	22	73	171/59	11(4)	43	Apolipoprotein A1
4402	Downregulated, p < 0.05	49/66	5	–	97/58	1(1)	4	Clusterin (Apo J)
4503	Downregulated, p < 0.05	93/66	13	33	72/59	6(2)	15	Haptoglobin
5503	Downregulated, p < 0.05	56/66	6	–	81/59	2(0)	4	Haptoglobin
7101	Upregulated, p < 0.05	74/66	6	20	99/56	2(1)	7	Haptoglobin
8101	**Upregulated, p < 0.05**	**55/66**	**5**	**–**	**73/56**	**2(1)**	**13**	**Haptoglobin**
9101	Upregulated, p < 0.05	49/66	3	–	105/55	1(1)	4	Haptoglobin

The second column shows the direction of the change observed in IR vs. non-IR. *Abbreviations: MS* Mass spectrometry, *MS-MS* Tandem mass spectrometry. Spots in bold remained significant after FDR analysis.

#9101 (r = +0.70; p < 0.01), both corresponding to low MW isoforms of haptoglobin. Serum visfatin levels were negatively correlated with the intensity of spot #3301 (clusterin/Apo J); r = -0.54; p < 0.05.

Effect of extensive weight reduction on the serum proteomic profile

The paired comparison of the serum proteomic profiles of 20 obese children (the Pros-OB group), at diagnosis (D) and after reducing their BMI in over 2 SDS (WL) (n = 20 at each time-point) allowed for the analysis of 237 protein spots. Comparison of protein spot intensities revealed that 8 of them showed significant differences with 5 proteins increasing after weight loss and the remaining 3 protein spots decreasing as a consequence of BMI reduction (Table 4, Figure 3).

Among the observed changes it was remarkable that weight loss in obese children ameliorated the obesity induced decrease in Apo-A1 by increasing the expression of two of its isoforms (#2201; #7201), as well as increasing transthyretin (#5103). No significant differences in HDL levels (45.83 ± 9.30 vs. 49.42 ± 11.78 mg/dl) were found

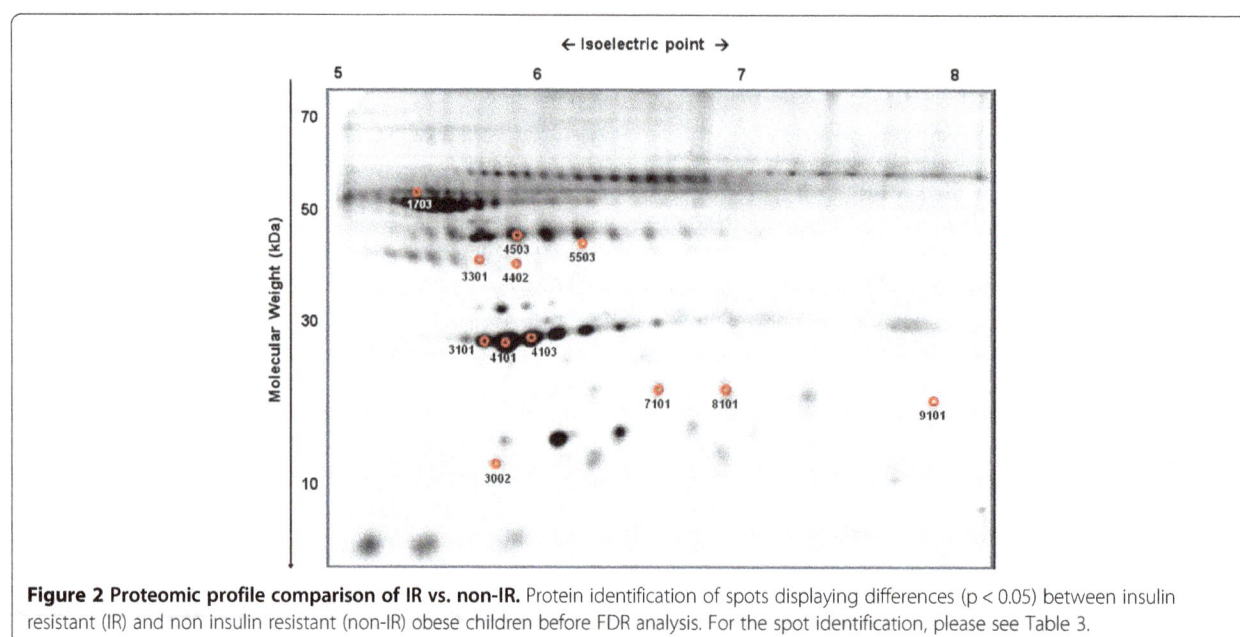

Figure 2 Proteomic profile comparison of IR vs. non-IR. Protein identification of spots displaying differences (p < 0.05) between insulin resistant (IR) and non insulin resistant (non-IR) obese children before FDR analysis. For the spot identification, please see Table 3.

Proteomic analysis allows for early detection of potential markers of metabolic impairment...

125

Table 4 Protein spot displaying intensity differences (p < 0.05) in pros-OB group after 2 SDS-BMI reduction

Spot	Spot intensity after weight loss	MS	MS	MS	MS-MS	MS-MS	MS-MS	Identification
	Significance level	Score/Cut.off	Matched fragments	Sequence coverage	Score/Cut-off	Matched fragments	Sequence coverage	
1704	Downregulated, p < 0.05	126/66	18	64	114/40	10(5)	37	*Alpha-1-Antitrypsin*
2201	Upregulated, p < 0.01	44/66	3	–	91/41	2(2)	12	*Apolipoprotein A1*
4801	Downregulated, p < 0.01	90/66	8	25	88/59	4(1)	12	*Alpha-1B-glycoprotein*
5103	Upregulated, p < 0.05	117/66	8	87	159/57	5(2)	79	*Transthyretin*
5503	Upregulated, p < 0.05	56/66	6	–	81/59	2(0)	4	*Haptoglobin*
7201	Upregulated, p < 0.01	106/66	16	66	76/59	3(2)	13	*Apolipoprotein A1*
7501	Upregulated, p < 0.05	55/66	4	–	86/59	2(2)	4	*Haptoglobin*
9101	Downregulated, p < 0.05	49/66	3	–	105/55	1(1)	4	*Haptoglobin*

The second column shows the direction of the change observed after weight loss. *Abbreviations: MS* Mass spectrometry, *MS-MS* Tandem mass spectrometry.

after weight loss when using standard assays, but Apo-A1 ELISA confirmed the increase in ApoA1 levels after weight reduction (242.6 ± 75.0 vs. 342.7 ± 83.9, p < 0.01). Similarly, no influence of weight loss on transthyretin (19.01 ± 3.95 vs. 19.66 ± 3.56 mg/dl) or RBP4 serum levels (572.5 ± 150.1 vs. 574.1 ± 127.6 mg/dl) were observed by kinetic nephelometry and ELISA, respectively.

Weight loss also decreased the expression of one isoform of low MW haptoglobin (#9101), whereas two haptoglobin isoforms with higher MW (#5503; #7501) were up-regulated after BMI reduction. In contrast, α1-AT (#1704) and α-1-BAGP (#4801) showed a decrease in their expression after weight loss. Standard assays were unable to detect significant changes after weight loss in serum levels of haptoglobin (177.5 ± 88.1 vs. 152.8 ± 55.6 mg/dl), α1-AT (120.2 ± 63.7 vs. 96.3 ± 71.1 mg/dl) or α-1-BAGP (156.0 ± 53.9 vs. 169.7 ± 43.8 mg/dl).

Discussion

In this study we have shown that obesity can result in changes in the circulating serum proteome even at young ages. The intensity of these changes depends upon the degree of BMI excess in some cases and could be, at least partially, ameliorated through weight loss. We have also demonstrated how insulin resistance, the first step in obesity associated impairment of carbohydrate metabolism, enhances these changes in the degree of expression of specific isoforms of proteins related to inflammation (haptoglobin) and metabolism (ApoA1), some of them correlating with serum levels of adipokines,

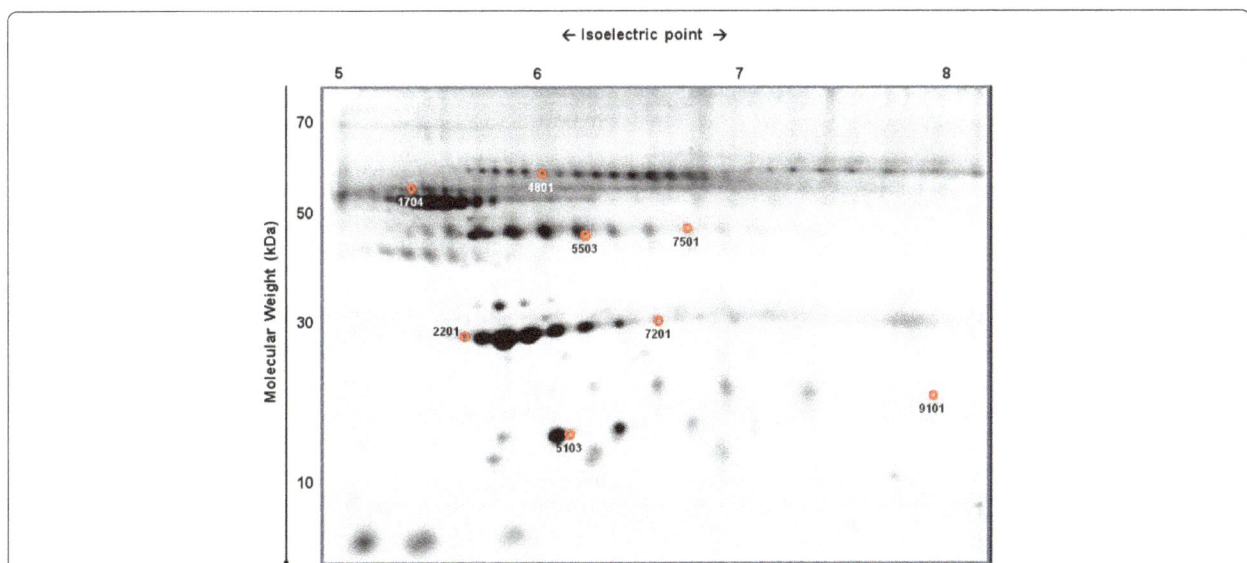

Figure 3 Proteomic profile comparison in Pros-OB: D *vs.* WL. Protein identification of spots displaying intensity differences (p < 0.05) in obese children (Pros-OB) between baseline (D) and after extensive BMI reduction (WL). For the spot identification, please see Table 4.

such as IL-6 and NAMPT/visfatin, with a known role in IR. Finally, we have demonstrated that serum proteomic analysis can complement the clinically used standard methodology in detecting these initial changes in the concentration of isoforms of circulating proteins associated with obesity related metabolic impairment and can identify new candidate biomarkers of early metabolic impairment.

One of the proteins significantly found to be affected in obesity associated IR is Apo-A1. There are two major classes of Apo-A; Apo-A1 and Apo-A2, with the former constituting the main component of HDL molecules [16]. Lipoprotein particles that contain only ApoA-1 (LpA-1 particles) can increase cellular cholesterol efflux from cultured cells *in vitro*, whereas LpA-1:A-2 particles do not [17]. Several studies support the fact that LpA-1 is more effective than LpA1:A-2 in promoting cellular cholesterol efflux, the first step in reverse cholesterol transport, leading to inhibition of dietary or genetically induced atherosclerosis [18]. Moreover, among the HDL molecules exclusively containing Apo-A1, several subclasses have been separated by gel filtration chromatography. These have been denoted large, medium and small LpA-1 and contain different amounts of lipids (much higher in large Lp-A1). This determines the differences in their cholesterol-reducing capacity, being lower in large LpA1 compared with medium and small LpA1 [19]. This huge variety of circulating HDL and ApoA1 molecules explains the different isoforms of ApoA1 differentiated by 2DE in our different comparison sets.

Our study affords three important observations regarding Apo-A1 dynamics in young obese children. First, the observation of the negative correlation found between BMI-SDS and most Apo-A1 isoforms in the whole cohort (OB + C) indicates that this is one of the initial derangements in lipid metabolism and that it can already be present at a very young age. Secondly, when obese children display IR, Apo-A1 production is more severely impaired. Finally, it is important to emphasize that the sensitivity of the standard methodology used in daily practice to determine HDL and Apo-A1 is insufficient to detect these initial changes in lipid metabolism demonstrated by 2DE under the presence of IR. As previously stated, this limited sensitivity can be influenced by the large variety of Apo-A1 and HDL isoforms [19] that can be selectively modified and/or change in different directions. In contrast, serum proteomic analysis by 2 DE is able to differentiate particular Apo-A1 isoforms and to detect the subtle and specific changes induced by obesity associated IR in very young obese children. Hence, this methodology could complement commonly used techniques in this subgroup of patients (insulin resistant obese).

Another apolipoprotein (J), also called clusterin, SGP2, TRPM-2, or CLI, has shown great variability in response to different pathological conditions. This is a plasma protein with cytoprotective and complement-inhibiting activities that acts through a specific receptor (megalin) and is also part of the HDL molecules. HDL molecules that contain Apo J and Apo A-I carry paraoxonase (PON1) that protects low-density lipoproteins from oxidative modification [20]. Since its discovery in the 80s, it has been proposed to influence inflammation and auto-immunity and to be involved in several pathophysiological processes such as carcinogenesis, kidney injury, senescence or Alzheimer disease [21].

To our knowledge, no data are available in the literature regarding serum clusterin dynamics in childhood obesity. Although the study by Kujiraoka et al. postulates that serum clusterin levels are unrelated to gender, BMI or age, it is reported to be increased in coronary heart disease with a postulated anti-atherogenic effect and its production enhanced by stress and in T2DM adults [22]. However, the elevation of clusterin in diabetes has been challenged, as it disappeared after adjusting for the level of glycemia [20]. Clusterin is known to accumulate in the artery wall during the development of atherosclerosis [22] and has been localized in the infarcted heart during myocardial infarction [23]. Moreover, a protective effect of exogenous clusterin has been demonstrated on ischemically challenged cardiomiocytes *in vitro* [24].

The differences between groups in clusterin levels observed in this study lost their significance after FDR analysis. However, the recurrent observation of these differences in every subset of comparisons established and the negative correlations with BMI-SDS, HOMA index and visfatin levels of some of its isoforms suggest an eventual relevance of this protein in the initial phase of metabolic impairment in obese children, differing from those observed in adults, not increasing but decreasing. This could suggest the loss of its postulated anti-atherogenic and lipid-lowering effects in direct relationship to of the degree of excess BMI and being further intensified with the onset of IR. It is possible that there is a lack of a stress stimulus powerful enough to induce the increase in serum clusterin described in adults as at these early ages gross metabolic impairment or arteriosclerotic changes are absent. The commercially available ELISA assay was unable to detect the trends to change in clusterin observed by 2DE, again reinforcing the need for validation of the changes in clusterin levels observed by 2DE in stages of initial metabolic derangement.

The third group of molecules where multiples changes were found is the set of haptoglobin isoforms. Obesity tended to decrease haptoglobin isoforms of higher MW and increase low MW isoforms, with this last change found to be significant after FDR analysis. This change was enhanced when comparing obese IR children with obese non-IR children, whereas weight loss causes the opposite effect, inducing an increase in higher MW haptoglobin isoforms and a decrease in the low MW ones. This could explain the limited ability of ELISA assays, which detect the different isoforms of haptoglobin as a pool, to discriminate these complex changes (as observed in the comparison between IR and non-IR).

Apart from the loss of significance of the differences between groups of several isoforms of haptoglobin after FDR analysis, two arguments can be raised to support the eventual pathophysiological relevance of these observations. These arguments include the abundance of haptoglobin isoforms in the serum proteome and the possible influence of inter-individual genetic variability. In effect, the two alleles for haptoglobin (1 and 2) give rise to three major phenotypes (Hp1-1, Hp2-2 and Hp2-1), each of them with different capacities to form homo- or hetero-polymers of haptoglobin [25]. However, the paired comparison performed after weight loss in the same set of children, determining an increase in the higher MW isoforms and a decrease in the low MW forms, supports a possible pathophysiological importance of our observation. Further support comes from the observed correlations between the excess of BMI and haptoglobin isoforms, positive for those with low MW and negative for those with high MW, and between HOMA index and the low MW isoforms of haptoglobin.

The increase in the synthesis of low MW isoforms of haptoglobin in obesity, and further when it associates IR, could be interpreted as a component of the low-degree inflammation state accompanying obesity, which is already present in early ages [6]. Haptoglobin is an acute phase protein exerting antioxidant activity through several mechanisms, including activation of neutrophils, maintenance of reverse cholesterol transport and inhibition of cyclooxygenase and lipooxygenase [26]. This antioxidant function is more pronounced in individuals with the Hp1-1 phenotype. Interestingly, this phenotype generates the smallest haptoglobin molecules (dimers), compared with the Hp2-1 (trimers and tetramers) and Hp2-2 (trimers, tetramers and polymers) phenotypes, with this last phenotype showing the lowest antioxidant capacity [25,26]. In this regard, the positive correlation found between serum IL-6 levels and the expression of two of the low MW isoforms of haptoglobin (including spot #8102) in our obese cohort suggests the feasibility of the proposed explanation, especially taking into account that IL-6 induces haptoglobin synthesis [25,27].

The lack of significance after FDR analysis of the increase in alpha 1 antitrypsin levels, another acute phase protein, as a consequence of IR in 2DE analysis as in ELISA does not allow any conclusion to be made, although its variations might be expected due to the existence of a proinflammatory environment. The increase in alpha-1-acid glycoprotein detected by ELISA and suggested by 2DE (although not reaching statistical significance after FDR) has been previously reported in obese adults [28] and T2DM [29], though its biological significance remains uncertain.

Decreased serum levels of some isoforms of two binding proteins, transthyretin and vD-BP, were observed in obese children, although they lost their significance after adjusting by FDR. Transtyretin is bound to RBP4 in plasma and an elevation in RBP4 is thought to contribute to the development of IR associated with obesity and T2DM [30] A decrease in transthyretin could result in increased free RBP4 levels contributing to IR in obese subjects, with weight loss improving this impairment. Similarly, low vitamin D levels have been consistently reported in obese patients of all ages [31]. Although vitamin D liposolubility seems to be the main determinant of its low serum levels in obese subjects, the detected decreases in vitamin D binding protein isoforms could also be involved. Again 2DE results for trend to change in these two proteins need further validation, but could confer 2DE a potential role in early detection of the decrease in specific isoforms of transtyretin and vD-BP, before changes in total transthyretin, RBP4 or vD-BP are observed.

Regarding the changes observed in protein spot intensity in the three sets of comparison, losing their significance after FDR analysis, it should be pointed that, although correction for multiple comparisons is considered statistically recommendable to avoid rejecting the null hypothesis too readily, some author postulate that it should be avoided. This is explained on the basis that reducing the type I error for null associations increases the type II error for those associations that are not null; thus suggesting that a policy of not making adjustments for multiple comparisons could be preferable because it will lead to fewer errors of interpretation when the data are actual observations on nature [32].

Conclusions

Our results suggest that changes in some isoforms of circulating peptides, mainly related to inflammation and lipid metabolism, accompany the early onset of obesity and IR in childhood. Furthermore, weight loss can ameliorate these modifications, at least partially. Some of these changes are undetectable by methods routinely used in the clinic under certain conditions, such as IR. Proteomic analysis, in particular, detection of isoforms of known proteins (ApoA1 and low MW haptoglobin) could be useful to complement them. In addition, this proteomic approach has allowed for the identification of several candidate proteins (including ApoJ/clustering, vitaminD binding protein, transthyretin) whose dynamics in childhood obesity and IR need further validation, but could result in novel biomarkers for the risk of development of obesity related metabolic complications.

Abbreviations
2-DE: Two dimension electrophoresis; α-1-BAGP: Alpha-1-acid glycoprotein; α1-AT: Alpha-1-acid antitrypsin; Apo-A1: Apolipoprotein A1; BMI: Body mass

index; C: Controls; D: Study time-point at diagnosis; FDR: False discovery rate analysis.; HDL: High density lipoprotein; HOMA: Homeostasis model assessment; HMW-adiponectin: High molecular weight adiponectin; IL-6: Interleukin 6; IR: Insulin resistance; LDL: Low density lipoprotein; MS: Mass spectrometry; MS-MS: Tandem mass spectrometry; OB: Obese; OGTT: Oral glucose tolerance test; Pros-OB: Prospectively followed obese cohort; RBP4: Retinol binding protein 4; SA: HMW to T adiponectin ratio; SDS: Standard deviation score; T2DM: Type 2 diabetes mellitus; T-adiponectin: Total adiponectin; TNF-α: Tumoral necrosis factor alpha; vD-BP: Vitamin D binding protein; VLDL: Very low density lipoprotein; WL: Study timepoint after weight loss.

Competing interests
The authors declare lack of any financial or non-financial competing interests.

Authors' contributions
GAMM and LSS carried out the proteomic studies, participated in data interpretation and drafted the manuscript. VB and SO carried out the immunoassays. DB participated in the result interpretation. JA and JJK conceived of the study, and participated in its design and coordination and helped to draft the manuscript. All authors read and approved the final manuscript.

Acknowledgements
The authors wish to thank Dr. Julie A. Chowen for the critical review of the manuscript, Dr. Julia Asensio for the clinical laboratory support and Prof. Wieland Kiess' group for his collaboration in visfatin and vaspin level determination. Gabriel A. Martos-Moreno is a recipient of a "Contrato Rio Hortega" from the "Instituto de Salud Carlos III" (FIS CM05/00100).. This work was supported by in part by the State of Ohio s Eminent Scholar Program that includes a gift from Milton and Lawrence Goll, by NIH Grants DK075436-01, AG019899-06, by the Diabetes Institute and the BioMolecular Innovation and Technology Partnership at Ohio University, by the CIBER Fisiopatología de la Obesidad y Nutrición (CIBERobn), Instituto de Salud Carlos III, the Fundación Endocrinología y Nutrición and Mutua Madrileña (AP2561/2008).

Author details
[1]Edison Biotechnology Institute, Ohio University, Konneker Research Laboratories, 1 Water Tower Drive, The Ridges, 45701 Athens, Ohio, USA. [2]Hospital Infantil Universitario Niño Jesús, Department of Endocrinology, Instituto de Investigación la Princesa, Universidad Autónoma de Madrid, Department of Pediatrics, Av. Menéndez Pelayo, 65, E-28009 Madrid, Spain. [3]CIBER Fisiopatología Obesidad y Nutrición (CIBERobn), Instituto de Salud Carlos III, Madrid, Spain. [4]Department of Biological Sciences, College of Arts and Sciences, Ohio University, Athens, Ohio, USA. [5]Molecular and Cellular Biology Program, Ohio University, Athens, Ohio, USA. [6]Department of Biomedical Sciences, College of Osteopathic Medicine, Ohio University, Athens, Ohio, USA.

References
1. Beilin L, Huang RC: **Childhood obesity, hypertension, the metabolic syndrome and adult cardiovascular disease.** *Clin Exp Pharmacol Physiol* 2008, **35:**409–411.
2. Camhi SM, Katzmarzyk PT, Broyles S, Srinivasan SR, Chen W, Bouchard C, Berenson GS: **Predicting adult body mass index-specific metabolic risk from childhood.** *Metab Syndr Relat Disord* 2010, **8:**165–172.
3. Mikhail N: **The metabolic syndrome: insulin resistance.** *Curr Hypertens Rep* 2009, **11:**156–158.
4. Martos-Moreno GÁ, Barrios V, Chowen JA, Argente J: **Adipokines in childhood obesity.** In *Vitamins & Hormones: "Obesity".* Edited by Litwack G. Burlington: Academic Press; 2013:107–142.
5. Haider DG, Holzer G, Schaller G, Weghuber D, Widhalm K, Wagner O, Kapiotis S, Wolzt M: **The adipokine visfatin is markedly elevated in obese children.** *J Pediatr Gastroenterol Nutr* 2006, **43:**548–549.

6. Martos-Moreno GÁ, Barrios V, Martínez G, Hawkins F, Argente J: **Effect of weight loss on high-molecular weight adiponectin in obese children.** *Obesity (Silver Spring)* 2010, **18:**2288–2294.
7. Martos-Moreno GA, Kratzsch J, Körner A, Barrios V, Hawkins F, Kiess W, Argente J: **Serum visfatin and vaspin levels in prepubertal children: effect of obesity and weight loss after behavior modifications on their secretion and relationship with glucose metabolism.** *Int J Obes (Lond)* 2011, **35:**1355–1362.
8. Tilg H, Moschen AR: **Inflammatory mechanisms in the regulation of insulin resistance.** *Mol Med* 2008, **14:**222–231.
9. Ding J, List EO, Okada S, Kopchick JJ: **Perspective: proteomic approach to detect biomarkers of human growth hormone.** *Growth Horm IGF Res* 2009, **19:**399–407.
10. Ding J, Okada S, Jørgensen JO, Kopchick JJ: **Novel serum protein biomarkers indicative of growth hormone doping in healthy human subjects.** *Proteomics* 2011, **11:**3565–3571.
11. Sackmann-Sala L, Ding J, Frohman LA, Kopchick JJ: **Activation of the GH/IGF-1 axis by CJC-1295, a long-acting GHRH analog, results in serum protein profile changes in normal adult subjects.** *Growth Horm IGF Res* 2009, **19:**471–477.
12. Cruz-Topete D, Jorgensen JO, Christensen B, Sackmann-Sala L, Krusenstjerna-Hafstrøm T, Jara A, Okada S, Kopchick JJ: **Identification of new biomarkers of low-dose GH replacement therapy in GH-deficient patients.** *J Clin Endocrinol Metab* 2011, **96:**2089–2097.
13. Sobradillo B, Aguirre A, Aresti U, Bilbao A, Fernández-Ramos C, Lizárraga A, Lorenzo H, Madariaga L, Rica I, Ruiz I, Sánchez E, Santamaría C, Serrano JM, Zabala A, Zurimendi B, Hernández M: **Curvas y tablas de crecimiento (estudio longitudinal y transversal).** In *Patrones de crecimiento y desarrollo en España. Atlas de gráficas y tablas.* Edited by Orbegozo F. Madrid: ERGON; 2004.
14. Eyzaguirre F, Mericq V: **Insulin resistance markers in children.** *Horm Res* 2009, **71:**65–74.
15. Martos-Moreno GÁ, Sackmann-Sala L, Berryman D, Blome DW, Argente J, Kopchick JJ: **The proteome of subcutaneous adipose tissue shows anatomical heterogeneity.** *An Ped (Barc)* 2013, **78:**140–148.
16. Boes E, Coassin S, Kollerits B, Heid IM, Kronenberg F: **Genetic-epidemiological evidence on genes associated with HDL cholesterol levels: a systematic in-depth review.** *Exp Gerontol* 2009, **44:**136–160.
17. Fruchart JC, Ailhaud G: **Apolipoprotein A-containing lipoprotein particles: physiological role, quantification, and clinical significance.** *Clin Chem* 1992, **38:**793–797.
18. Duriez P, Fruchart JC: **High-density lipoprotein subclasses and apolipoprotein A-I.** *Clin Chim Acta* 1999, **286:**97–114.
19. Ohta T, Saku K, Takata K, Nakamura R, Ikeda Y, Matsuda I: **Different effects of subclasses of HDL containing apoA-I but not apoA-II (LpA-I) on cholesterol esterification in plasma and net cholesterol efflux from foam cells.** *Arterioscler Thromb Vasc Biol* 1995, **15:**956–962.
20. Kujiraoka T, Hattori H, Miwa Y, Ishihara M, Ueno T, Ishii J, Tsuji M, Iwasaki T, Sasaguri Y, Fujioka T, Saito S, Tsushima M, Maruyama T, Miller IP, Miller NE, Egashira T: **Serum apolipoprotein J in health, coronary heart disease and type 2 diabetes mellitus.** *J Atheroscler Thromb* 2006, **13:**314–322.
21. Falgarone G, Chiocchia G: **Chapter 8: Clusterin: a multifacet protein at the crossroad of inflammation and autoimmunity.** *Adv Cancer Res* 2009, **104:**139–170.
22. Trougakos IP, Poulakou M, Stathatos M, Chalikia A, Melidonis A, Gonos ES: **Serum levels of the senescence biomarker clusterin/apolipoprotein J increase significantly in diabetes type II and during development of coronary heart disease or at myocardial infarction.** *Exp Gerontol* 2002, **37:**1175–1187.
23. Krijnen PA, Cillessen SA, Manoe R, Muller A, Visser CA, Meijer CJ, Musters RJ, Hack CE, Aarden LA, Niessen HW: **Clusterin: a protective mediator for ischemic cardiomyocytes?** *Am J Physiol Heart Circ Physiol* 2005, **289:**H2193–H2202.
24. van Dijk A, Vermond RA, Krijnen PA, Juffermans LJ, Hahn NE, Makker SP, Aarden LA, Hack E, Spreeuwenberg M, van Rossum BC, Meischl C, Paulus WJ, Van Milligen FJ, Niessen HW: **Intravenous clusterin administration reduces myocardial infarct size in rats.** *Eur J Clin Invest* 2010, **40:**893–902.
25. Asleh R, Levy AP: **In vivo and in vitro studies establishing haptoglobin as a major susceptibility gene for diabetic vascular disease.** *Vasc Health Risk Manag* 2005, **1:**19–28.
26. Quaye IK: **Haptoglobin, inflammation and disease.** *Trans R Soc Trop Med Hyg* 2008, **102:**735–742.

27. Kalmovarin N, Friedrichs WE, O'Brien HV, Linehan LA, Bowman BH, Yang F: **Extrahepatic expression of plasma protein genes during inflammation.** *Inflammation* 1991, **15**:369–379.

28. Benedek IH, Blouin RA, McNamara PJ: **Serum protein binding and the role of increased alpha 1-acid glycoprotein in moderately obese male subjects.** *Br J Clin Pharmacol* 1984, **18**:941–946.

29. Galazis N, Afxentiou T, Xenophontos M, Diamanti-Kandarakis E, Atiomo W: **Proteomic biomarkers of type 2 diabetes mellitus risk in women with polycystic ovary syndrome.** *Eur J Endocrinol* 2013, **168**:33–43.

30. Frey SK, Spranger J, Henze A, Pfeiffer AF, Schweigert FJ, Raila J: **Factors that influence retinol-binding protein 4-transthyretin interaction are not altered in overweight subjects and overweight subjects with type 2 diabetes mellitus.** *Metabolism* 2009, **58**:1386–1392.

31. Codoñer-Franch P, Tavárez-Alonso S, Simó-Jordá R, Laporta-Martín P, Carratalá-Calvo A, Alonso-Iglesias E: **Vitamin D status is linked to biomarkers of oxidative stress, inflammation, and endothelial activation in obese children.** *J Pediatr* 2012, **161**:848–854.

32. Rothman KJ: **No adjustments are needed for multiple comparisons.** *Epidemiology* 1990, **1**:43–46.

18

Deferring surgical treatment of ambiguous genitalia into adolescence in girls with 21-hydroxylase deficiency: a feasibility study

Pierre Bougnères[1*], Claire Bouvattier[1], Maryse Cartigny[2] and Lina Michala[3]

Abstract

Background: Genital surgery in Disorders of Sex Development (DSD) has been an area of debate over the past 20 years. Emerging scientific evidence in the late 1990s defied the then routine practice to surgically align genitalia to the sex of rearing, as early as possible. However, despite multitude of data showing detrimental effects to genital sensation and sexuality, few patients born with ambiguous genitalia have remained unoperated into adolescence.

Methods: We followed up girls with 21 hydroxylase deficiency (21- OHD) in genital morphology during childhood and acceptability among patients and parents of such an approach.

Results: Preliminary results from 7 children, aged 1–8 years (median 4.5 years), suggest that it is acceptable among patients and families to defer genital operation in 21-OHD. All patients had a Prader stage III and above. Median clitoral length at birth was 24 mm (20-28 mm) and had diminished to a median of 9 mm (5-15 mm) at their last visit. Height and weight have remained strictly normal in all patients. So far girls and their parents have not expressed significant concerns regarding genital ambiguity.

Conclusions: With this encouraging data at hand, we propose to formally address levels of anxiety, adaptation and quality of life during childhood, with an ultimate goal to assess long term satisfaction and effects on sexuality through deferring genital surgery for adolescence.

Keywords: 21-hydroxylase deficiency, Ambiguous genitalia, Congenital adrenal hyperplasia, Genital surgery

Background

Surgical management in Disorders of Sex Development (DSD) remains an area of controversy, even following the 2005 Chicago consensus, which attempted to delineate treatment guidelines and advocated a more cautious approach to genital surgery [8]. For years, the norm in DSD, was to align genitalia with the assigned gender as early as possible. Supporters of early surgery have based their practice on a need to reinforce sex of rearing, while relieving parental tension regarding the ambiguity of the genitalia [13]. Early surgery, when assessed in the immediate postoperative period was thought to provide ideal cosmetic and anatomical results, with the additional benefit that a procedure performed early enough in infancy would be forgotten by the patient.

It was not until the 1990s that this practice was challenged by patients themselves, who came forward with significant problems in adulthood, including anatomical difficulties in penetrative sexual intercourse and decreased genital sensation or ability to reach orgasm [15].

Multiple scientific voices have joined those of patients and support groups to question long term results of early genital surgery [5, 6, 12, 14]. Decreased genital sensitivity and need for further surgery in adulthood, as well as poor cosmetic results in the long run have been proven by studies in multiple institutions, suggesting dissatisfaction in a significant proportion of patients irrespective of geographical provenance [2, 6, 11, 14].

* Correspondence: pierre.bougneres@inserm.fr
[1]Pediatric Endocrinology, Bicêtre Hospital, Paris South University, 78 Avenue du Général Leclerc, Kremin Bicêtre, 94270 Paris, France
Full list of author information is available at the end of the article

Despite concerns, inertia has perpetuated the practice of early genital surgery into the present, and, to date, there have been no series of patients left unoperated until adolescence or adulthood so as to form a basis for comparison. Current practice still favours early genital surgery, usually based on nebulous and unproven scientific facts, as shown by national statistics [7], audits of practice among pediatric surgeons [16], and the paucity of data on unoperated patients in series of 21-OHD patients. Nevertheless, the handful of DSD patients that have remained unoperated, seem to have similar genital sensation to normal controls, with numbers however remaining too small to draw firm conclusions on [4]. With evidence on long term outcomes lacking, it is impossible to formulate a well-supported scientific argument for deferring genital operation.

Methods

During the last decade, our institution, a tertiary referral centre for complex paediatric endocrinological disorders, has had a policy of offering unbiased information regarding the pros and cons of genital operation to all parents of children born with 21- hydroxylase deficiency and Prader III-IV stages. Parents are given the opportunity to discuss the care of their child with a paediatric endocrinologist, a gynaecologist with expertise in paediatric and adolescent care and if requested, a paediatric urologist. The child and parents are followed at regular intervals irrespective of whether they have opted for surgery or not. During visits, we assess the child's behaviour, her interaction with her parents, evaluate for the presence of parental anxiety and note down any evidence of disruption to everyday activities due to the ambiguous appearance of the genitalia, urinary symptoms or clitoral erections.

Results

We are currently following seven 21-OHD girls with a median age of 4.5 years (range 1–8 years) whose operation has been deferred.

The first girl, named GK, was born 8 years ago. She was left unoperated following a decision from the parents and PB. After observing the girl during one year, it was clear that the length of the clitoris could be minimized with 50 mg hydrocortisone/m2 daily in four divided doses, bring serum testosterone and delta-4-androstenedione levels to under 0.02 ng/ml. Over the following years, GK's parents did not express any concern regarding the psychological or physical well-being of their child, despite episodic clitoral erections.

Since GK's experience was encouraging, this pilot 2-year observation was shared with CB and MC who used it to inform other parents. From 2010 to 2015, CB and MC have been following 6 more girls with 21-OHD, born with Prader III-IV stages, who were left unoperated. These girls

are followed up closely, with regards to their growth pattern, the degree of change in clitoral size and their psycho-developmental adjustment. So far all girls and their parents have not expressed significant concerns regarding genital ambiguity, despite episodic clitoral erections. There have been no cases of urinary track infections. Median clitoral length in this group of patients at birth was 25 mm (range 20-28 mm), whereas at their last visit median length was 9 mm (range 5-15 mm $p < 0.001$, Wilcoxon signed rank test). Growth rate, height and weight have remained strictly normal in all patients (Fig. 1). The main characteristics of the seven girls are depicted in Table 1. Figures 2 and 3 shows the results of the treatment at age 1 month in girl ON followed by MC. Treatment in all girls was started at a dosage of 50 mg/m2 daily in four divided doses, a higher dosage than usually recommended, for the first year of life and 50 μg fludrocortisone administered twice daily, and 2gr NaCL daily divided in four doses.. Thereafter, the daily dosage of hydrocortisone was gradually reduced to an average of 40 mg/m2 for the second year of life and 10-25 mg/m2 from the third year of life onwards. The doses of hydrocortisone that we used are closer to the Japanese [9] than to the European or American guidelines [10].

Discussion

The audit of our small series demonstrates that, at least in childhood, and with appropriate medical care and psychological support, it is possible to defer genital surgery. Whilst so far no major concerns have been reported from patients and their families, it remains unclear whether patients will continue to accept their diversity as they grow.

Clitoromegaly may be obvious enough to peers and may become the element and basis of bullying. One would have to put this in context of the current vogue among 'normal' women (with no genital ambiguity) to readily explore their genital area and opt for plastic surgery to their normal labia minora or clitoral prepuce, in order to diminish tissue that protrudes in the genital region [3]. In this current trend, a girl growing with clitoromegaly and ambiguous genitalia should be under frequent psychological support to enable better understanding of the condition and reinforce strategies to cope with being diverse.

Nevertheless, the degree of clitoromegaly may not be accurately assessed at birth as the newborn's genitals are under the full influence of adrenal androgens and maternal oestrogens. Although clitoromegaly is not reversible, anecdotal reports and our experience suggest that the clitoris could decrease in size as higher doses of glucocorticoid and mineralocorticoid replacement are instituted for the first year of life. Furthermore, as the child grows the relative larger size of the clitoris might become less evident.

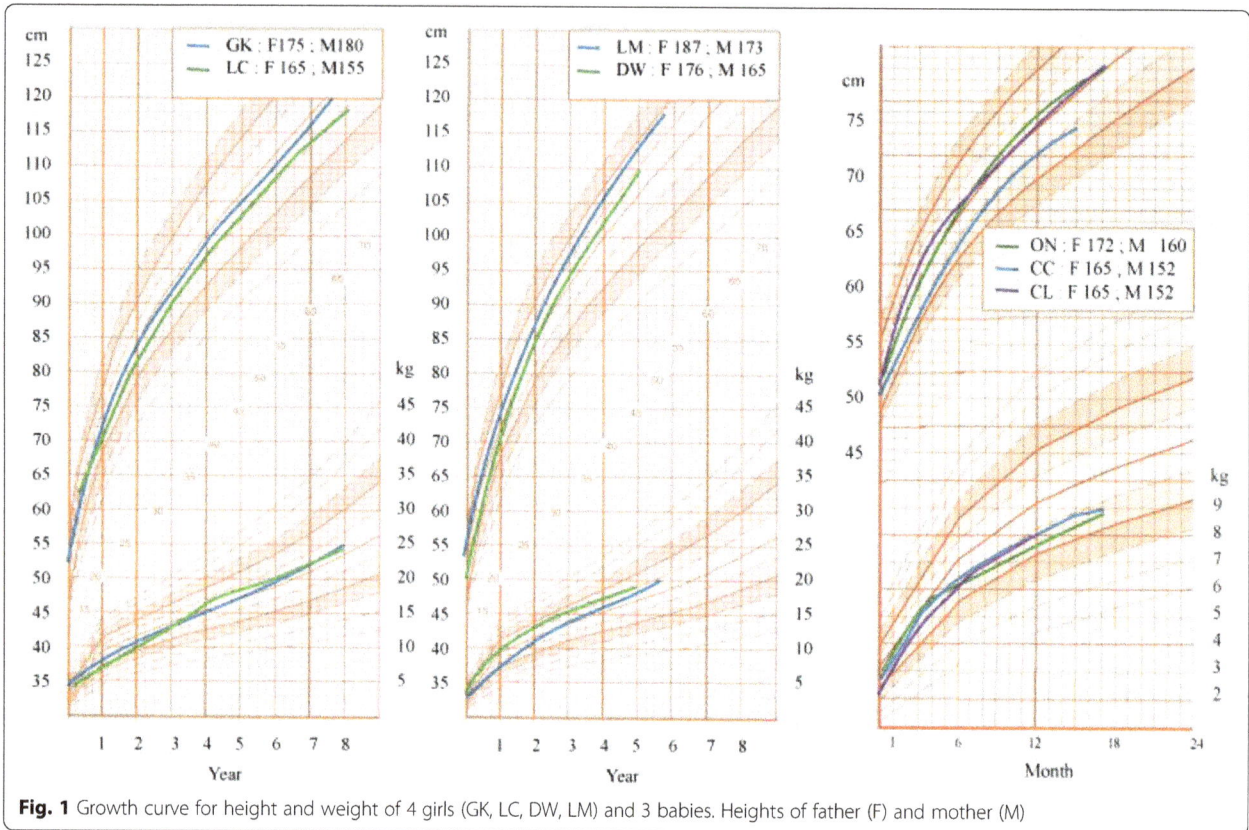

Fig. 1 Growth curve for height and weight of 4 girls (GK, LC, DW, LM) and 3 babies. Heights of father (F) and mother (M)

A personalized regimen of glucocorticoids needs to be defined within the therapeutic window, maintaining complete suppression of androstenedione and testosterone production and avoiding the unwanted effects of chronic hypercorticism. Individualized dosage and daily administration timing should be defined pragmatically in each patient instead of a per kg dogmatic prescription expected to fit all cases.

Compliance to medication is a reported concern in 21-OHD, particularly when adolescents start to be more rebellious and independent, omitting dosages or resisting and resenting treatment all together. This explains why a proportion of patients operated in childhood may need revisions to the clitoris in adolescence because of regrowth of tissue in puberty, due to a resurgence of androgens. With this in mind a stricter control with more frequent visits and better psychological support would be required in adolescence [1].

When the girl reaches adolescence, an examination under anaesthesia, a cystoscopy and vaginoplasty will allow for an accurate evaluation of the girl's genitalia, including measuring the width and length of the clitoris and assessing the distance of the urethral and vaginal confluence to the perineum and the caliber of the vagina. This examination is usually organized on a day surgery basis and can easily be accommodated around school commitments, so as to interfere to a minimum with the lifestyle of the girl.

Table 1 Main characteristics of the 7 girls with 21-OHD left unoperated in the current feasibility study

	Prenatal diagnosis	Prader stage at birth	Clitoris length at birth (mm)	17OHP diagnosis ng/ml	T at diagnosis (ng/ml)	Age at last examination (yrs)	Clitoris length at last examination (mm)	Height at last examination[a] (SD)
GK	yes	3-4	25	257	8	8	15	+0.2
LC	yes	3-4	20	119	9.8	7	7	−0.3
LM	no	3-4	20	414	14	5.5	5	+0.3
DW	yes	3-4	20	150	9	4.5	5	+0.4
CL	no	3-4	25	49	14	1	10	+0.4
CC	no	3-4	25	14	6.5	1	15	0
ON	yes	4	28	230	14.8	1	9	0

[a]SD departure from height for age calculated from mid-parental target height

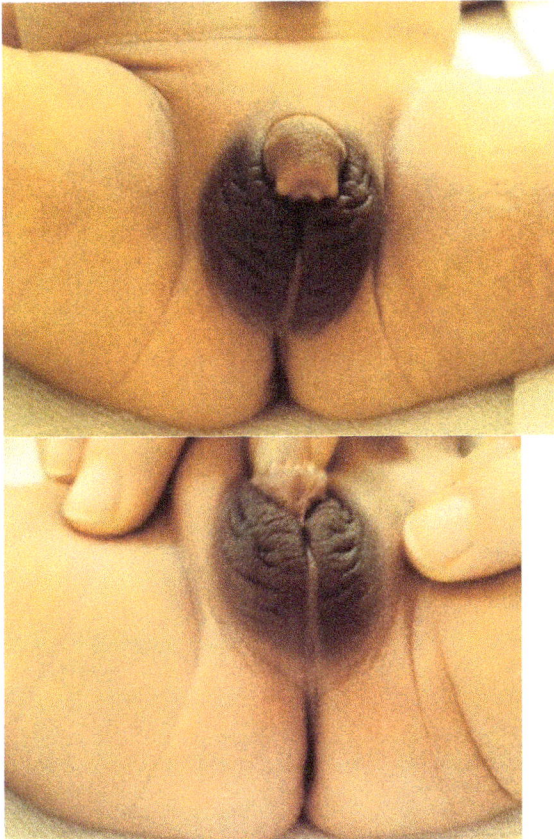

Fig. 2 Aspects of external genitalia of ON at birth

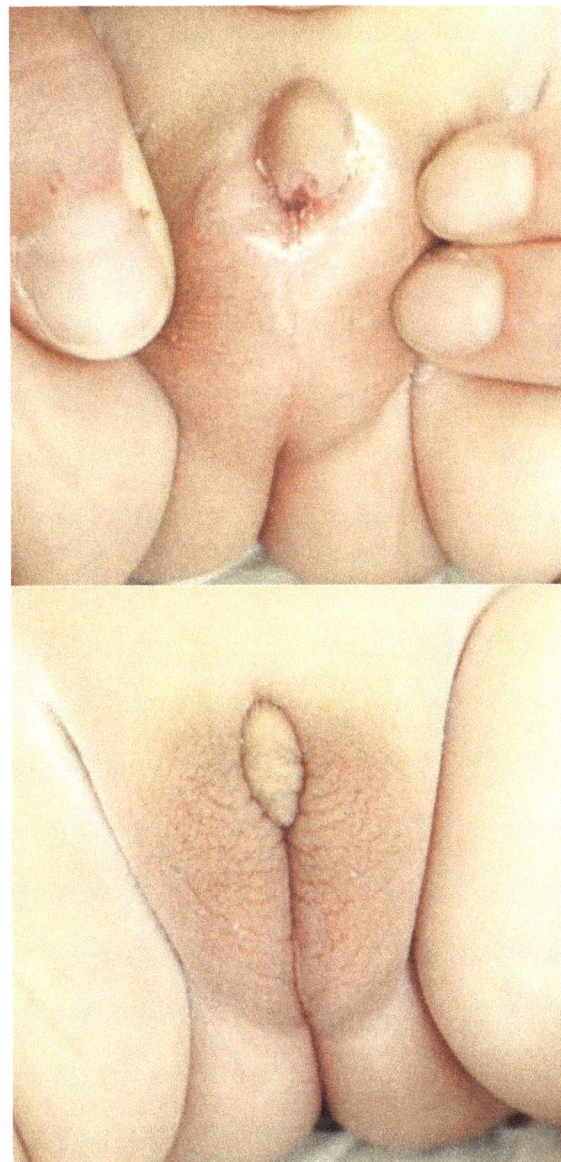

Fig. 3 External genitalia at two months of age

A vaginoplasty performed in adolescence is technically similar to the one performed in infancy. Advantages in adolescence are the larger caliber of the proximal vagina, allowing for a better end result at the level of anastomosis. Certainly the presence of oestrogens should allow for easier tissue plane identification and postoperative healing. Further to these technical advantages, an adolescent is in a better position to perform postoperative vaginal dilation, which will be required to avoid the formation of strictures, a complication often reported in the literature in as high as 50% of patients having had a vaginoplasty in childhood [2, 5, 6, 11].

Irrespective of potential technical benefits of performing surgery later in life, a major ethical advantage stems from the fact that the patient herself can be involved in the decision to proceed or not with an operation to the clitoris, taking into account the implications of surgery, the benefits to appearance and the possible risks to genital sensation and sexual function. It is perceived that a number of patients may opt against surgery all together as they grow, either because of a decreased size of the clitoris (relative or true) or because of a concern of effects of surgery on genital sensitivity. In either case it can be her choice to proceed to a clitoral reduction, even if the parent or guardian still has the legal responsibility for the operation.

We will collect preliminary results over the next few years, regarding concerns stemming from the ambiguity of the genitalia during childhood. However, the final outcome of a study should be long term adjustment, both with regards to sexuality and quality of life. It is obvious that these results will be available fifteen to twenty years from now, when current infants with 21-OHD will be entering adolescence and adulthood. Development of a prospective study with long follow up needs planning not only with regards to a well-designed protocol and measures to decrease dropout rates and patients lost to follow up. We also need to provide continuity of care within our service, to the next generation of researchers and clinicians, the current trainees or young specialists that will be gathering and analyzing results in the future.

Conclusions

Preliminary results in 7 young girls now aged 1–8 years affected with 21-OHD and born with Prader III-IV stages suggest that deferring genital operation is acceptable among patients and families. A careful medical treatment allowed the decrease of median clitoral length from 24 mm at birth to 9 mm at their last visit. So far girls and their parents have not expressed significant concerns regarding genital ambiguity.

With these encouraging data at hand, we propose to formally address levels of anxiety, adaptation and quality of life during childhood, with an ultimate goal to assess long- term satisfaction and effects on sexuality through deferring genital surgery for adolescence. These observations may pave the way for a new management of the disease in a subset of patients.

Abbreviations
17-OH- P: 17-hydroxyprogesterone; 21-OH-D: 21- hydroxylase deficiency; CAH: Congenital adrenal hyperplasia; DSD: Disorder of sex development

Acknowledgements
PB acknowledges AG and JG, the parents of GK, for making the initial decision that paved the way for this study.

Funding
The current study was part of the usual care of children with 21-OH-D, thus required no funding.

Authors' contributions
PB made the initial decision of offering to defer surgical correction, had the first patient in this series left unoperated and drafted the manuscript. CB and MC followed the other 6 patients. LM drafted the manuscript. All authors read and approved the final manuscript.

Competing interests
The authors declare that they have no competing interests.

Author details
[1]Pediatric Endocrinology, Bicêtre Hospital, Paris South University, 78 Avenue du Général Leclerc, Kremin Bicêtre, 94270 Paris, France. [2]Pediatric Endocrinology, Jeanne de Flandre Hospital, Lille University, Lille, France. [3]First Department of Obstetrics and Gynaecology, University of Athens, Alexandra Hospital, Athens, Greece.

References
1. Arlt W, Willis DS, Wild SH, Krone N, Doherty EJ, Hahner S, Han TS, Carroll PV, Conway GS, Rees DA, Stimson RH, Walker BR, Connell JM, Ross RJ, (CaHASE), United Kingdom Congenital Adrenal Hyperplasia Adult Study Executive. Health status of adults with congenital adrenal hyperplasia: a cohort study of 203 patients. J Clin Endocrinol Metab. 2010;95:5110–21.
2. Creighton SM, Minto CL, Steel SJ. Objective cosmetic and anatomical outcomes at adolescence of feminising surgery for ambiguous genitalia done in childhood. Lancet. 2001;358:124–5.
3. Crouch NS, Deans R, Michala L, Liao LM, Creighton SM. Clinical characteristics of well women seeking labial reduction surgery: a prospective study. BJOG. 2011;118:1507–10.
4. Crouch NS, Liao LM, Woodhouse CRJ, Conway GS. Sexual function and genital sensitivity following feminizing genitoplasty for congenital adrenal hyperplasia. J Urol. 2008;179:634–8.
5. Fagerholm R, Santtila P, Miettinen PJ, Mattila A, Rintala R, Taskinen S. Sexual function and attitudes toward surgery after feminizing genitoplasty. J Urol. 2011;185:1900–4.
6. Gastaud F, Bouvattier C, Duranteau L, Brauner R, Thibaud E, Kutten F, Bougneres P. Impaired sexual and reproductive outcomes in women with classical forms of congenital adrenal hyperplasia. J Clin Endocrinol Metab. 2007;92:1391–6.
7. HES. Hospital Episode Statistics. www.hscic.gov.uk/hes. [Online].
8. Hughes IA, Houk C, Ahmed SF, Lee PA, LWPES1/ESPE2 Consensus Group. Consensus statement on management of intersex disorders. Arch Dis Child. 2006;91:554–63.
9. Ishii T, Anzo M, Adachi M, Onigata K, Kusuda S, Nagasaki K, Harada S, Horikawa R, Minagawa M, Minamitani K, Mizuno H, Yamakami Y, Fukushi M, Tajima T. Guidelines for diagnosis and treatment of 21-hydroxylase deficiency. Clin Pediatr Endocrinol. 2015;24:77–105.
10. LWPES/ESPE, Joint CAH Working Group. Consensus stateent on 21-hydroxylase deficiency from the Lawson Wilkins Pediatric Endocrine Society and the European Society for Paediatric Endocrinology. J Clin Endocrinol Metab. 2002;87:4048–53.
11. Michala L, Liao LM, Wood D, Conway GS, Creighton SM. Practice changes in childhood surgery for ambiguous genitalia? J Pediatr Urol. 2014;10:934–9.
12. Minto CL, Liao LM, Woodhouse CR, Ransley PG, Creighton SM. The effect of clitoral surgery on sexual outcome in indivicuals who have intersex conditions with ambiguous genitalia: a cross sectional study. Lancet. 2003;361:1252–7.
13. Money J, Hampson JG, Hampson JL. Hermaphroditism: Recommendations concerning assignment of sex, change of sex and psychologic management. Bull Johns Hopkins Hosp. 1955;97:284–300.
14. Nordenstrom A, Frisen L, Falhammar H, Filipsson H, Holmadahl G, Janson PO, Thoren M, Hagenfeldt K, Nordenskjold A. Sexual function and surgical outcome in women with congenital adrenal hyperplasia due to CYP21A2 deficiency. Clinical perspective and patient's perception. J Clin Endocrinol Metab. 2010;95:3633–40.
15. Intersex Soeciety of North America. www.isna.org.
16. Yancovic F, Cherian A, Steven L, Mathur A, Cuckow P. Current practice in feminising surgery for congenital adrenal hyperplasia; a specialist survey. J Pediatr Urol. 2013;9:1100–7.

19

GPS suggests low physical activity in urban Hispanic school children: a proof of concept study

Aaron L Carrel[1*], Jeffrey S Sledge[2], Stephen J Ventura[2], Jens C Eickhoff[1] and David B Allen[1]

Abstract

Background: Urban environments can increase risk for development of obesity, insulin resistance (IR), and type 2 diabetes mellitus (T2DM) by limiting physical activity. This study examined, in a cohort of urban Hispanic youth, the relationship between daily physical activity (PA) measured by GPS, insulin resistance and cardiovascular fitness.

Methods: Hispanic middle school children (n = 141) were assessed for body mass index (BMI), IR (homeostasis model [HOMA-IR]), cardiovascular fitness (progressive aerobic cardiovascular endurance run [PACER]). PA was measured (GPS-PA) and energy expenditure estimated (GPS-EE) utilizing a global positioning mapping device worn for up to 7 days.

Results: Students (mean age 12.7 ± 1.2 years, 52% female) spent 98% of waking time in sedentary activities, 1.7% in moderate intensity PA, and 0.3% in vigorous intensity. GPS analysis revealed extremely low amounts of physical movement during waking hours. The degree of low PA confounded correlation analysis with PACER or HOMA-IR.

Conclusions: Levels of moderate and vigorous intensity PA, measured by GPS, were extremely low in these urban Hispanic youth, possibly contributing to high rates of obesity and IR. Physical movement patterns suggest barriers to PA in play options near home, transportation to school, and in school recess time. GPS technology can objectively and accurately evaluate initiatives designed to reduce obesity and its morbidities by increasing PA.

Keywords: Hispanic, GPS, School assessment, Exercise, School, Child

Background

Built environments can impede, or encourage active lifestyles for children [1,2]. Social environments influence how children choose, or are permitted, to interact with the environment. Reduced daily physical movement is one factor contributing to overweight/obesity, now the most common medical condition of childhood in the US. Certain ethnic minority populations, including Hispanic children, are at greater risk for obesity and its related morbidities [3-5]. Increasing numbers of children also fail to meet minimum recommendations for physical activity [6]. Both poor physical fitness and obesity are risk factors for T2DM and cardiovascular disease [7-12]. In fact, cardiovascular fitness (CVF) is a stronger predictor of

mortality than obesity [13,14]. Increased physical activity and fitness in children is associated with reduced risk for diabetes and other improved health outcomes. Thus, identifying and altering modifiable barriers to physical activity and lifestyle behaviors during childhood is paramount [15,16,17]. Successful public health interventions often utilize the Social Ecological Model (SEM) to address interacting environments at the individual, home, school, community, and society levels [18,19]. GPS offers the technology to document where, when, and how much activity is taking place.

One particularly attractive target for assessment and potential improvement of physical activity for children and adolescents is the school-day routine: travel to/from, recess movement, and after-school activities [16,17]. Since school attendance is an experience shared by the vast majority of children, the school environment and routine can potentially address low levels of physical

* Correspondence: alcarrel@wisc.edu
[1]Department of Pediatrics, University of Wisconsin, 600 Highland Avenue, H4-436, Madison, WI 53792-4108, USA
Full list of author information is available at the end of the article

activity (PA) and higher levels of sedentary behaviors, both of which are associated with IR. Most studies of childhood PA have relied on recall or physical activity logs, and very little objectively measured data is available regarding physical activity patterns of minority youth, including Hispanic children, who have a high rate of obesity, T2DM, and low fitness [20]. In this study, we utilize GPS to measure daily physical activity outside of classroom time in urban Hispanic youth and its relationship to BMI, cardiovascular fitness, and insulin resistance.

Methods

Children (n = 141) from the Bruce-Guadalupe middle school (grades 5–8) in Milwaukee, Wisconsin, were invited to participate. Human Subjects Committee at the University of Wisconsin approved all procedures, and informed written consent was obtained from student and parent before study enrollment. All consenting was done with both Spanish and English speaking investigators to allow families the best opportunity to ask questions. All students were Hispanic (78% Mexican and 21% Puerto Rican) children. Students had a mean age of 12.7 (±1.2), and 52% were females. Students underwent assessment of cardiovascular fitness measured by the progressive aerobic cardiovascular endurance run (PACER), calculation of body mass index (BMI), and a subset (n = 55) underwent fasting blood work performed for insulin and glucose (HOMA-IR) after a 12 hour fast.

Children wore Global Positioning (GPS) receivers (QStarz 1300S carried in pocket, backpack or worn on a lanyard) to track and record daily physical and sedentary activity. GPS receivers with unique unit identifiers were assigned to students, who were asked to keep the GPS unit on their person and wear at all times outside of school classroom time, with the exception of sleeping and showering for a 7-day time period. The intent was to capture activity before or after school, or on weekends, rather than "in classroom" time. Each receiver was cleared and set to record time and position at a one second intervals using WAAS enabled satellite signal detection. Theoretical position resolution at this standard was less than three meters.

School staff received training, software, and support for performing Fitnessgram® testing including PACER and BMI determination at the school. Staff was trained to download and store data and to recharge and clear GPS units. Installation of GPS download and viewer software was accomplished by installation in the school's information technology system.

PA was assessed using a geospatial model to equate GPS-recorded movement with energy expenditure. Using ArcGIS 9.X software, a community level "map" of movement by type (e.g., walking, running, motorized transport) was created to predict children's energy expenditure (EE; in kilojoules) as they move through the community. For each child, energy expenditures were predicted from position (e.g., GPS) and movement, producing highly accurate records of spatio-temporally placed EE. GPS recordings were considered evaluable for analysis if the GPS unit was active for at least 90 minutes on a given day. In order to determine the daily average over the 7-day recording period for each participant, the mean values for each GPS measure (energy expenditure, distribution, minutes and percent time spent on activity) across the recording period were calculated and analyzed.

Levels of EE were defined by velocity as recorded by the GPS units. The units automatically stopped recording when motionless for extended periods, thus only time spent in activity was included in "GPS active time." GPS data were processed into motion tracks in ArcGIS 9.x, using a standard spline function over three second intervals to smooth data spikes. Mode of travel was distinguished by acceleration signature coupled with peak and or sustained velocity. Time segments were manually interpreted from tracks and entered into a database for subsequent analysis.

Sedentary was defined as either lack of significant motion, or motion at rates and track patterns indicating travel in a motorized vehicle. Lack of motion was defined as less than 0.45 m/s (about 1 mile/per hour). Moderate intensity of activity was between 0.45 and 1.35 m/s, and vigorous activity was greater than 1.35 m/s in track patterns that did not correspond to vehicular travel. These distinctions are based on accepted definitions of NHANES datasets. Additionally, these GPS units included accelerometer triggers that helped us distinguish between the unit being at rest and unused, as opposed to being worn but with no positional change.

Cardiovascular fitness (CVF) was assessed using the PACER test, in which subjects run back and forth along a 20-meter shuttle run, and each minute the pace required to run the 20 meters quickens. The pace is set from a prerecorded audio file or CD. The initial running speed is 8.5 km/hour, and the speed increases by 0.5 km/hour every minute. The test is finished when the subject fails to complete the 20-meter run in the allotted time twice. The PACER is expressed as number of laps completed [21]. PACER Z-score were calculated based upon Wisconsin references [22]. A single teacher performed all PACER testing after undergoing certified training in PACER testing procedures.

A 5 ml fasting blood sample was obtained for insulin and glucose levels on a single 12 hour fasting blood specimen. Glucose was determined by hexokinase method and insulin by chemiluminescent immunoassay (University of Wisconsin Hospitals and Clinics Laboratory, Madison, WI). HOMA-IR was calculated from glucose and insulin values (fasting glucose (mg/dL) × fasting insulin (μU/ml)/405).

All analyses were performed using SAS software version 9.2 (SAS Institute, NC). Demographic variables were summarized in terms of means ± standard deviations or as percentages. The distribution of GPS measures was highly skewed so that medians and ranges were used to summarize these measures. In order to account for the daily variability in the GPS measures across the 7 days recording period, the analyses of GPS measures were weighted using the inverse of the standard errors of the estimated mean GPS values as weights. Nonparametric, partial Spearman's rank correlation coefficients were calculated to evaluate the associations between each GPS measures and BMI, fitness and insulin resistance measures. Since there was a large variation in the time for which the GPS device was active, the correlation analysis was adjusted by the median daily time the GPS device was active. Fisher's z-transformation was used to construct 95% confidence intervals for the correlation coefficients. A two-sided 5% significance level was used for all statistical tests.

Results

Complete data was collected on 141 students. A subset of 55 underwent fasting blood work; no differences were found comparing the group obtaining blood work with respect to mean BMI z-score, HOMA-IR, or PACER z-score. Mean BMI z-score was 0.91 (±1.0), mean HOMA-IR was 4.2 (±2.9), and mean PACER z-score was 0.31 (±0.98), based on age and gender (Table 1). Forty-nine percent of students had a BMI >85th-94th percentile (overweight), and 29% of students had a BMI >95th percentile (obese). PACER z-score was negatively correlated with BMI z-score (r = −0.47, 95% CI: −0.58 − -0.33;

p < 0.00001) and with HOMA-IR (−0.60, 95% CI: −0.70 − -0.48; (p < 0.0001).

There was a total of 519 days with evaluable (at least 90 minutes of active recording) GPS measurements across the 7-day period. The mean number of days with evaluable GPS measurements per student was 3.6 (±1.6).

The GPS device was activated daily with a median duration of 310 minutes (range 97 − 1086). Students spent a median time of 6 minutes (range 1 − 318 minutes) on moderate intensity PA, 0 minute (range 0 − 65 minutes) on vigorous intensity PA and 294 minutes (range 94 − 780 minutes) on sedentary activities (Table 2, and Figure 1). The median daily time spent in a motorized state was 18 minutes (range 0 − 316 minutes). Seventy seven percent of participants spent ≤10% of waking time on moderate intensity activities, 90% spent <5% of the time on vigorous intensity activities, and 77% spent no time in vigorous intensity activity (Figure 1). Forty-five percent of the participants spent at a daily average of least 20 minutes in a motorized vehicle.

Discussion

Daily physical activity, objectively measured by GPS, was extremely low in this school-based cohort of urban Hispanic youth. Most subjects engaged in almost no vigorous activity during the study period, only 22% spent >10% of waking time (~90 minutes) in moderate activity, and the median percentage time spent in sedentary state was 98%. Median energy expenditure attributed to moderate and vigorous PA was 18 and 0 calories/day, respectively. GPS analysis revealed extremely low amounts of physical

Table 1 Demographics of study population

	N	Mean	SD
Age (yrs)	141	12.7	1.2
BMI	141	23.0	5.1
BMI z-score	141	0.91	1.03
PACER (laps)	124	39.7	20.2
PACER z-score	122	0.31	0.98
Insulin	55	20.0	15.7
Glucose	55	89.4	6.7
HOMA IR	55	4.2	2.9
		N	%
Gender	141		
Male		73	48%
Female		68	52%
Overweight (BMI percentile ≥85th)	136	66	49%
Obese (BMI percentile ≥95th)		39	29%

Table 2 Summary statistics of daily average GPS measures

	Median[†]	Range
GPS active time (minutes)	310	97 − 1086
Time (minutes)		
Moderate intensity	6	1 − 318
Vigorous intensity	0	0 − 65
Sedentary	294	94 − 780
% Time spent		
Moderate intensity	2	0 − 42
Vigorous intensity	0	0 − 16
Sedentary	97	58 − 100
Energy (kcal expended)		
Moderate intensity	19	0 − 559
Vigorous intensity	0	0 − 205
Distribution		
Moderate intensity	1	0 − 31
Vigorous intensity	0	0 − 10

[†]Weighted using the inverse of the standard error of the estimated mean value across the 7-day study period.

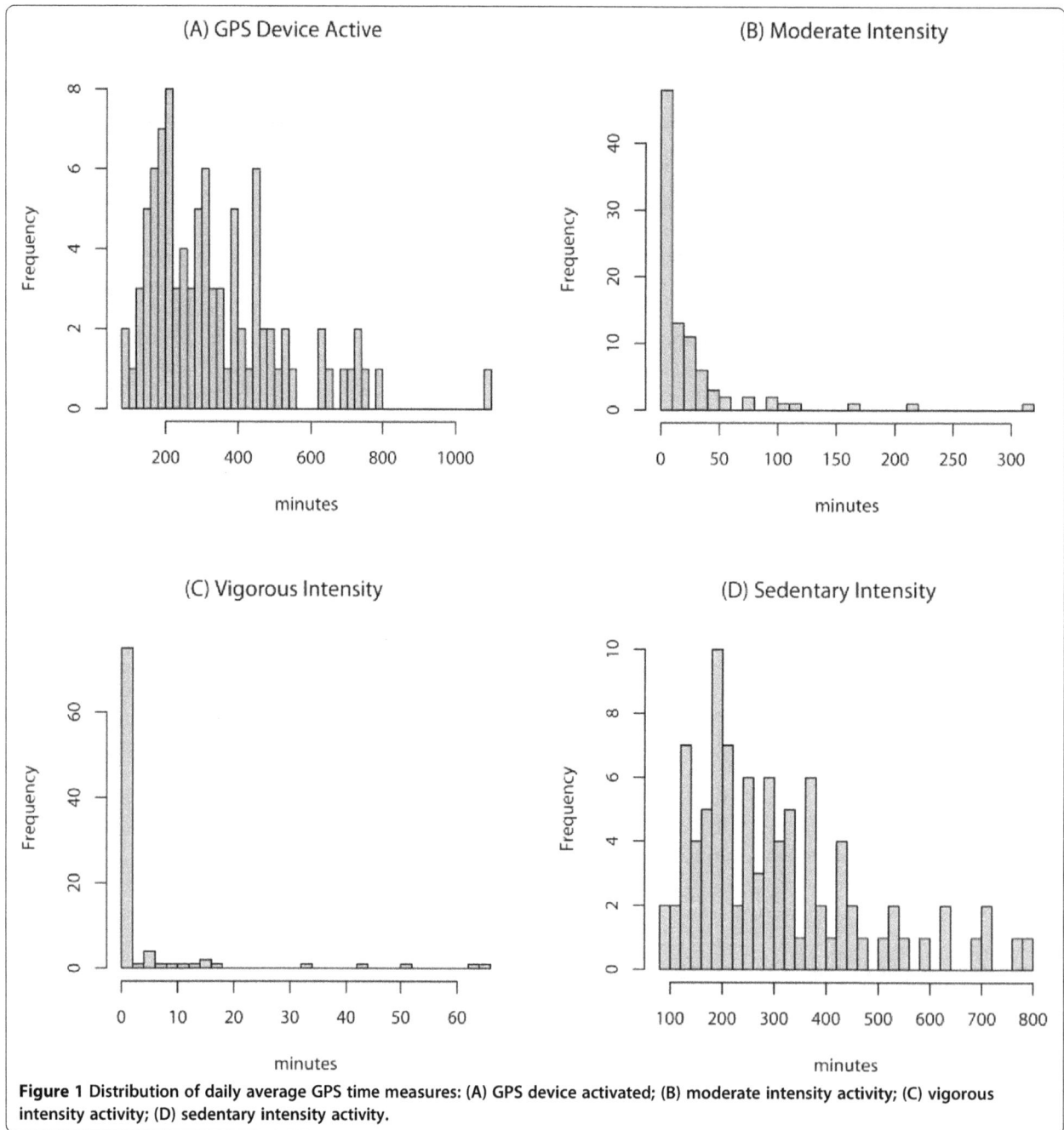

Figure 1 Distribution of daily average GPS time measures: (A) GPS device activated; (B) moderate intensity activity; (C) vigorous intensity activity; (D) sedentary intensity activity.

movement. The degree of low PA confounded correlation analysis with PACER or HOMA-IR. High levels of time were spent in motorized transport and low amounts of PA occurred both at the school and home environment. Since current national guidelines recommend a daily total of 60 minutes of moderate-to-vigorous activity (MVPA) for children [23], these data indicate that for many urban youth, there is a large gap between such recommendations and the realities of their daily life.

To evaluate the impact of public health interventions designed to increase physical activity, reliable measurements

of movement are essential. This study demonstrates that GPS can provide reliable and objective measures of duration, distance, and intensity of physical movement. In addition, specific GPS-generated time-activity patterns can suggest barriers to movement and targeted interventions to address them. Students generally viewed using GPS very positively, and use of GPS enabled analysis of their specific physical activity behaviors and transportation choices and routes. This study provides proof-of-concept data that GPS tracking can be an effective research tool to accurately document duration of physical activity, intensity of physical activity, and specific location of physical activity [23]. For future intervention studies, linking GPS data to metabolic measurements in children provides an opportunity to objectively and accurately evaluate the impact of physical activity changes on metabolic health.

Factors influencing children's lifestyle options and choices can generate differences in physical activity and energy expenditure which, over time, lead to health-altering decreases in movement and fitness, and increases in adiposity. While there is agreement that socioeconomic and built environment conditions can promote or inhibit physical activity, there are inconsistencies in the association of built environments and physical activity [24]. These may be due in part to challenges of accurately measuring and recording physical activity [25]. The data from this study suggest (but do not show) that children in urban settings confront physical, cultural, and attitudinal barriers that severely limit physical activity. The urban built environment near the school in this study (i.e. high crime area abutting a major highway) could markedly impede children's unstructured activity (play). The extremely low levels of PA observed in the study group were particularly concerning in light of ongoing efforts at the school, involving parents and older generation family members, to promote healthy lifestyle changes. Instead, GPS data demonstrated that children were driven for almost all trips to and from school, that they moved little during the school day, and that they spent very little time moving in outdoor recreational facilities such as public parks after school.

The large proportion of students demonstrating little to no amounts of physical activity raises questions about adherence to use of the GPS device. Most of the assessment occurred with the help of the school staff, and while parents were included during consenting procedures, it is possible that parents were not supportive of students wearing GPS devices. Thus if children did not wear their GPS during times of physical activity, "capturing" that activity data could conceivably have been lost. This resulted in a large variability in the GPS measures and, consequently, in low statistical power when correlating the GPS measures with weight, fitness and insulin resistance measures. We set a minimum "threshold" of ninety minutes per day of GPS usage to be included in the activity analysis. While this threshold may be considered somewhat arbitrary, this was done to eliminate data from GPS devices that were unused, or idle, so as not to falsely lower the amount of activity "measured". Additionally, these data were collected in a single school, with its own distinctive built and cultural environment, and the findings may not be generalizable to other Hispanic communities or other urban communities.

Promoting physical activity during childhood and developing active patterns of moving through one's daily environment are positive steps toward reducing health consequences associated with obesity and poor fitness [26]. Hispanic youth show unique risks for obesity related illness [3,27] and, as suggested by the findings of this study of an urban environment, often display extremely low levels of PA which fall far short of federally recommended amounts of physical activity per day. These data provide evidence that reduced movement-associated energy expenditure is one factor contributing to susceptibility for obesity and T2DM risk in this group of children. If environmental interventions designed to increase physical activity can be envisioned and implemented, follow-up studies utilizing GPS will enable accurate assessment of their effect on children's movement, levels of physical activity, and energy expenditure.

Conclusion

Utilization of GPS to measure physical activity and its associated energy expenditure revealed that physical activity and EE were extremely low in a group of urban Hispanic children, far below recommendations for health during childhood. Analysis of movement at home, between home and school, and after school showed low levels of physical activity in all settings, indicating that previous school-based measures thus far have not increased PA, and suggesting limited outdoor play options and/or choices near home. This study strengthens the notion that there is need and opportunity for public health interventions that focus on environmental changes in the home, school, and community settings that facilitate daily physical activity for children living in an urban setting. Tools for accurately tracking physical activity are greatly needed. To provide objective documentation of changes in movement associated with and correctly attributable to such interventions, use of GPS technology may be helpful.

Abbreviations

HOMA: Homeostasis model assessment of insulin resistance; PACER: Progressive aerobic cardiovascular endurance run; CVF: Cardiovascular fitness; T2DM: Type 2 diabetes mellitus; GPS: Global positioning system; EE: Energy expenditure; PA: Physical activity.

Competing interests

The authors have no financial relationships relevant to this article to disclose. Potential conflicts of interest: The authors have no conflicts of interest relevant to disclose.

Authors' contributions

ALC: was principal investigator of the study, conceptualized and designed the study, recruited subjects for the study, drafted the initial manuscript, and approved the final version. JSS: helped with conception and design of the GPS methodology for this study, was the primary GPS analyst for the study, analyzed the GPS data, edited the manuscript, and approved the final version. SJV: helped with conception and design of the GPS methodology for this study, helped supervise the GPS analysis for the study, edited the manuscript, and approved the final version. JCE: helped design the study including power analysis and analysis plan, did the bio-statistical analyses for the study, edited the manuscript, and approved the final version. DBA: conceptualized and designed the study, recruited subjects for the study, edited the initial manuscript, and approved the final version. All authors read and approved the final manuscript.

Authors' information
Supported by the University of Wisconsin-Madison Wisconsin Partnership Program and College of Agricultural and Life Science. The sponsors had no involvement in the design, data collection or analysis.

Acknowledgements
Funding for this project was provided by the UW School of Medicine and Public Health from the Wisconsin Partnership Program with additional support from the UW College of Agricultural and Life Sciences. The study sponsors had no role in 1) study design; 2) the collection, analysis, and interpretation of data; 3) the writing of the report; and 4) the decision to submit the manuscript for publication.
The community engaged research project required a partnership among staff from the Community Research Office and Bruce Guadalupe Community School at the United Community Center, Milwaukee and researchers from the University of Wisconsin-Madison who are members of the Wisconsin Prevention for Obesity and Diabetes (WiPOD) network. Also contributing were staff from the UW Collaborative Center for Health Equity, home to a NIH/NIMHD funded Center of Excellence in Minority Health and Health Disparities (5 P60 MD003428). Special thanks to Andrea Maser MS and Margarita Santiago PhD.

Author details
[1]Department of Pediatrics, University of Wisconsin, 600 Highland Avenue, H4-436, Madison, WI 53792-4108, USA. [2]Land Information and Computer Graphics Facility, University of Wisconsin, 600 Highland Avenue, H4-436, Madison, WI 53792-4108, USA.

References
1. Berke EM, Koepsell T, Vernez A, Moudon RB, Larson EB: Association of the built environment with physical activity and obesity in older persons. *Am J Public Health* 2007, **97**(3):486–492.
2. Norman GJ, Nutter SK, Ryan S, Sallis JF, Patrick K: Community design and access to recreational facilities as correlates of adolescent physical activity and body-mass index. *J Phys Act Health* 2006, **3**(1):s118–s128.
3. Curtis VA, Carrel AL, Eickhoff JC, Allen DB: Gender and race influence metabolic benefits of fitness in children: a cross-sectional study. *Int J Pediatr Endocrinol* 2012, **2012**(1):4.
4. Lind C, Mirchandani GG, Castrucci BC, Chavez N, Handler A, Hoelscher DM: The effects of acculturation on healthy lifestyle characteristics among hispanic fourth-grade children in Texas Public Schools, 2004–2005. *J Sch Health* 2012, **82**(4):166–174.
5. Cong Z, Feng D, Liu Y, Esperat MC: Sedentary behaviors among Hispanic children: influences of parental support in a school intervention program. *Am J Health Promot* 2012, **26**(5):270–280.
6. Pate RR, Wang CY, Dowda M, Farrell SW, O'Neill JR: Cardiorespiratory fitness levels among us youth 12 to 19 years of age. *Arch Pediatr Adolesc Med* 2006, **160**:1005–1012.
7. Ortega FB, Ruiz JR, Castillo MJ, Sjostrom M: Physical fitness in childhood and adolescence: a powerful marker of health. *Int J Obes* 2008, **32**:1–11.
8. Katzmarzyk PT, Gagnon J, Leon AS, Skinner JS, Wilmore JH, Rao DC, Bouchard C: Fitness, fatness, and estimated coronary heart disease risk: the HERITAGE family study. *Med Sci Sports Exerc* 2001, **33**(4):585–590.
9. Must A, Strauss RS: Risks and consequences of childhood and adolescent obesity. [Review]. *Int J Obes Relat Metab Disord* 1999, **23**(Suppl 11):2–11.
10. Freedman DS, Srinivasan GL, Burke CL, Shear CL, Smoak CG, Harsha DW, Webber LS, Berenson GS: Relation of body fat distribution to hyperinsulinemia in children and adolescents. The Bogalusa Heart Study. *Am J Clin Nutr* 1987, **46**:403–410.
11. Brambilla P, Pozzobon G, Pietrobelli A: Physical activity as the main therapeutic tool for metabolic syndrome in childhood. *Int J Obes* 2011, **35**:16–28.
12. Dietz WH: Health consequences of obesity in youth: childhood predictors of adult disease. *Pediatrics* 1998, **101**:518–525.
13. Blair SN, Cheng Y, Holder JS: Is physical activity or physical fitness more important than defining health benefits? *Med Sci Sports Exerc* 2001, **33**:S379–S399.
14. Lee CD, Blair SN, Jackson AS: Cardiorespiratory fitness, body composition, and all-cause and cardiovascular disease mortality in men. *Am J Clin Nutr* 1999, **69**(3):373–380.
15. Morrison JA, Friedman LA, Gray-McGuire C: Metabolic syndrome in childhood predicts adult cardiovascular disease 25 years later: the Princeton lipid research follow-up study. *Pediatrics* 2007, **120**:340–345.
16. Centers for Disease Control and Prevention (CDC): Obesity in K-8 students - New York City, 2006–07 to 2010–11 school years. *MMWR Morb Mortal Wkly Rep* 2011, **60**(49):1673–1678.
17. Dobbins M, De Corby K, Robeson P, Husson H, Tirillis D: School-based physical activity programs for promoting physical activity and fitness in children and adolescents aged 6–18. *Cochrane Database Syst Rev* 2009, **21**(1):1–112.
18. Kumanyika SK, Obarzanek E, Stettler N, Poston WC: Population-based prevention of obesity: the need for comprehensive promotion of healthful eating, physical activity, and energy balance. *Circulation* 2008, **22**(118):428–464.
19. Stokols D, Misra S, Moser RP, Hall KL, Taylor BK: The ecology of team science: understanding contextual influences on transdisciplinary collaboration. *Am J Prev Med* 2008, **35**(2):s96–s115.
20. Ogden CL, Carroll MD, Kit BK, Flegal KM: Prevalence of obesity and trends in body mass index among US children and adolescents, 1999–2010. *JAMA* 2012, **307**:483–490.
21. Zhu W, Mahar MT, Welk GJ, Going SB, Cureton KJ: Approaches for development of criterion-referenced standards in health-related youth fitness tests. *Am J Prev Med* 2011, **41**(4 Suppl 2):S68–S76.
22. Carrel AL, Bowser J, White D, Moberg DP, Weaver B, Hisgen J, Eickhoff JC, Allen DB: Standardized childhood fitness percentiles derived from school-based testing. *J Pediatr* 2012, **161**:120–124.
23. Strong WB, Malina RM, Blimkie CJR: Evidence based physical activity for school-age youth. *J Pediatr* 2005, **146**(6):732–737.
24. Carroll-Scott A, Gilstad-Hayden K, Rosenthal L, Peters SM, McCaslin C, Joyce R, Ickovics JR: Disentangling neighborhood contextual associations with child body mass index, diet, and physical activity: the role of built, socioeconomic, and social environments. *Soc Sci Med* 2013, **95**:106–114.
25. Rainham DG, Bates CJ, Blanchard CM, Dummer TJ, Kirk SF, CSchearer CL: Spatial classification of youth physical activity patterns. *Am J Prev Med* 2012, **42**(5):e87–e96.
26. Allen DB: TODAY- a stark glimpse of tomorrow. *N Engl J Med* 2012, **366**:2315–2316.
27. Santiago-Torres M, Adams AK, Carrel AL, La Rowe TL, Schoeller DA: Home food availability, parental dietary intake, and family eating habits influence the diet quality of urban Hispanic children. *Child Obes* 2014, **10**(5):1–8.

20

Etiological and clinical characteristics of central diabetes insipidus in children: a single center experience

Janel D. Hunter and Ali S. Calikoglu[*]

Abstract

Background: Central diabetes insipidus (CDI) results from a number of conditions affecting the hypothalamic-neurohypophyseal system to cause vasopressin deficiency. Diagnosis of CDI is challenging, and clinical data and guidelines for management are lacking. We aim to characterize clinical and radiological characteristics of a cohort of pediatric patients with CDI.

Methods: A chart review of 35 patients with CDI followed at North Carolina Children's Hospital from 2000 to 2015 was undertaken. The frequencies of specific etiologies of CDI and characteristic magnetic resonance imaging (MRI) findings were determined. The presence of additional hormone deficiencies at diagnosis and later in the disease course was ascertained. Patient characteristics and management strategies were evaluated.

Results: The cohort included 14 female and 21 male patients with a median age of 4.7 years (range, less than 1 month to 16 years) at diagnosis. Median duration of follow-up was 5 years (range, 2 months to 16 years). The cause of CDI was intracranial mass in 13 patients (37.2 %), septo-optic dysplasia in 9 patients (25.7 %), holoprosencephaly in 5 patients (14.2 %), Langerhans cell histiocytosis in 3 patients (8.6 %), isolated pituitary hypoplasia in 2 patients (5.7 %), and encephalocele in 1 patient (2.9 %). Patients were symptomatic for a mean of 6.3 months (range, less than 1 month to 36 months) prior to diagnosis of CDI. Growth hormone (GH), thyrotropin (TSH), adrenocorticotropic hormone (ACTH), and gonadotropin deficiencies were present at diagnosis in 34, 23, 23, and 6 % of patients, respectively. GH, TSH, ACTH, and gonadotropin deficiencies were diagnosed during follow-up in 23, 40, 37, and 14 % of patients, respectively. In patients with structural CNS abnormalities, development of additional hormone deficiencies occurred anywhere from 2 months to 13 years after the time of initial presentation.

Conclusions: All patients in our cohort had an underlying organic etiology for CDI, with intracranial masses and CNS malformations being most common. Therefore, MRI of the brain is indicated in all pediatric patients with CDI. Other pituitary hormone deficiencies should be investigated at diagnosis as well as during follow-up.

Keywords: Diabetes insipidus, Hypopituitarism, Vasopressin, Magnetic resonance imaging

Background

Central diabetes insipidus (CDI) is characterized by polyuria, polydipsia, and the inability to concentrate urine as a result of arginine vasopressin deficiency. Maintenance of normal tonicity of extracellular fluids is vital to cellular function and is regulated by the complex interaction of fluid intake, vasopressin secretion, and urine output. Dysfunction of the system that maintains water homeostasis may result in life-threatening hypernatremia, seizures, dehydration, and failure to thrive. Vasopressin is synthesized by neurons of the hypothalamic paraventricular and supraoptic nuclei and secreted by the posterior pituitary gland [1]. Therefore, malformation or damage to midline cerebral and cranial structures may result in the absence of vasopressin production or secretion. Known etiologies of CDI include central nervous system (CNS) tumors, post-neurosurgical or accidental trauma, autoimmune disease, or infiltrative diseases. Genetic mutations resulting in abnormal synthesis of vasopressin precursor hormones

* Correspondence: ali_calikoglu@med.unc.edu
Division of Pediatric Endocrinology, University of North Carolina at Chapel Hill, Campus Box #7039, Medical School Wing E, Chapel Hill, NC 27599, USA

may occur rarely [2]. In a large Danish study in 2014, the annual incidence of CDI overall was 3 to 4 patients per 100,000 with an incidence of 2 cases of congenital CDI per 100,000 infants [3].

CDI presents a number of diagnostic and therapeutic challenges. The diagnosis may be delayed during evaluation for more common etiologies of polydipsia and polyuria, and often requires formal water deprivation testing [1]. After the diagnosis of CDI is confirmed, further work-up to determine the etiology of CDI and to assess for additional pituitary hormone deficiencies is necessary; however, clear guidelines for which laboratory and imaging studies to obtain and at what intervals to repeat these investigations are lacking.

The mainstay of therapy for CDI is desmopressin (DDAVP), a synthetic analog of arginine vasopressin with an extended duration of action; however, education of patients and caregivers regarding the safe use of DDAVP is essential to minimize risks of water-intoxication and hyponatremia. Risks of DDAVP-associated hyponatremia are increased in neonates, in patients without an intact thirst mechanism, and in patients requiring high-volume intravenous fluid hydration for chemotherapy. Given the number of diagnostic and therapeutic challenges associated with CDI, we performed a retrospective chart review of a cohort of pediatric patients with CDI followed at the North Carolina Children's Hospital (NCCH) in order to describe our experience and to contribute further to generalizable knowledge about the diagnosis and management of CDI.

Methods

The study was approved by the University of North Carolina Institutional Review Board, and conducted in compliance with the Helsinki Declaration. The NCCH electronic medical record was reviewed in order to identify all patients with CDI followed in pediatric endocrinology clinic. All patients that have been evaluated for management or diagnosis of CDI in the past year were included. Extracted data included patient characteristics (age, gender, race), duration of clinical symptoms prior to diagnosis in those presenting with CDI, pituitary hormone laboratory evaluation, family history, neuroimaging study results, and pathology findings. Management strategies were also reviewed.

The frequencies of various etiologies of CDI as well as characteristic magnetic resonance imaging (MRI) findings were determined. CDI was diagnosed either by water deprivation testing or by the presence of concurrent polyuria, hypernatremia, elevated serum osmolality, low urine osmolality, and low urine specific gravity. The prevalence of additional anterior pituitary hormone deficiencies at each patient's presentation and the incidence of hormone deficiencies acquired later in the disease

course were also evaluated. The presence of a hormone deficiency was confirmed by laboratory evidence of insufficient hormone production.

Results

The cohort included 21 male patients and 14 female patients whose median age at diagnosis of CDI was 4.8 years (range, less than 1 month to 16 years). In the patients with CDI at their initial presentation, mean duration of symptoms prior to diagnosis was 6.3 months (range, less than 1 week to 36 months). Characteristics of the cohort and etiologies of CDI are reported in detail in Table 1. Etiologies included CNS malformations in 17 patients (48.5 %), intracranial masses in 13 patients (37.2 %), and Langerhans cell histiocytosis (LCH) in 3 patients (8.6 %). The underlying cause of CDI remains unclear in 2 patients (5.7 %) but both had abnormal MRI findings. Their cases are discussed in detail later in the article. No patients had a family history of DI. Median duration of follow-up was 5 years (range, 2 months to 16 years).

All patients underwent MRI of the brain. Thirty-three patients had neuroimaging performed at NCCH, and reports from referring hospitals were available for the remaining 2 patients. All but one had abnormalities on MRI of the brain including CNS malformations, intracranial masses, pituitary gland or stalk abnormalities. The one patient with a normal MRI of the brain was diagnosed with LCH (biopsy-proven) after presenting with

Table 1 Patient demographics and etiologies of central diabetes insipidus

Demographics	
Total Number of Patients, n	35
Female patients, n	14
Average Age of CDI Diagnosis, months	57.6 (0.73–192)
Time from Symptom Onset to CDI Diagnosis, months	6.4 (0.03–36)
Duration of Follow Up, months	60 (2.4–192)
Etiology	n (%)
Central Nervous System Malformation	*17 (48.5 %)*
Septo-Optic Dysplasia	9 (25.7 %)
Holoprosencephaly	5 (14.2 %)
Pituitary Hypoplasia	2 (5.7 %)
Encephalocele	1 (2.9 %)
Intracranial Mass	*13 (37.2 %)*
Craniopharyngioma	6 (17.1 %)
Astrocytoma	3 (8.6 %)
Germinoma	3 (8.6 %)
Pituitary Adenoma	1 (2.9 %)
Langerhans Cell Histiocytosis	*3 (8.6 %)*
Unknown	*2 (5.7 %)*

a posterior auricular mass. Of the 17 patients with CNS malformations on MRI, 9 (25.7 %) had septo-optic dysplasia (SOD), 5 (14.2 %) had holoprosencephaly, 2 (5.7 %) had isolated pituitary hypoplasia, and 1 (2.9 %) had a large encephalocele. MRI revealed intracranial masses in 13 patients (37.2 %), including craniopharyngioma (6 patients, 17.1 %), astrocytoma (3 patients, 8.6 %), germ cell tumor (3 patients, 8.6 %), and pituitary adenoma (1 patient, 2.9 %). Four patients had pituitary stalk thickening. Of these patients, 2 were diagnosed with LCH, 1 was diagnosed with a germ cell tumor, and 1 has not yet undergone biopsy to determine a definitive diagnosis. One patient had absence of the posterior pituitary bright spot alone, without other structural abnormalities on MRI.

Six of 35 patients required formal water deprivation testing for diagnosis of CDI. The remaining patients already fulfilled the diagnostic criteria. All patients who required water deprivation test had abnormal findings on MRI of the brain, and etiologies for CDI included LCH, ectopic pituitary gland, pituitary hypoplasia, SOD, astrocytoma, and pituitary adenoma. Two of 6 patients had ADH deficiency alone at the time of diagnosis while the remainder had concurrent hormone deficiencies at presentation.

Twenty-one patients (60 %) had CDI at their initial presentation and 10 patients (29 %) developed CDI as a result of neurosurgical management of intracranial masses (6 with craniopharyngioma, 2 with astrocytoma, 1 with germinoma, and 1 with adrenocorticoptropic hormone (ACTH) secreting pituitary adenoma). Four patients (2 with SOD and 2 with ectopic posterior pituitary glands) did not have CDI at presentation but developed it during the follow-up period. One of the patients with SOD was diagnosed with thyrotropin (TSH), ACTH, and growth hormone (GH) deficiencies at birth but did not

develop symptoms of CDI until 2 months of age. The second patient was diagnosed with SOD at 4 months of age but did not develop CDI until 12 years of age. One patient with an ectopic pituitary gland was diagnosed with panhypopituitarism except CDI at 2 months of age and developed CDI 1 year later. The other patient with an ectopic pituitary gland presented with GH deficiency and delayed puberty at 12 years of age and was diagnosed with CDI at 15 years of age.

GH deficiency was the most common concurrent hormone deficiency at presentation in patients with CDI and occurred in 12 patients (34 %). TSH, ACTH, and gonadotropin deficiencies were present at the time of diagnosis in 23 %, 23 %, and 6 % of patients, respectively. TSH deficiency was subsequently diagnosed in an additional 40 % of patients during follow-up. ACTH deficiency and gonadotropin deficiencies were later diagnosed in 37 % and 14 % of patients, respectively (Figure 1). Eighteen patients (51 %) were prepubertal in age so that the presence of gonadotropin deficiencies could not be assessed accurately. All 3 patients with LCH had CDI at presentation, and 1 developed subsequent hormone deficiencies as a result of disease progression and neurosurgery for diagnosis. Of the 5 patients with CDI as a result of holoprosencephaly, only 1 developed an additional hormone deficiency over time. The development of additional anterior hormone deficiencies occurred over time in 44 % of patients with SOD. Time from diagnosis of SOD to onset of subsequent hormone deficiencies ranged from months to years, with one patient having a normal pituitary evaluation at 4 months of age who did not develop subsequent hormone deficiencies until 12 years of age (see Table 2).

There were 2 patients with CDI of unclear etiology. The first patient has been followed at NCCH for 6 years. He has undergone MRI of the brain on an annual basis

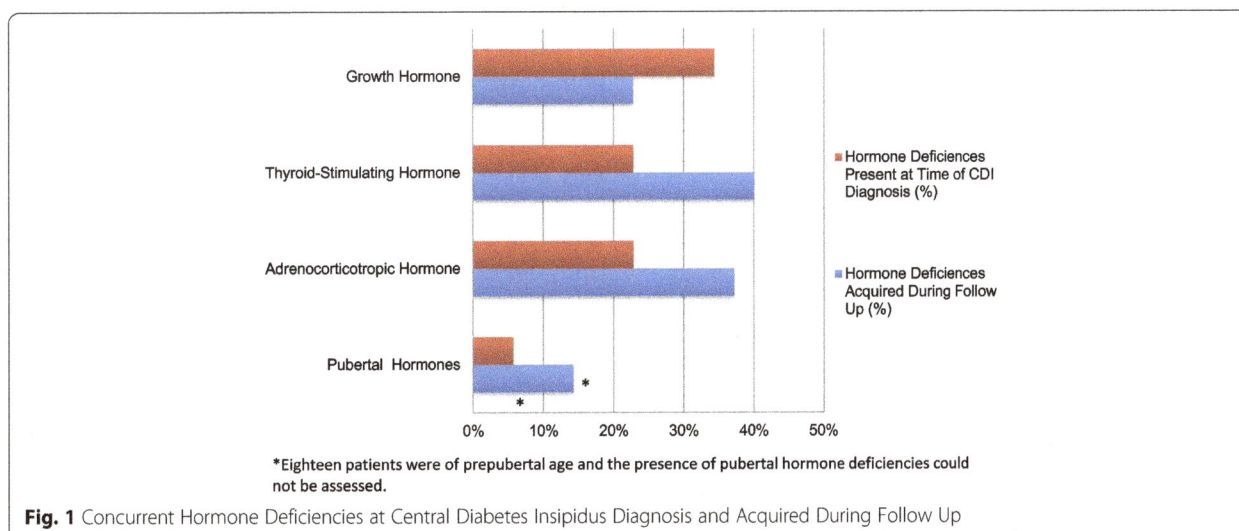

*Eighteen patients were of prepubertal age and the presence of pubertal hormone deficiencies could not be assessed.

Fig. 1 Concurrent Hormone Deficiencies at Central Diabetes Insipidus Diagnosis and Acquired During Follow Up

Table 2 Timing of development of pituitary hormone deficiencies in patients with cns malformations

Etiology	Age at diagnosis of CNS abnormality	Time from diagnosis of CNS abnormality to diagnosis of hormone deficiencies
Ectopic Pituitary	2 months	ACTH, GH, TSH, at presentationADH, 1 year
Holoprosencephaly	3 months	ADH, at presentationTSH, 2 years
Pituitary Hypoplasia	13 years	GH, at presentationTSH, 9 monthsADH, 2 yearsFSH, LH, 3 years
Septo-Optic Dysplasia	2 days	ACTH, GH, TSH, at presentationADH, 2 months
Septo-Optic Dysplasia	4 months	GH,12 yearsACTH, ADH, TSH, 13 years
Septo-Optic Dysplasia	8 months	ADH, GH, at presentationTSH, 1 year
Septo-Optic Dysplasia	22 months	ADH, GH, at presentationACTH, 2 years

which has demonstrated a stable 4 mm focus of hypoenhancement within his right pituitary gland which may represent a Rathke's cleft cyst or adenoma; however, he continues to follow-up with oncology given the possibility of LCH or germ cell tumor. He has had a total of two osseous surveys (2 years apart) that have failed to demonstrate evidence of LCH. He has undergone pituitary hormone screening every 6 to 12 months without development of subsequent hormone deficiencies. The other patient with CDI of unknown etiology is 13 year old female who presented for evaluation secondary amenorrhea, rapid weight gain, polydipsia and polyuria. She has been followed in our clinic for nearly 1 year, and her evaluation is significant for evidence of pituitary stalk thickening with absence of the posterior pituitary bright spot on MRI as well as TSH, GH, and gonadotropin deficiencies. A skeletal survey was normal. Neurosurgery has not yet agreed to obtain a biopsy for definitive diagnosis.

CDI in 31 patients was successfully managed with DDAVP. Chlorothiazide was used in 3 patients during infancy. One patient was managed with oral free water intake alone per the family's preference. One patient with an astrocytoma had resolution of CDI after four years as a result of surgical intervention and chemotherapy.

Discussion

In our series of pediatric patients with CDI, nearly all patients (97 %) had abnormalities on MRI of the brain, with CNS malformations and intracranial masses being the most common findings. Our findings are consistent with a recent study by Werny at al [4] that reports a higher prevalence of CNS malformations in patients with CDI than previously reported, as well as fewer idiopathic cases. We identified tumors or LCH in nearly half (46 %) of our patients with CDI, which is similar to the rate of tumors and infiltrative processes (56 %) found by Werny et al [4]. We did not identify any cases of familial/genetic, autoimmune, or idiopathic CDI, which is inconsistent with other previous studies citing familial causes in 7 % [4] and 6 % [5] and idiopathic etiology in 12 % [4] and 52 % [5]. These findings are likely a result

of our small sample size. Despite traumatic causes of CDI being reported in 3 % of cases overall [5], we did not identify any cases. This is likely due to the fact that patients may have had either nonsurvivable brain injuries or transient CDI, and we included only patients followed in our outpatient clinic. Also congruent with the Werny study, our patients with pituitary stalk thickening were likely to be diagnosed with LCH or germ cell tumor [4-6]. Given the high likelihood of identifying an underlying etiology, it is of utmost importance to obtain neuroimaging promptly in patients diagnosed with CDI. In our cohort of patients with CDI, there was a high incidence of concurrent anterior pituitary hormone deficiencies. Hormone insufficiencies evolved over time in many of our patients with CNS malformations, particularly in those with SOD, or occurred abruptly as a result of neurosurgical intervention in patients with intracranial masses. Multiple pituitary hormone insufficiencies were identified at the time of diagnosis in 89 % of patients with SOD. Forty-four percent of patients with SOD developed additional hormone deficiencies anywhere from 2 months to 13 years after initial diagnosis [7], highlighting the importance of regular screening. This is in contrast to our patients with holoprosencephaly who were less likely to demonstrate evolution of anterior pituitary hormone deficiencies over time. These patients, who may have abnormal osmoreceptor function (previously termed "essential hypernatremia"), as a result of hypothalamic, rather than pituitary dysfunction [8, 9], may warrant less diligent hormonal screening evaluations over time compared to those with SOD; however, larger studies are needed to identify appropriate time intervals for repeat screening. The requirement for water deprivation testing to achieve the diagnosis of CDI was not associated with a specific underlying etiology or with the presence or absence of concurrent hormone deficiencies in our cohort.

CDI was managed successfully with DDAVP in the majority of patients in our cohort; however, patients in the neonatal period present a particular therapeutic challenge [8]. In our experience, DDAVP titration was problematic in such young patients and often resulted in wide fluctuations in sodium levels, including severe hyponatremia that occasionally resulted in seizures. In agreement with previous reports, we have been able to maintain acceptable sodium concentrations using chlorothiazide and low solute formula in infants up to 6 months of age, after which DDAVP doses may be titrated more easily [10, 11].

There are some limitations to our study that should be considered. First, the retrospective nature of our study results in inter-patient variability in the diagnosis of pituitary hormone deficiencies (random laboratory values versus provocative testing) and evaluation of hormone deficiencies over time. Furthermore, diagnostic laboratory data was limited in patients that had begun hormone replacement therapy prior to referral to our clinic. It is also likely that the incidence of gonadotropin deficiency is underreported given that many of our patients are too young to manifest symptoms of delayed puberty. Additionally, variability in MRI interpretation may result in under or over reporting of pituitary abnormalities. Finally, our population may not be representative of all children with CDI because we included only patients followed in the outpatient setting, excluding those with nonsurvivable CNS insults or transient CDI.

Conclusions

Most children with CDI have abnormal findings on MRI of the brain, with intracranial masses and CNS malformations being most common. Therefore, the diagnosis of idiopathic CDI should be made with extreme caution in children, and only after extensive evaluation, including MRI of the brain, has been obtained. GH deficiency was the most common concurrent hormone deficiency at presentation in patients with CDI. TSH and ACTH deficiencies were more commonly diagnosed during follow-up evaluation; however, the development of additional hormone deficiencies in patients who did not undergo surgical intervention remains unpredictable, especially in those with SOD. Continued screening for endocrine dysfunction is warranted though further studies are needed to determine the most appropriate screening interval.

Abbreviations
ACTH: Adrenocorticotropic hormone; CDI: Central diabetes insipidus; CNS: Central nervous system; DDAVP: Desmopressin; GH: Growth hormone; LCH: Langerhans cell histiocytosis; MRI: Magnetic resonance imaging; NCCH: North Carolina children's hospital; SOD: Septo-optic dysplasia; TSH: Thyroid-stimulating hormone.

Competing interests
The authors declare that they have no competing interests.

Author's contributions
JDH acquired and interpreted the data, drafted the initial manuscript, and approved the final manuscript as submitted. ASC conceptualized the study, critically reviewed the manuscript, and approved the final manuscript as submitted.

Acknowledgement
We thank to Dr. Elizabeth Estrada for critical review of the article.

References
1. Muglia LH, Majzoub JA. Disorders of the posterior pituitary. In: Sperling M, editor. Pediatric endocrinology. 3rd ed. Philadelphia: Saunders Elsevier; 2008. p. 335–73.
2. Di Iorgi N, Napoli F, Allegri AE, Olivieri I, Bertelli E, Gallizia A, et al. Diabetes insipidus—diagnosis and management. Horm Res Paediatr. 2012;77(2):69–84.
3. Juul KV, Schroeder M, Rittig S, Norgaard JP. National Surveillance of Central Diabetes Insipidus (CDI) in Denmark: results from 5 years registration of 9309 prescriptions of desmopressin to 1285 CDI patients. J Clin Endocrinol Metab. 2014;99(6):2181–7.
4. Werny D, Elfers C, Perez FA, Pihoker C, Roth CL. Pediatric central diabetes insipidus: brain malformations are common and few patients have idiopathic disease. J Clin Endocrinol Metab. 2015;100:3074–80.
5. Leger J, Velasquez A, Garel C, Hassan M, Czernichow P. Thickened pituitary stalk on magnetic resonance imaging in children with central diabetes insipidus. J Clin Endocrinol Metab. 1999;84:1954–60.
6. Maghnie M, Cosi G, Genovese E, Manca-Bitti ML, Cohen A, Zecca S, et al. Central diabetes insipidus in children and young adults. N Engl J Med. 2000; 343:998–1007.
7. Oatman OJ, McClellan DR, Olson ML, Garcia-Filion P. Endocrine and pubertal disturbances in optic nerve hypoplasia, from infancy to adolescence. Int J Pediatr Endocrinol. 2015;8:1–6.
8. Suneja M, Makki N, Kuppachi S. Essential hypernatremia: evidence of reset osmostat in the absence of demonstrable hypothalamic lesions. Am J Med Sci. 2014;347(4):341–2.
9. Oh MS, Carroll HJ. Essential hypernatremia: is there such a thing? Nephron. 1994;67(2):144–5.
10. Pogacar PR, Mahnke S, Rivkees SA. Management of central diabetes insipidus in infancy with low renal solute load formula and chlorothiazide. Curr Opin Pediatr. 2000;12(4):405–11.
11. Rivkees SA, Dunbar N, Wilson TA. The management of central diabetes insipidus in infancy: desmopressin, low renal solute load formula, thiazide diuretics. J Pediatr Endocrinol Metab. 2007;20(4):459–69.

21

Body mass index in girls with idiopathic central precocious puberty during and after treatment with GnRH analogues

A. J. Arcari[*], M. G. Gryngarten, A. V. Freire, M. G. Ballerini, M. G. Ropelato, I. Bergadá and M. E. Escobar

Abstract

Background: In girls with Idiopathic Central Precocious Puberty (ICPP) concern has been raised by the potential impact of GnRH-analogues (GnRHa) treatment on body weight. We evaluated the effect of GnRHa on Body Mass Index (BMI) in girls with ICPP according to weight status at diagnosis.

Methods: One hundred seventeen ICPP girls were divided according to pretreatment weight status in: normal weight (NW), overweight (OW) and obese (OB). BMI at one and two years of treatment was assessed. BMI-SDS of 60 patients who reached adult height (AH) was compared to that of 33 ICPP untreated girls.

Results: NW girls significantly increased their baseline BMI-SDS at 1 and 2 years of treatment. OW girls only had a significant increment at one year of treatment while OB girls showed no BMI-SDS change. Patients evaluated at AH (at least four years after GnRHa withdrawal) showed a significant decrease on BMI compared to baseline and a significantly lower BMI than the untreated group.

Conclusion: In ICPP girls the BMI increase under GnRHa was inversely related to the pretreatment weight status. In the long term follow-up, no detrimental effect of GnRHa on body weight was observed. BMI-SDS was lower in treated than in untreated girls.

Keywords: Central Precocious Puberty, BMI, GnRH analogues

Background

Central Precocious Puberty (CPP) results from the premature activation of the hypothalamo-pituitary-ovarian axis. In girls, it is defined as the onset of secondary sexual development before the age of 8 with further progression, accompanied by increased growth velocity and bone age acceleration usually leading to adult height impairment.

Gonadotropin-releasing hormone analogues (GnRHa) are the treatment of choice in CPP and their effectiveness on adult height (AH) improvement has been widely recognized. However, concern has been raised by the potential impact of this treatment on body weight. While some studies have reported association between GnRHa treatment and Body Mass Index (BMI) increase [1–7],

others have found no influence of GnRHa treatment on weight status [8–13] or even some decrease in BMI under therapy [14–16]. It has been demonstrated that girls with CPP are prone to developing obesity (8). A few reports have analyzed the influence of GnRHa on body weight according to BMI status at onset of treatment. However, in some of these studies follow-up was limited to a period under treatment or to a short time after withdrawal [17–19], whereas studies with a long-term follow-up did not categorize patients according to pre-treatment BMI status [20, 21].

The aim of the present study was to evaluate the impact of GnRHa therapy on BMI in girls with Idiopathic CPP (ICPP) according to weight status at diagnosis up to adult height (AH). The subgroup of patients who achieved AH was compared to a control group of untreated ICPP girls.

* Correspondence: aarcari@cedie.org.ar; ajarcari@hotmail.com
Centro de Investigaciones Endocrinológicas "Dr. César Bergadá" (CEDIE),
CONICET – FEI – División de Endocrinología, Hospital de Niños Ricardo
Gutiérrez, Gallo 1330, C1425EFD Buenos Aires, Argentina

Patients and methods

Patients

This retrospective study was done reviewing the clinical charts of 117 girls with ICPP referred to the Division of Endocrinology of the Hospital de Niños Ricardo Gutiérrez (Buenos Aires, Argentina) from 1985 to 2010. All patients were treated for at least two years with intramuscular depot GnRHa (Triptorelin acetate), at a dose of 100–120 ug/kg, every 28 days for 2.8 ± 0.2 years; no patient received additional medications.

Inclusion criteria: patients with diagnosis of ICPP according to the following criteria: (1) onset of breast development before 8 years of chronological age (CA), (2) height velocity above the 97 centile for age and bone age (BA) advancement by at least one year over CA, (3) pubertal LH response to GnRH (≥ 6 mUI/ml), (4) uterine length $\geq$ to 35 mm. Exclusion criteria: organic central precocious puberty, congenital adrenal hyperplasia and any other underlying condition or medication that might affect body weight.

Patients were divided into three groups according to weight status at start of therapy: normal weight (NW); overweight (OW) and obese (OB). BMI at the end of first and second year of GnRH treatment was assessed. No specific life style intervention was recommended to any patient. At the time of reaching AH, auxological parameters in 60 patients were compared to those of a control group of 33 girls with ICPP who had not received treatment (age of menarche 9.5 ± 0.3).

Methods

Clinical and auxological features were assessed as follows: pubertal stage according to Marshall and Tanner criteria [22]; height in cm measured by a Harpenden stadiometer; weight using a calibrated scale; bone age according to Greulich and Pyle [23].

Weight status was determined as BMI and it was expressed as BMI-SDS using the software Auxology version 1.0 b 17 Copyright® 2003 Pfizer. Overweight was defined as BMI > 85th centile and obesity as BMI > 95th centile according to Cole criteria [24].

AH was defined when two successive height measurements six months apart were equal or less than 0.5 cm, and/or when BA was equal or greater than 15 years. This study fulfilled the requirements defined by the Ethical Committee of Hospital de Niños Ricardo Gutiérrez for retrospective studies. Reference number CEI 11.053.

Statistical analyses were performed using GraphPad Prism version 5.00 for Windows (GraphPad Software, San Diego, CA). Changes on BMI were analyzed by ANOVA for repeated measurements. *Post hoc* Tukey's multiple comparison test was performed when differences were detected by ANOVA. Chi square test was used to compare the percentage of NW, OW and OB girls in the whole group at treatment start vs the percentage of NW, OW and OB girls in those who reached AH. The comparison between patients and control girls who reached AH was done using Mann Whitney test. $P < 0.05$ was considered statistically significant. Data is expressed as mean $\pm$ SD.

Results

A total of 117 girls with ICPP were studied. At treatment start all patients had breast development Grade II-III (Tanner) and three of them have had menarche. CA was 7.6 ± 1.3 years, BA 9.6 ± 0.16 years, height SDS 1.71 ± 0.08. The uterine length was 37.2 ± 0.7 mm.

Before treatment, BMI in the whole group was 18.5 ± 2.4 (SDS 1.1 ± 1). BMI distribution by groups showed: 48 % girls NW, 37 % OW and 15 % OB. No significant difference in chronological age was observed among groups, p: ns (Table 1).

The whole cohort of patients significantly increased their baseline BMI-SDS (1.1 ± 1) at year one (1.35 ± 0.95, $p < 0.001$) and year two (1.26 ± 0.1 $p < 0.01$) of treatment. When changes in BMI were analyzed according to the initial weight status, NW patients showed a significant increase in BMI-SDS from 0.3 ± 0.7 to 0.7 ± 0.8 at one year of treatment and 0.6 ± 0.8 at two years ($p < 0.001$). In OW girls a significant increase was only observed between baseline (1.5 ± 0.2) and one year of treatment (1.7 ± 0.5) ($p < 0.05$). OB girls showed no BMI-SDS changes during treatment (baseline 2.4 ± 0.3, year one 2.4 ± 0.4 and year two 2.3 ± 0.6) (Fig. 1).

A subset of 60 girls were followed up to AH [160.4 ± 0.7 cm (SDS -0.01 ± 0.14)], which was achieved at 4.4 ± 0.4 years after GnRHa withdrawal. BMI composition at beginning of treatment of the group of girls who attained AH was not different from that of the whole group (NW 47 % vs 48 %, OW 33 % vs 37 %, OB 20 % vs 15 %, respectively, p = ns). All girls in the AH group showed a significant decrease on BMI-SDS at the moment of reaching AH (0.5 ± 1.1) compared to BMI-SDS at start (1.0 ± 1.1), $p < 0.001$. A similar pattern was observed when the BMI status was analyzed in each subgroup (Table 2) (Fig. 2). The BMI-SDS of the 60 treated patients who reached adult height was 0.5 ± 1.1, significantly lower

Table 1 Auxological characteristics of the whole group at start of treatment

	Age (years)	BMI at start (kg/m^2)	BMI-SDS at start
All patients ($n = 117$)	7.6 ± 1.3	18.5 ± 2.4	1.1 ± 1
Normal Weight ($n = 56$)	7.53 ± 1.3	16.5 ± 1.3	0.3 ± 0.7
Overweight ($n = 43$)	7.33 ± 1.5	19.3 ± 4.7	1.5 ± 0.3
Obese ($n = 18$)	7.74 ± 0.8	22.4 ± 1.2	2.4 ± 0.3

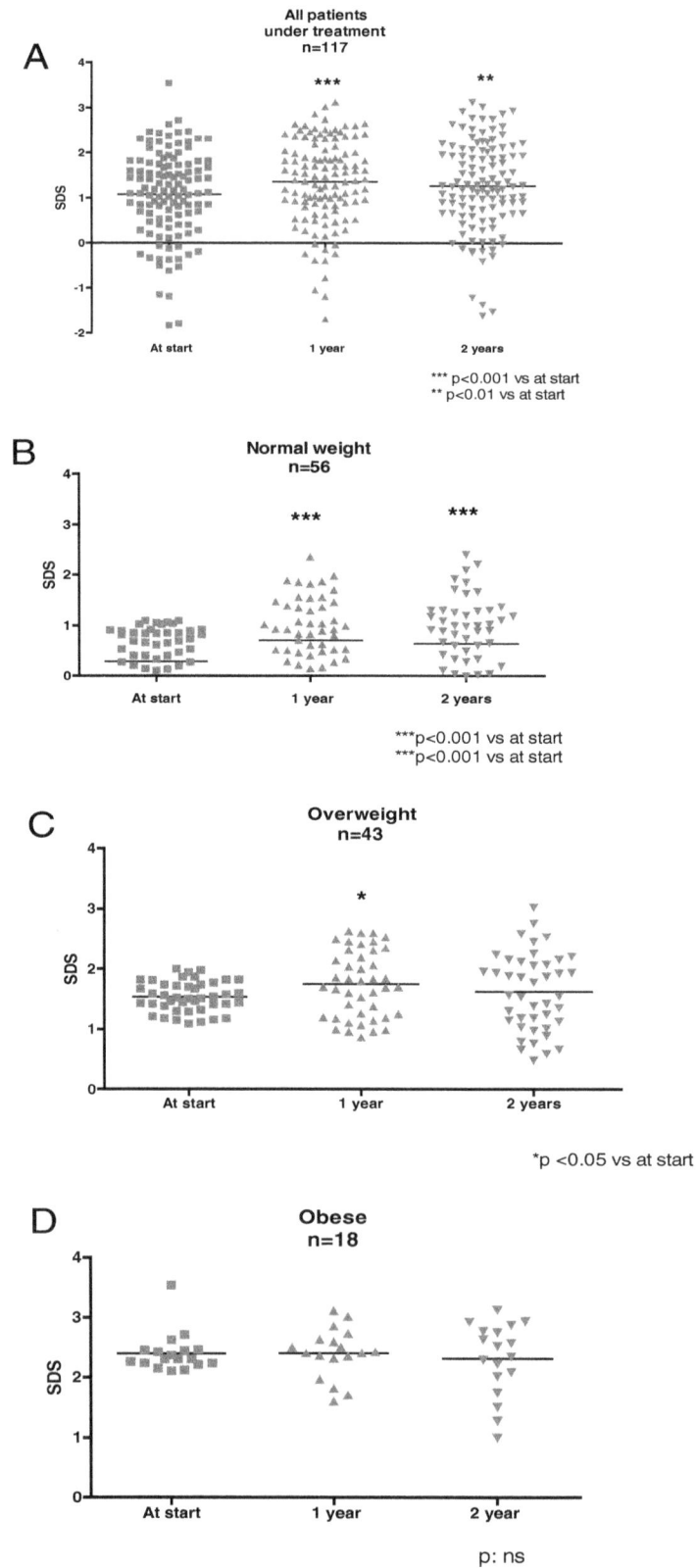

Fig. 1 BMI evolution of patients with ICPP during treatment with GnRHa. **a** All, **b** Normal weight, **c** Overweight, **d** Obese

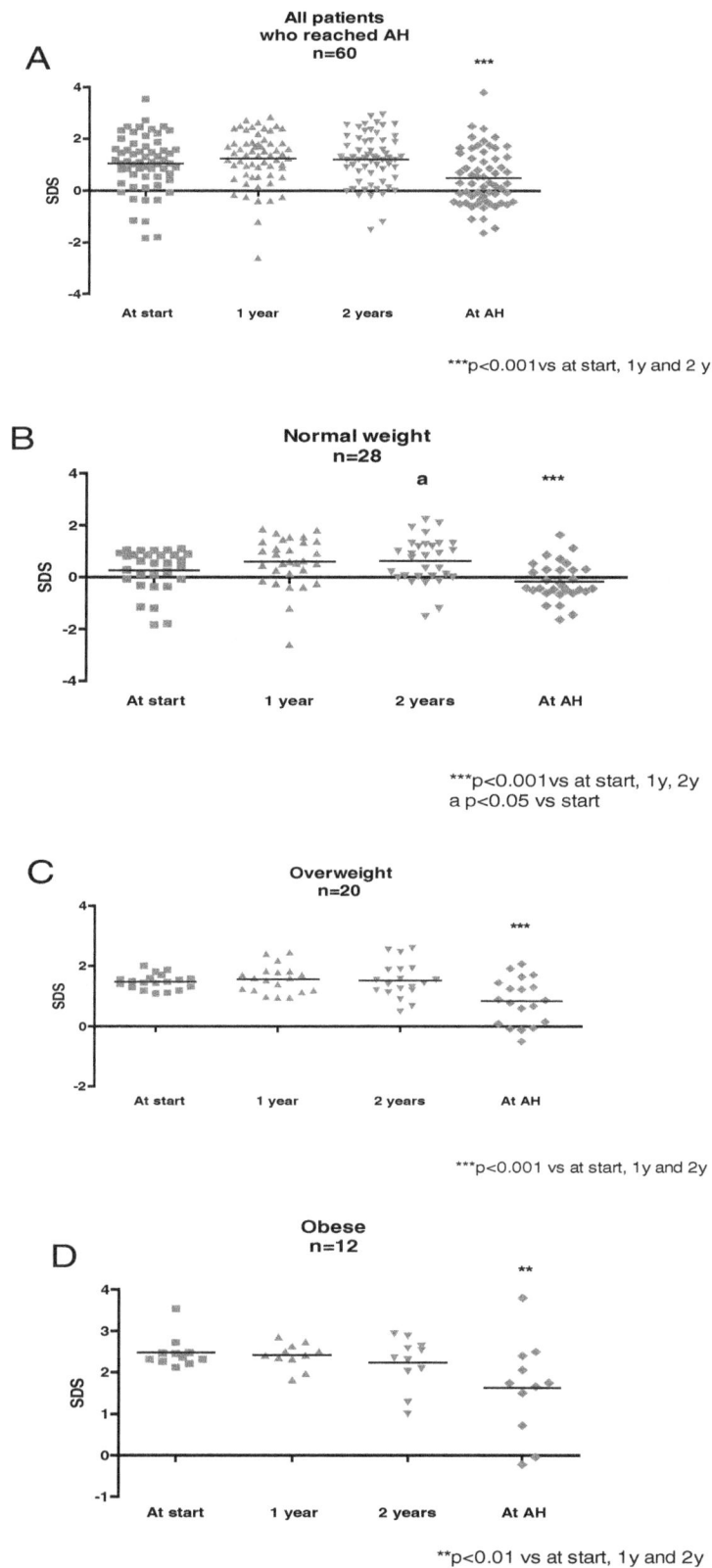

A All patients who reached AH n=60

***p<0.001vs at start, 1y and 2 y

B Normal weight n=28

***p<0.001vs at start, 1y, 2y
a p<0.05 vs start

C Overweight n=20

***p<0.001 vs at start, 1y and 2y

D Obese n=12

**p<0.01 vs at start, 1y and 2y

Fig. 2 BMI evolution during treatment in 60 patients at the time of reaching Adult Height. **a** All, **b** Normal weight, **c** Overweight, **d** Obese

Table 2 Auxological characteristics in girls who reached adult height (AH)

	BMI at start (SDS)	BMI at AH (SDS)
All patients ($n = 60$)	1.0 ± 1.1	0.5 ± 1.1
Normal Weight ($n = 28$)	0.25 ± 0.8	-0.19 ± 0.7
Overweight ($n = 20$)	1.4 ± 0.2	0.7 ± 0.7 b,c
Obese ($n = 12$)	2.4 ± 0.4	1.57 ± 1.1 a

ANOVA a < 0.0001 vs NW, b 0.001 vs NW, c 0.03 vs OB. Unpaired *t* Test start vs at AH: All patients *p* 0.004, NW *p* 0.07, OW *p* 0.0004, OB *p* 0.03

Table 3 Evolution of BMI category during follow-up in each subgroup

At start	At Adult Height (N° of patients)
NW $n = 28$	NW 27
	OW 1
	OB 0
OW $n = 20$	NW 14
	OW 5
	OB 1
OB $n = 12$	NW 4
	OW 4
	OB 4

than the BMI-SDS of the untreated control group, 1.3 $\pm$ 1.00 ($p = 0.0004$) (Fig. 3).

The evolution of the weight status from start to AH in each category is shown in Table 3.

Discussion

The present study evaluates the long-term effect of a monthly depot GnRHa therapy on BMI in a large cohort of 117 girls with ICPP from a single endocrine pediatric center in relation to weight status at diagnosis, along treatment and at AH in a subset of 60 patients.

Girls with ICPP at the moment of diagnosis usually have a high prevalence of overweight and obesity [17–19, 25], although if early puberty is the cause or the consequence of the increased body fat remains unclear. In agreement with the literature, before treatment our patients had an elevated proportion of overweight and obesity, 37 and 15 % respectively, these rates are higher than those of average Argentinian girls of the same age, 20.8 and 5.4 % [26].

The impact of GnRHa treatment on body weight in our patients was clearly related to the pretreatment condition. Although the whole cohort of ICPP patients showed a BMI increase along treatment, the negative effect of the GnRHa seemed to decrease as the pretreatment weight was higher. Girls in the NW subgroup showed an increase of BMI at one and two years of treatment while OW girls had a higher BMI only at year

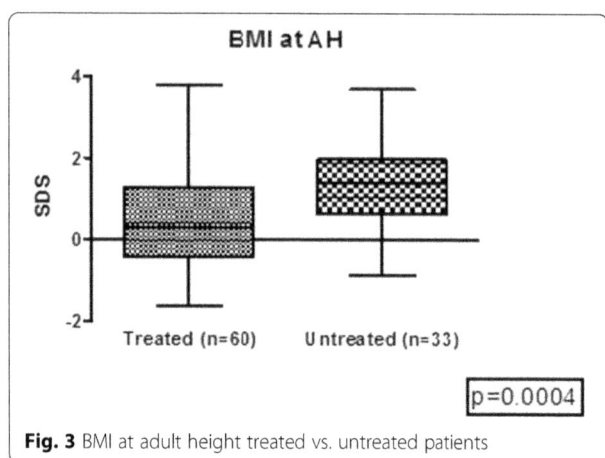

Fig. 3 BMI at adult height treated vs. untreated patients

one, while no changes were observed in OB girls along the treatment.

The inconsistency in the results about the effect of GnRHa on body weight found in the literature could be related to differences in the studied populations, i.e., mixed early and precocious puberty, idiopathic and organic CPP, and/or comparison with heterogeneous control groups.

While some authors found no changes in body weight on ICPP patients under GnRHa [8–13], few studies categorized patients according to pretreatment BMI to analyze the effect of treatment. Some reports showed that OW/OB girls at baseline remained unchanged or increased at the end of treatment, without any reference to NW patients [27, 28].

Lee et al. studied a group of girls with CPP (including 3 with organic CPP) during 18 months on treatment with GnRHa, and showed a significant BMI increase in the whole group, higher although not significant, in NW than in OW patients [18].

Wolters et al. evaluated a mixed group of girls with early or precocious puberty treated with GnRHa during one year according to pretreatment weight status and compared the OW subgroup to an OW untreated control group. In agreement with our study, their whole population of girls with CPP had a significant BMI increase along treatment, as well as the NW subset patients, whereas OW girls showed no changes in BMI while the OW control group showed a BMI increase [17].

Colmenares et al. analyzed 37 girls with ICPP and 34 girls with early puberty under GnRHa treatment, compared to a heterogeneous control group of untreated girls (3 with CPP who refused treatment, 2 with slowly progressive CPP and 20 with early slowly progressive puberty). In this study 72.9 % of the girls with ICPP were OW or OB, a percentage significantly higher than that of OW/OB girls with early puberty (35.3 %). The entire group of treated ICPP girls showed no changes in BMI at one and two years of treatment, whereas an increase at year three was observed compared to the control group. However, no individual analysis was performed in relation to the weight status at baseline [19].

The few reports evaluating body weight status in ICPP patients after GnRHa treatment showed return to pre-treatment values [27] or no differences in BMI when compared to untreated control girls [20, 29]. Lazar et al. analyzed the evolution of a large cohort of CPP treated patients at the third to fifth decades of life and found that although the BMI was increased at start and during early treatment, it normalized thereafter [30]. None of the studies with a long-term follow-up analyzed BMI in relation to the weight status at the beginning of treatment.

Our subgroup of 60 patients evaluated at least four years after GnRHa withdrawal, when they had reached AH, showed a significant decrease in BMI compared to pre-treatment BMI. The same pattern was observed when BMI status was analyzed for each subgroup. Approximately 2/3 of OW and 2/3 of OB patients showed a decrease in weight status, whereas only 1 /28 NW girls had become OW at AH. Furthermore, this subgroup with a long-term follow-up had a significantly lower BMI than the control group of untreated CPP girls, both compared at AH.

Categorizing our patients according to their weight status at start, along and after treatment allowed us to observe that only NW girls increased their BMI during treatment, while OW and OB girls did not, despite no changes in dietary habits or exercise were prescribed. Wolters et al. found a similar BMI behavior in CPP treated patients. The BMI of their OW girls (authors did not categorize between OW and OB) remained stable while a control group of untreated girls showed a significant BMI increase during follow-up, and they suggested a positive effect of GnRHa on weight status in OW children [17]. We did not have a control group of untreated patients evaluated as from the moment of diagnosis, but the comparison between our treated CPP girls with our group of untreated patients at AH status showed a significantly lower BMI among treated girls, thus seeming to confirm Wolters´s suggestion.

A limitation in our study was that we were able to analyze the body composition as a marker of nutritional status only on a small group of girls. There are a few reports evaluating the changes in body composition in CPP under GnRHa treatment. Van der Sluis et al. observed an increase of fat mass (estimated by DEXA) during treatment and a normalization after withdrawal. Chiocca et al. analyzed a cohort of CPP girls after GnRHa treatment at near final height and found no changes in BMI but an increase of total fat mass compared to a control group. Both authors suggested that the body fat accumulation was related to the estrogen depletion produced by GnRHa, as a "menopausal effect" [5, 14].

At present, there is no clear explanation of the different effects produced by GnRHa treatment on lean and

overweight ICPP girls. Although no specific prescription on life style was given to our patients, it is not possible to rule out that the fact that OW/OB girls did not increase their BMI under treatment could have been related to a family concern about weight gain leading to changes in dietary or physical activity.

Although in the present study, we did not systematically analyze the metabolic profile of our patients, Colmenares et al. found no differences for glucose and lipids at baseline and during follow-up among treated children [19].

Conclusions

In conclusion, in our study, although a moderate increase in BMI was observed throughout the first and second year on GnRHa treatment, mainly in NW girls, such increase did not lead to further obesity since a significant improvement on BMI was observed when girls achieved adult height. Furthermore, the fact that treated girls had a lower BMI than untreated girls at adult height allowed us to rule out a long-term detrimental effect of GnRHa treatment on body mass in girls with Central Precocious Puberty. Further studies analyzing changes in body composition are desired.

Abbreviations
AH, adult height; BA, bone age; BMI, Body Mass Index; CA, chronological age; CPP, Central Precocious Puberty; GnRHa, GnRH-analogues; ICPP, Idiopathic Central Precocious Puberty; NW, normal weight; OB, obese; OW, overweight

Acknowledgements
Not applicable.

Funding
This research has no sources of funding.

Authors' contributions
All authors made substantial contributions to the conception and design of this data. All authors read and approved the final manuscript.

Authors' information
All authors work at the Endocrinology Division of Hospital de Niños Ricardo Gutiérrez.

Competing interests
The authors declare that they have no competing interests.

References
1.   Boot AM, De Muinck K-SS, Pols HA, Krenning EP, Drop SL. Bone mineral density and body composition before and during treatment with

gonadotropin-releasing hormone agonist in children with central precocious and early puberty. J Clin Endocrinol Metab. 1998;83(2):370–3.

2. Feuillan P, Jones J, Barnes K, Oerter-Klein K, Cutler Jr G. Reproductive axis after discontinuation of gonadotropin-releasing hormone analog treatment of girls with precocious puberty: long term follow-up comparing girls with hypothalamic hamartoma to those with idiopathic precocious puberty. J Clin Endocrinol Metab. 1999;84(1):44–9.

3. Chiumello G, Brambilla P, Guarneri MP, Russo G, Manzoni P, Sgaramella P. Precocious puberty and body composition: effects of GnRH analog treatment. J Pediatr Endocrinol Metab. 2000;13 Suppl 1:791–4.

4. Traggiai C, Perucchin P, Zerbini K, Gastaldi R, De Biasio P, Lorini R. Outcome after depot gonadotrophin-releasing hormone agonist treatment for central precocious puberty: effects on body mass index and final height. Eur J Endocrinol. 2005;153(3):463–4.

5. Chiocca E, Dati E, Baroncelli GI, Mora S, Parrini D, Erba P, Bertelloni S. Body mass index and body composition in adolescents treated with gonadotropin-releasing hormone analogue triptorelin depot for central precocious puberty: data at near final height. Neuroendocrinology. 2009; 89(4):441–7. doi:10.1159/000197862. Epub 2009 Jan 29.

6. Taşcilar ME, Bilir P, Akinci A, Köse K, Akçora D, Inceoğlu D, Fitöz SO. The effect of gonadotropin-releasing hormone analog treatment (leuprolide) on body fat distribution in idiopathic central precocious puberty. Turk J Pediatr. 2011;53(1):27–33.

7. Anık A, Çatlı G, Abacı A, Böber E. Effect of gonadotropin-releasing hormone agonist therapy on body mass index and growth in girls with idiopathic central precocious puberty. Indian J Endocrinol Metab. 2015;19(2):267–71.

8. Palmert MR, Mansfield MJ, Crowley Jr WF, Crigler Jr JF, Crawford JD, Boepple PA. Is obesity an outcome of gonadotropin-releasing hormone agonist administration? Analysis of growth and body composition in 110 patients with central precocious puberty. J Clin Endocrinol Metab. 1999; 84(12):4480–8.

9. Heger S, Partsch CJ, Sippell WG. Long-term outcome after depot gonadotropin-releasing hormone agonist treatment of central precocious puberty: final height, body proportions, body composition, bone mineral density, and reproductive function. J Clin Endocrinol Metab. 1999;84(12):4583–90.

10. Lazar L, Kauli R, Pertzelan A, Phillip M. Gonadotropin-suppressive therapy in girls with early and fast puberty affects the pace of puberty but not total pubertal growth or final height. J Clin Endocrinol Metab. 2002;87(5):2090–4.

11. Glab E, Barg E, Wikiera B, Grabowski M, Noczyńska A. Influence of GnRH analog therapy on body mass in central precocious puberty. Pediatr Endocrinol Diabetes Metab. 2009;15(1):7–11.

12. Ko JH, Lee HS, Lim JS, Kim SM, Hwang JS. Changes in bone mineral density and body composition in children with central precocious puberty and early puberty before and after one year of treatment with GnRH agonist. Horm Res Paediatr. 2011;75:174–9.

13. Arani KS, Heidari F. Gonadotropin-releasing hormone agonist therapy and obesity in girls. Int J Endocrinol Metab. 2015;13(3):e23085. doi:10.5812.

14. van der Sluis IM, Boot AM, Krenning EP, Drop SL, de Muinck Keizer-Schrama SM. Longitudinal follow-up of bone density and body composition in children with precocious or early puberty before, during and after cessation of GnRH agonist therapy. J Clin Endocrinol Metab. 2002;87(2):506–12.

15. Arrigo T, De Luca F, Antoniazzi F, Galluzzi F, Segni M, Rosano M, Messina MF, Lombardo F. Reduction of baseline body mass index under gonadotropin-suppressive therapy in girls with idiopathic precocious puberty. Eur J Endocrinol. 2004;150:533–7.

16. Poomthavorn P, Suphasit R, Mahachoklertwattana P. Adult height, body mass index and time of menarche of girls with idiopathic central precocious puberty after gonadotropin-releasing hormone analogue treatment. Gynecol Endocrinol. 2011;27:524–8.

17. Wolters B, Lass N, Reinehr T. Treatment with gonadotropin-releasing hormone analogues: different impact on body weight in normal-weight and overweight children. Horm Res Paediatr. 2012;78(5–6):304–11. doi:10.1159/000346145. Epub 2012 Dec 2.

18. Lee SJ, Yang EM, Seo JY, Jong KC. Effects of gonadotropin-releasing hormone agonist therapy on body mass index and height in girls with central precocious puberty. Chonnam Med J. 2012;48:27–31.

19. Colmenares A, Gunczler P, Lanes R. Higher prevalence of obesity and overweight without an adverse metabolic profile in girls with central precocious puberty compared to girls with early puberty, regardless of GnRH analogue treatment. Int J Pediatr Endocrinol. 2014;2014:5. P 1–7.

20. Alessandri SB, Pereira Fde A, Villela RA, Antonini SR, Elias PC, Martinelli Jr CE, Castro MD, Moreira AC, Paula FJ. Bone mineral density and body composition in girls with idiopathic central precocious puberty before and after treatment with a gonadotropin-releasing hormone agonist. Clinics (Sao Paulo). 2012;67(6):591–6.

21. Magiakou MA, Manousaki D, Papadaki M, Hadjidakis D, Levidou G, Vakaki M, Papaefstathiou A, Lalioti N, Kanaka-Gantenbein C, Piaditis G, Chrousos G, Dacou-Voutetakis C. The efficacy and safety of gonadotropin-releasing hormone analog treatment in childhood and adolescence: a single center, long-term follow-up study. J Clin Endocrinol Metab. 2010;95(1):109–17.

22. Marshall WA, Tanner JM. Variations in the pattern of pubertal changes in girls. Arch Dis Child. 1969;44:291–303.

23. Greulich WW. Radiographic atlas of skeletal development of the hand and wrist, Pyle SI. 2nd ed. Palo Alto: Standford University Press; 1959.

24. Cole TJ, Bellizi MC, Fiegal KM, Dietz WH. Establishing a standard definition for child overweight and obesity worldwide: international survey. Brit Med J. 2000;320:1240–3.

25. Carel J-C, Eugster E, Mogol A, Ghizzoni L, Palmert MR, on behalf of the members of the ESPE-LWPES GnRH Analogs Consensus Conference Group, on behalf of the members of the ESPE-LWPES GnRH Analogs Consensus Conference Group. Consensus statement on the use of gonadotropin-releasing hormone analogs in children. Pediatrics. 2009;123:752–62. doi:10.1542/peds.2008-1783. Epub 2009 Mar 30.

26. Consenso sobre factores de riesgo de enfermedad cardiovascular en Pediatría. Obesidad. Subcomisión de Epidemiología y Comité de Nutrición. Coordinadores: Durán P, Piazza N y Trifone L. Arch Argent Pediatr. 2005; 103(3):262–81.

27. Paterson WF, McNeill E, Young D, Donaldson MDC. Auxological outcome and time to menarche following long-acting goserelin therapy in girls with central precocious or early puberty. Clin Endocrinol. 2004;61:626–34.

28. Pasquino AM, Pucarelli I, Accardo F, Demiraj V, Segni M, Di Nardo R. Long-term observation of 87 girls with idiopathic central precocious puberty treated with gonadotropin-releasing hormone analogs: impact on adult height, body mass index, bone mineral content, and reproductive function. J Clin Endocrinol Metab. 2008;93(1):190–5. Epub 2007 Oct 16.

29. Cassio A, Bal MO, Orsini LF, Balsamo A, Sansavini S, Gennari M, De Cristofaro E, Cicognani A. Reproductive outcome in patients treated and not treated for idiopathic early puberty: long-term results of a randomized trial in adults. J Pediatr. 2006;149:532–6.

30. Lazar L, Lebenthal Y, Yackobovitch-Gavan M, Shalitin S, de Vries L, Phillip M, Meyerovitch J. Treated and untreated women with idiopathic precocious puberty: BMI evolution, metabolic outcome, and general health between third and fifth decades. J Clin Endocrinol Metab. 2015;100(4):1445–51. doi:10.1210/jc.2014-3748. Epub 2015 Feb 4.

22

Early menarche and childhood adversities in a nationally representative sample

Kimberly L Henrichs[1], Heather L McCauley[2,3], Elizabeth Miller[2,3], Dennis M Styne[4*], Naomi Saito[5] and Joshua Breslau[6]

Abstract

Background: Epidemiological evidence suggests that early menarche, defined as onset of menses at age 11 or earlier, has increased in prevalence in recent birth cohorts and is associated with multiple poor medical and mental health outcomes in adulthood. There is evidence that childhood adversities occurring prior to menarche contribute to early menarche.

Methods: Data collected in face-to-face interviews with a nationally representative sample of women age 18 and over (N = 3288), as part of the National Comorbidity Survey-Replication, were analyzed. Associations between pre-menarchal childhood adversities and menarche at age 11 or earlier were estimated in discrete time survival models with statistical adjustment for age at interview, ethnicity, and body mass index. Adversities investigated included physical abuse, sexual abuse, neglect, biological father absence from the home, other parent loss, parent mental illness, parent substance abuse, parent criminality, inter-parental violence, serious physical illness in childhood, and family economic adversity.

Results: Mean age at menarche varied across decadal birth cohorts ($\chi^2_{(4)} = 21.41$, p < .001) ranging from a high of 12.9 years in the oldest cohort (age 59 or older at the time of interview) to a low of 12.4 in the second youngest cohort (age 28-37). Childhood adversities were also more common in younger than older cohorts. Of the 11 childhood adversities, 5 were associated with menarche at age 11 or earlier, with OR of 1.3 or greater. Each of these five adversities is associated with a 26% increase in the odds of early menarche (OR = 1.26, 95% CI 1.14-1.39). The relationship between childhood sexual abuse and early menarche was sustained after adjustment for co-occurring adversities. (OR = 1.77, 95% CI 1.21-2.6).

Conclusions: Evidence from this study is consistent with hypothesized physiological effects of early childhood family environment on endocrine development. Childhood sexual abuse is the adversity most strongly associated with early menarche. However, because of the complex way that childhood adversities cluster within families, the more generalized influence of highly dysfunctional family environments cannot be ruled out.

Background

Among industrialized nations, and the United States in particular, the average age of menarche has decreased over the past century [1-3]. This trend is of public health concern as early menarche, commonly defined as onset of menses before age 12, is associated with multiple poor health outcomes in adults from increased cardiovascular and metabolic diseases to breast cancer and all-cause mortality [4-6]. Early menarche has also been linked to increased health risk behaviors, earlier sexual debut, and depression [7-9].

Early menarche is likely the result of multiple influences on early endocrine development. Epidemiological studies have found that early menarche is associated with multiple inter-related social and environmental factors, including nutrition and obesity [10-12], genetic factors [13,14], and general health status [15], with differences noted by race/ethnicity and familial socioeconomic status [16-18]. Among social factors with potential influence on early menarche, a growing body of literature points to exposure to childhood adversities as a risk factor for early menarche, including childhood sexual abuse [9,19-34]. The adverse impacts of biological father absence and the presence of non-related males in the home have also been suggested, though the evidence remains mixed [26,35-41]. To the best of our knowledge,

* Correspondence: dennis.styne@ucdmc.ucdavis.edu
[4]University of California Davis, 2516 Stockton Blvd, Sacramento, CA 95817, USA
Full list of author information is available at the end of the article

studies to date have not considered the effects of a broader range of related childhood adversities on menarche. As adversities tend to cluster together, identifying specific adversities associated with early menarche could help identify particular environmental influences on endocrine pathways, should they exist. Elucidating the types of adversities associated with early onset of menarche is critical not only for guiding research on the impact of stressors on neuroendocrine development but also informing the design of targeted interventions for children exposed to specific adversities and potentially mitigating the impact of early pubertal development. This study assesses the joint predictive effects on age of menarche of a broad range of childhood adversities, including absence of biological father in the home and childhood sexual abuse, utilizing a large nationally representative sample from the United States, the National Comorbidity Survey Replication (NCS-R).

Methods

Sample

The NCS-R is a multi-stage clustered area probability survey (respondents selected into the sample were clustered within selected geographic units [42]) representative of the adult (ages 18+), non-institutionalized, civilian, English speaking population of the continental US focused on the prevalence and correlates of mental disorders [43,44]. Non-clinician interviewers conducted computer assisted face-to-face structured interviews between February 2001 and April 2003. The NCS-R interview schedule was the version of the World Health Organization (WHO) Composite International Diagnostic Interview (CIDI) developed for the WHO World Mental Health Survey Initiative [38,44,45]. The Human Subjects Committees of both Harvard Medical School and the University of Michigan approved the NCS-R recruitment, consent and field procedures. All NCS-R data and documentation are publically available at http://www.icpsr.umich.edu/CPES.

All respondents (N = 8098) completed a Part I core diagnostic interview. To reduce respondent burden, a subsample (selected with known probabilities) received a Part II interview, which included assessments of risk factors, consequences, services and other correlates of the core disorders. The Part II sample included all Part I respondents age 25 or younger, all Part I respondents meeting initial criteria for a mental disorder, and a random sample of Part I respondents over the age of 25 who did not meet criteria for a mental disorder. Sample weights accounted for differential probability of selection and non-response. Additional weights helped match demographic characteristics of the sample to those of the target population [43,44]. Of the 3,310 women completing the Part II interview, 22 provided no information

on age at menarche and were excluded from the analysis, leaving a sample of 3288 women.

Measures

Early menarche

Age at menarche was the self-reported age at first menstrual period. Early menarche was defined as occurrence of menarche at 11 years of age or less, consistent with values equal to or less than the 25th percentile for age as published from national estimates of menarche timing for non-Hispanic White U.S. girls in the National Health and Nutrition Examination Survey III (1988-1994) [46]. Missing values for age of menarche were imputed for 40 participants who did not recall their exact age using information from questions about whether their first period occurred about the same time as, earlier than, or much earlier than their peers. Ages were imputed using the average age intervals associated with these categories among the large majority of respondents who provided their exact age at menarche.

Childhood adversities

Eleven childhood adversities were included in the analyses – (1) physical abuse, (2) sexual abuse, (3) neglect, (4) biological father absence from the home, (5) other parent loss, (6) parent mental illness, (7) parent substance abuse, (8) parent criminality, (9) inter-parental violence, (10) serious physical illness in childhood, and (11) family economic adversity. Physical abuse and inter-parental violence were coded as moderate physical violence towards the respondent by the parent or adult caregiver or between parents or adult caregivers, respectively, using the revised Conflict Tactics Scale [47]. Sexual abuse was assessed with questions developed for the baseline National Comorbidity Survey about rape, sexual assault and molestation [48]. Neglect was assessed with a five-item scale developed for child welfare studies [49].

Absence of biological father was defined using a series of questions about respondents' family structure during childhood. Respondents were first asked whether they had lived their entire childhood up to age 16 with both biological parents in their household. Respondents who answered 'no' to this question were considered to have had an absent biological father if they had more than one adult male living in their household for at least six months during childhood, the male head of household for most of their childhood was not their biological father, their biological father died prior to their age at menarche, they lived in foster care or with an adoptive family, or they had no male head of household for most of their childhood.

Parent mental illness and substance use disorders were assessed using the family history research diagnostic criteria, for either male or female adult caregiver [50,51]. Parental criminality was assessed through questions about whether the respondent's parents were involved in criminal activities, arrested or sent to prison. Economic adversity was defined as having received welfare or not having a working parent as head of household. Information on the timing of parental death, divorce, separation, serious physical illness, inter-parental violence and sexual abuse was used to determine whether these childhood adversities began before the initiation of menstruation.

Additional covariates

Body mass index at time of interview was calculated from self-reported height and weight. Z-scores for variation in an individual's BMI (body mass index) from the mean of their birth cohort were calculated and used to adjust statistically for BMI, given the relative stability of BMI within cohorts over time [52,53]. Race-ethnic categories were defined as mutually exclusive categories based on self-report. Age groups were defined to produce five birth cohorts of approximately equal size.

Statistical analysis

Prevalence of early menarche was calculated as the proportion of respondents who reported that their first menstrual period occurred at 11 years of age or younger. Discrete time survival models with time-varying covariates were used to estimate associations of childhood adversities with early menarche. Survival models were adjusted statistically for age, race/ethnicity and BMI. Data were arranged by person-year (from age 6 to age 11 or age of menarche, whichever came first) with time-varying indicators for each childhood adversity. The survival models include one observation per year of age starting with age 6. If a respondent reported an adversity occurring prior to age 6, then that adversity was coded as present at age 6 (and all subsequent ages). Associations between childhood adversities and early menarche were calculated as adjusted odds ratios. Confidence intervals and statistical tests were calculated using the Taylor series linearization method as implemented in the SUDAAN software package to account for the complex sample design of the NCS-R [54]. Statistical significance was assessed using two-sided .05 level tests.

Results

Sample characteristics and cohort variation in age at menarche and childhood adversities

The mean age of the sample was 45.7 years (se = 0.60). 72% were White, 13% non-Hispanic Black, 10% Hispanic, and 4% other race/ethnicity. Mean BMI was 27.

The mean age at menarche was highest (12.9 years) in the oldest birth cohort, those age 59 and over at the time of interview, but the decline was not monotonic across birth cohorts (Table 1). Variation in the prevalence of childhood adversities across birth cohorts follows a similar pattern. Just over half (52.8%) of the eldest cohort reported no adversities in contrast to 38.2% of the youngest cohort (i.e. those ages 18-27). In particular, younger cohorts reported increased frequency of biological father absence ($\chi^2 = 84.01$, p <0.001), a childhood adversity theorized to have a particularly strong connection to early menarche. The proportion of girls not living with their biological fathers was more than twice as high in youngest versus oldest birth cohorts. Childhood sexual abuse was reported with greater frequency among the two younger cohorts ($\chi^2 = 25.13$, p < 0.001). The 28-37 year old cohort reported the highest prevalence of early menarche (24.9%, CI 21.3-28.8), the youngest mean age of menarche (12.4 years), the greatest exposure to adversities (66.5%), and the highest prevalence of multiple co-occurring adversities.

Figure 1 shows the prevalence of early menarche across groups defined by the number of pre-menarchal childhood adversities. The prevalence of early menarche is close to 20% among people reporting no adversities, 1 or 2 adversities and 3 or 4 adversities. Elevated prevalence of early menarche is limited to the group with 5 or more adversities among whom it reaches 34%.

Associations of pre-menarchal childhood adversities with early menarche

An initial set of models was specified to identify the adversities most strongly associated with early menarche, adjusting for age, ethnicity and BMI, but without adjustment for co-occurring adversities (Table 2). Of the 11 childhood adversities tested, only 4 were significantly associated with early menarche at the p = .05 level. Odds ratios for these four adversities (physical abuse, sexual abuse, parental mental illness and family violence) ranged from 1.36 to 2.19. The odds ratio associated with parental substance use was of similar magnitude, 1.3, but did not reach statistical significance (95% CI 0.91-1.91). Absence of the biological father from the home was not associated with early menarche (OR = 1.08 95% CI 0.86- 1.36).

The five childhood adversities most strongly associated with early menarche were entered into two models to determine the joint effects of co-occurring adversities on early menarche (Table 3). In the first model, a simple count of adversities was entered as a continuous variable, with statistical adjustment for age, ethnicity, and BMI. Each adversity was associated with a statistically significant 26% increase in the odds of early menarche. In the second model, to examine the relative impact of specific adversities on early menarche, all five adversities were entered as simultaneous predictors (main effects model), with no interactions among the adversities. All

Table 1 Age of menarche, absence of bio-father, childhood sexual abuse (prior to menarche), and number of childhood adversities across birth cohorts

Age	N	AOM Mean (SD)	Early menarche % (n)	Not Lived with Bio-father % (n)	Childhood sexual abuse % (n)	Number ACE				Number ACE Mean (SD)
						0 % (n)	1,2 % (n)	3,4 % (n)	4 < % (n)	
18-27y/o	654	12.5 (1.57)	20.2 (158)	37.1 (243)	15.8 (133)	38.2 (221)	40.2 (266)	15.4 (104)	6.2 (63)	1.4 (1.55)
28-37y/o	655	12.4 (1.31)	24.9 (163)	33.4 (206)	18.7 (144)	33.5 (210)	44.0 (286)	15.9 (99)	6.7 (60)	1.6 (1.50)
38-47y/o	697	12.7 (1.62)	20.4 (152)	21.1 (149)	14.8 (128)	47.9 (290)	40.0 (281)	8.1 (80)	4.2 (46)	1.0 (1.36)
48-58y/o	636	12.6 (1.52)	22.5 (146)	15.5 (112)	14.8 (118)	49.4 (276)	37.0 (249)	9.1 (73)	5.0 (38)	1.1 (1.42)
59-98y/o	646	12.9 (1.84)	17.7 (126)	16.2 (104)	7.3 (57)	52.8 (331)	38.6 (250)	7.6 (52)	0.9 (13)	0.8 (1.21)
Wald chi-square		$\chi^2_{(4)} = 21.41$	$\chi^2_{(4)} = 9.43$	$\chi^2_{(4)} = 84.01$	$\chi^2_{(4)} = 25.13$	$\chi^2_{(12)} = 123.62$				$\chi^2_{(4)} = 46.46$
P-value		<0.001	0.051	<0.001	<0.001	< 0.001				<0.001

Birth cohorts divided by decade of birth; percentages are weighted.
AOM = age of menarche.
ACE = adverse childhood experiences.

odds ratios in the second model exceeded 1, but only sexual abuse reached statistical significance (OR = 1.77, 95% CI 1.21-2.60). Tests of statistical interactions between co-occurring adversities, including tests for diffuse interactions, were not statistically significant. In addition, tests for statistical interactions between race/ethnicity and childhood adversities were not statistically significant.

Discussion

Childhood adversities predict earlier onset of menarche in this large national sample of women, after statistical adjustment for BMI and race/ethnicity. The prevalence of early menarche is elevated at high levels of co-occurring adversities, specifically in the 5% of the population with more than five adversities. Among respondents reporting between one and four adversities (51% of the sample), the prevalence of early menarche was not significantly higher than those reporting no adversities (44% of the sample).

While risk for early menarche appears to increase with a greater number of childhood adversities, the variable for the count of adversities (Model 1 in Table 3) imposes an assumption that each adversity is associated with an

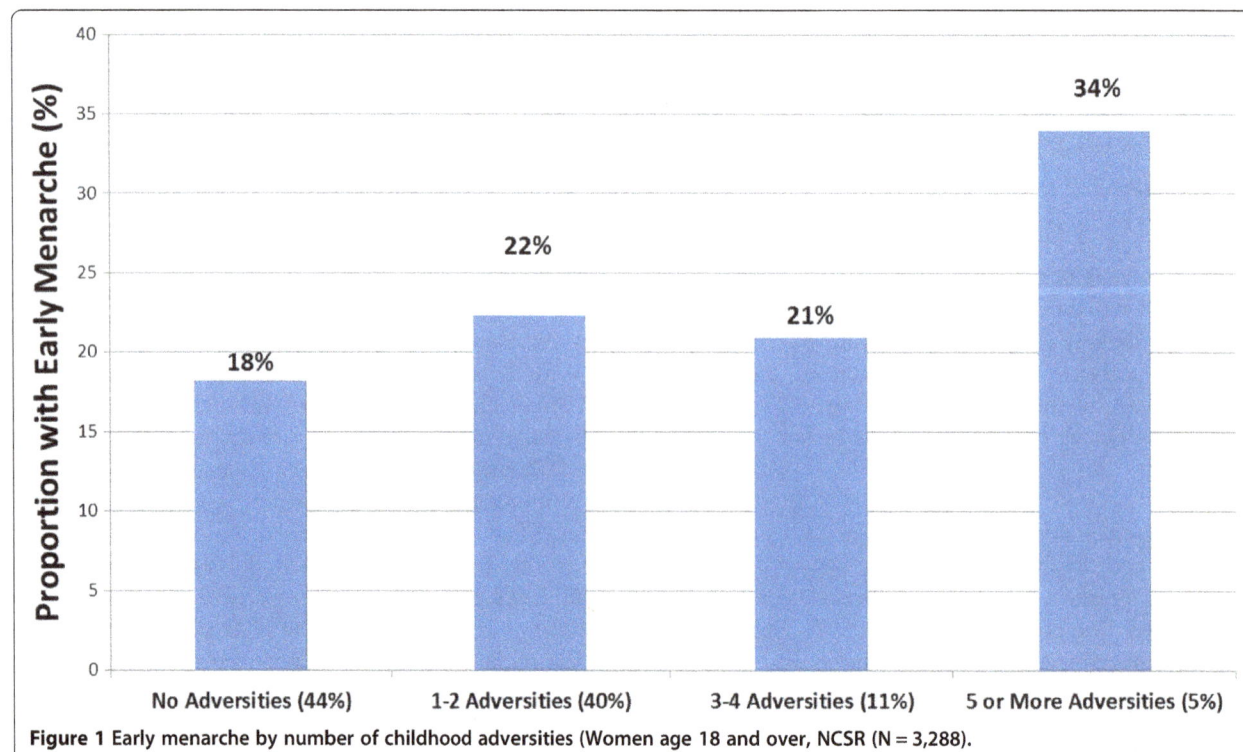

Figure 1 Early menarche by number of childhood adversities (Women age 18 and over, NCSR (N = 3,288).

Table 2 Associations of individual adverse childhood experiences with early menarche

	Odds ratio	95% CI	Wald ChiSq
Neglect	1.03	(0.63, 1.67)	0.01
Parent criminality	1.05	(0.77, 1.43)	0.10
Bio-father absent	1.08	(0.86, 1.36)	0.48
Physical illness	1.08	(0.71, 1.64)	0.13
Other parent loss	1.15	(0.63, 2.09)	0.23
Economic adversity	1.23	(0.88, 1.73)	1.53
Parent substance abuse	1.30	(0.91, 1.91)	2.15
Parent mental illness	1.36	(1.08, 1.71)	7.32**
Family violence	1.40	(1.03, 1.89)	4.97***
Physical abuse	1.81	(1.32, 2.48)	14.59*
Sexual abuse	2.19	(1.54, 3.12)	20.22*

*p < 0.001. **p < 0.01. ***p < 0.05.
Each odds ratio estimated in a separate model with statistical adjustment for age and race/ethnicity.

identical increase in the risk for early menarche. The 26% increase found with Model 1 is an average across all the adversities. Figure 1, in contrast, does not make this assumption. This apparent contradiction demonstrates the difficulty in selecting between different models of the association between adversities and early menarche. The findings appear to go against a simple, linear relationship and suggest that a threshold model is a better fit to the overall pattern in the data. That is, risk for

early menarche appears to increase above a certain number of adversities.

These analyses were also designed to identify contributions of specific childhood adversities on early menarche (Model 2 in Table 3); findings are consistent with the suggestion in the literature that childhood sexual abuse is associated with earlier onset of menarche. As observational studies have limited ability to distinguish between effects of specific adversities and more generalized effects of childhood environment in the context of highly clustered adversities, this study included a much broader range of childhood adversities than prior studies. Specifically, of the 11 adversities, childhood sexual abuse had the strongest association with early menarche when each adversity was examined in a separate model. In models adjusting for co-occurrence among the five adversities most strongly associated with early menarche, only childhood sexual abuse remained associated with early menarche at a statistically significant level. Absence of biological father during childhood, theorized to affect early menarche due to early triggering of sexual development, was not associated with early menarche in this study.

These results are consistent with prior studies in finding that stressors in childhood may have biological influences on endocrine development resulting in early menarche, a key developmental milestone with important social and biological consequences that extend

Table 3 Adjusted associations of number of adversities and individual types of adversities with early menarche

		Model 1		Model 2	
		Adjusted odds ratio	95% CI	Adjusted odds ratio	95% CI
Age (years)	18-27	1		1	
	28-37	1.22	(0.90, 1.66)	1.23	(0.90, 1.67)
	38-47	0.94	(0.67, 1.32)	0.94	(0.67, 1.33)
	48-58	1.13	(0.84, 1.54)	1.14	(0.83, 1.56)
	59-98	0.97	(0.68, 1.39)	0.98	(0.68, 1.41)
Ethnicity	White	1		1	
	Hispanic	1.49	(1.02, 2.15)	1.47	(1.00, 2.15)
	Black	1.45	(0.94, 2.22)	1.44	(0.94, 2.21)
	Other	0.61	(0.33, 1.16)	0.61	(0.31, 1.20)
BMI (standardized)		1.22	(1.12, 1.33)	1.22	(1.12, 1.33)
Number of adversities		1.26	(1.14, 1.39)	–	–
Type of adversities	Parent substance abuse	–	–	1.06	(0.74, 1.50)
	Parent mental illness	–	–	1.18	(0.91, 1.55)
	Family violence	–	–	1.14	(0.87, 1.50)
	Physical abuse	–	–	1.35	(0.98, 1.88)
	Sexual abuse	–	–	1.77	(1.21, 2.60)

Model 1: Number (count) of adversities as a continuous predictor with statistical adjustment for age, ethnicity, and BMI (i.e. ORs in model 1 are adjusted for all variables in the first column).
Model 2: Main effects of the five childhood adversities with the strongest associations with early menarche with statistical adjustment for age, ethnicity, and BMI (i.e. ORs in model 2 are adjusted for all variables in the second column).

across adulthood. However, the evidence regarding specific mechanisms is mixed. Theories related to paternal investment, suggested by Draper and Harpending [55] as well as Belsky [56], hypothesizing that the absence of the biological father during childhood would trigger early sexual development have received some support. However, in this study, absence of the biological father was not associated with early menarche. The current findings are congruent with those of Ellis [36,37], in that the impact of early father absence on early menarche does not exist independent of other moderating factors in the environment. At the same time, the finding that sexual abuse prior to menarche is the strongest predictor of early menarche may implicate a related pathway. Several previous studies have also found that childhood sexual abuse is associated with early menarche [19,28,30,31,57,58], including a recent study showing links between childhood sexual abuse and early menarche in a large sample of African-American women [29] as well as a study suggesting a dose-response relationship between severity of sexual abuse and early menarche [34]. None of these studies including the current study, however, has included information on timing of pre-menarchal development of secondary sexual characteristics, which may contribute to increased risk for sexual abuse. Similarly, while beyond the scope of this study, examination of the differential impact of childhood adversities such as absence of biological father at different developmental stages (i.e., early childhood versus early adolescence) would help elucidate the specific pathways for the influence of childhood adversities on pubertal development.

This study has several limitations. Most importantly, we rely on retrospective reporting of both childhood adversities and age of menarche. A large literature examining associations of recalled childhood adversities with health outcomes has proven valuable despite the known limitation of retrospective assessment [59]. However, it is possible that certain adversities such as sexual abuse will be recalled more readily than others. Previous studies on recalled age of menarche found participant recall to be accurate within one year in 90% of cases between the teenage years and 30 years after the event [60,61]. As some of the study participants were in their 50s and 60s, it is possible that there is more recall bias with underreporting of childhood adversities and inaccurate timing of menarche among the older birth cohorts. In addition, data on BMI were available only from the time of interview as an adult, not from the period preceding menarche. This limitation is partially addressed by including participants' BMI at the time of the interview in final analyses, as adult obesity and childhood obesity are highly correlated [62,63]. However, the self-reported adult height and weight to calculate BMI add an additional potential inaccuracy to these

data (i.e., BMI is likely to be underestimated). Finally, information on the exact timing was not available for all adversities considered in the analysis, in particular for absence of biological father. It is possible in these cases that the adversity occurred after menarche and was misclassified in this study. Definitions have been constructed in these cases to minimize the possible impact of misclassification. It is unlikely that the remaining misclassification would result in bias in any particular direction.

Interpretation of the findings should also consider the absence of information on maternal age at menarche in this study and in most other studies of this topic. As noted by Moffitt and colleagues [24], early menarche may lead to early sexual debut and early marriage. Given that early age at marriage is a strong predictor of divorce, children of mothers with early age at marriage may be more likely to grow up in disadvantaged settings, in which they are at risk for a wide variety of childhood adversities. In this scenario, genetic transmission of age at menarche may underlie the observed associations between childhood adversities and early menarche. A study by Wise and colleagues included statistical control for maternal age at marriage, which would adjust in part for this pathway [29]. In that study, sexual abuse and physical abuse remained significantly associated with early menarche, although with associations of lesser magnitude than identified in this study.

Conclusions

These findings are consistent with the theory that adverse family environments have physiologic effects on endocrine development and, through these effects, may impact mental and physical health outcomes in adulthood. Childhood sexual abuse is the adversity most strongly associated with early menarche. However, because of the complex way that childhood adversities cluster within families, the more generalized influence of highly dysfunctional family environments cannot be ruled out. More detailed studies that address gene-environment correlations as well as the possibility of confounding by pre-menarchal development are needed to advance towards more solid evidence that the associations observed here reflect a distinct bio-social etiology.

Abbreviation
NCS-R: National Comorbidity Survey Replication.

Competing interests
The authors declared that they have no competing interests.

Authors' contributions
KH conceptualized the study, conducted the literature review, participated in the design and analyses, drafted the initial manuscript, and approved the final manuscript as submitted. HLM participated in review of the analyses, critically reviewed and revised the manuscript, and approved the final manuscript as submitted. EM conceptualized and designed the study, reviewed and revised the manuscript, and approved the final manuscript as

submitted. DS assisted in conceptualizing and designing the study, reviewed and revised the manuscript, and approved the final manuscript as submitted. NS participated in the design of the study, carried out the analyses, reviewed and revised the manuscript, and approved the final manuscript as submitted. JAB designed the study, directed the analyses, reviewed and revised the manuscript, and approved the final manuscript as submitted. All authors read and approved the final manuscript.

Acknowledgments
This research was supported by a Children's Miracle Network Grant. We appreciate the additional support from the Department of Pediatrics at the University of California Davis. We also acknowledge the Honorable Donna Petre for her encouragement to examine the role of absent biological father on development.

Author details
[1]University of Wisconsin School of Medicine and Public Health, 600 Highland Avenue, Madison, WI 53792-4108, USA. [2]University of Pittsburgh School of Medicine, 3420 Fifth Avenue, Pittsburgh, PA 15213, USA. [3]Children's Hospital of Pittsburgh, University of Pittsburgh Medical Center, 3420 Fifth Avenue, Pittsburgh, PA 15213, USA. [4]University of California Davis, 2516 Stockton Blvd, Sacramento, CA 95817, USA. [5]University of California Davis, 1616 DaVinci Court, Davis, CA 95618, USA. [6]RAND Corporation, 4570 Fifth Avenue, Suite 600, Pittsburgh, PA 15213, USA.

References
1. Thomas F, Renaud F, Benefice R, de Meeus T, Guegan JF: International variability of ages at menarche and menopause: patterns and main determinants. *Hum Biol* 2001, 73(2):271–290.
2. Ong KK, Ahmed ML, Dunger DB: Lessons from large population studies on timing and tempo of puberty (secular trends and relation to body size): the European trend. *Mol Cell Endocrinol* 2006, 254-255:8–12. Epub 2006 Jun 6.
3. Melmed S, Polonsky KS, Larsen PR, Kronenberg HM: *Williams Textbook of Endocrinology*. 12th edition. Philadelphia, PA: Saunders and Elsevier Inc; 2011.
4. Jacobsen BK, Oda K, Knutsen SF, Fraser GE: Age at menarche, total mortality and mortality from ischaemic heart disease and stroke: the Adventist Health Study, 1976-88. *Int J Epidemiol* 2009, 38(1):245–252.
5. Lakshman R, Forouhi NG, Sharp SJ, Luben R, Bingham SA, Khaw KT, Wareham NJ, Ong KK: Early age at menarche associated with cardiovascular disease and mortality. *J Clin Endocrinol Metab* 2009, 94(12):4953–4960.
6. Remsberg KE, Demerath EW, Schubert CM, Chumlea WC, Sun SS, Siervogel RM: Early menarche and the development of cardiovascular disease risk factors in adolescent girls: the Fels Longitudinal Study. *J Clin Endocrinol Metab* 2005, 90(5):2718–2724. Epub 2005 Feb 22.
7. Black SR, Klein DN: Early Menarcheal Age and Risk for Later Depressive Symptomatology: The Role of Childhood Depressive Symptoms. *J Youth Adolesc* 2012, 41(9):1142–50.
8. Downing J, Bellis MA: Early pubertal onset and its relationship with sexual risk taking, substance use and anti-social behaviour: a preliminary cross-sectional study. *BMC Public Health* 2009, 9:446.
9. Belsky J, Steinberg L, Houts RM, Halpern-Felsher BL, NICHD Early Child Care Research Network: The development of reproductive strategy in females: early maternal harshness – earlier menarche – increased sexual risk taking. *Dev Psychol* 2010, 46(1):120–128.
10. Rosell M, Appleby P, Key T: Height, age at menarche, body weight and body mass index in life-long vegetarians. *Public Health Nutr* 2005, 8(7):870–875.
11. Lee JM, Appugliese D, Kaciroti N, Corwyn RF, Bradley RH, Lumeng JC: Weight status in young girls and the onset of puberty. *Pediatrics* 2007, 119(3):e624–e630.
12. Ahmed ML, Ong KK, Dunger DB: Childhood obesity and the timing of puberty. *Trends Endocrinol Metab* 2009, 20(5):237–242. Epub 2009 Jun 21.
13. Elks CE, Ong KK: Whole genome associated studies for age at menarche. *Brief Funct Genomics* 2011, 10(2):91–97.
14. Manuck SB, Craig AE, Flory JD, Halder I, Ferrell RE: Reported early family environment covaries with menarcheal age as a function of polymorphic variation in estrogen receptor-alpha. *Dev Psychopathol* 2011, 23(1):69–83.
15. Umlawska W, Krzyzanowska M: Puberty in certain chronic illness. *Pediatr Endocrinol Diabetes Metab* 2009, 15(3):216–218.
16. Anderson SE, Dallal GE, Must A: Relative weight and race influence average age at menarche: results from two nationally representative surveys of US girls studied 25 years apart. *Pediatrics* 2003, 111(4 Pt 1):844–850.
17. Braithwaite D, Moore DH, Lustig RH, Epel ES, Ong KK, Rehkopf DH, Wang MC, Miller SM, Hiatt RA: Socioeconomic status in relation to early menarche among black and white girls. *Cancer Causes Control* 2009, 20(5):713–720. Epub 2008 Dec 25.
18. Freedman DS, Khan LK, Serdula MK, Dietz WH, Srinivasan SR, Berenson GS: Relation of age at menarche to race, time period, and anthropometric dimensions: the Bogalusa Heart Study. *Pediatrics* 2002, 110(4):e43.
19. Vigil JM, Geary DC, Byrd-Craven J: A life history assessment of early childhood sexual abuse in women. *Dev Psychol* 2005, 41(3):553–561.
20. Boynton-Jarrett R, Ryan LM, Berkman LF, Wright RJ: Cumulative violence exposure and self-rated health: longitudinal study of adolescents in the United States. *Pediatrics* 2008, 122(5):961–970.
21. Greenfield EA: Child abuse as a life-course social determinant of adult health. *Maturitas* 2010, 66(1):51–55. Epub 2010 Mar 6.
22. Boynton-Jarrett R, Rich-Edwards JW, Jun HJ, Hibert EN, Wright RJ: Abuse in childhood and risk of uterine leiomyoma: the role of emotional support in biologic resilience. *Epidemiology* 2011, 22(1):6–14.
23. Boynton-Jarrett R, Rosenberg L, Palmer JR, Boggs DA, Wise LA: Child and Adolescent Abuse in Relation to Obesity in Adulthood: The Black Women's Health Study. *Pediatrics* 2012, 130(2):245–253.
24. Moffitt TE, Caspi A, Belsky J, Silva PA: Childhood experience and the onset of menarche: a test of a sociobiological model. *Child Dev* 1992, 63(1):47–58.
25. Wierson M, Long PJ, Forehand RL: Toward a new understanding of early menarche: the role of environmental stress in pubertal timing. *Adolescence* 1993, 28(112):913–924.
26. Belsky J, Steinberg LD, Houts RM, Friedman SL, DeHart G, Cauffman E, Roisman GI, Halpern-Felsher BL, Susman E, NICHD Early Child Care Research Network: Family rearing antecedents of pubertal timing. *Child Dev* 2007, 78(4):1302–1321.
27. Herman-Giddens ME, Sandler AD, Friedman NE: Sexual precocity in girls. An association with sexual abuse? *Am J Dis Child* 1988, 142(4):431–433.
28. Romans SE, Martin JM, Gendall K, Herbison GP: Age of menarche: the role of some psychosocial factors. *Psychol Med* 2003, 33(5):933–939.
29. Wise LA, Palmer JR, Rothman EF, Rosenberg L: Childhood abuse and early menarche: findings from the black women's health study. *Am J Public Health* 2009, 99(Suppl 2):S460–S466. Epub 2009 May 14.
30. Zabin LS, Emerson MR, Rowland DL: Childhood sexual abuse and early menarche: the direction of their relationship and its implications. *J Adolesc Health* 2005, 36(5):393–400.
31. Brown J, Cohen P, Chen H, Smailes E, Johnson JG: Sexual trajectories of abused and neglected youths. *J Dev Behav Pediatr* 2004, 25(2):77–82.
32. Turner P, Runtz M, Galambos N: Sexual abuse, pubertal timing, and subjective age in adolescent girls: A research note. *J Reprod Infant Psychol* 1993, 17:111–118.
33. Mendle J, Leve LD, Van Ryzin M, Natsuaki MN, Ge X: Associations between early life stress, child maltreatment, and pubertal development among girls in foster care. *J Res Adolesc* 2011, 21(4):871–880.
34. Boynton-Jarrett R, Wright RJ, Putnam FW, Hibert EL, Michels KB, Forman MR, Rich-Edwards J: Childhood abuse and age at menarche. *J Adolesc Health* 2013, 52(2):241–247.
35. Campbell BC, Udry JR: Stress and age at menarche of mothers and daughters. *J Biosoc Sci* 1995, 27(2):127–134.
36. Deardorff J, Ekwaru JP, Kushi LH, Ellis BJ, Greenspan LC, Mirabedi A, Landaverde EG, Hiatt RA: Father absence, body mass index, and pubertal timing in girls: differential effects by family income and ethnicity. *J Adolesc Health* 2011, 48(5):441–447.
37. Tither JM, Ellis BJ: Impact of fathers on daughters' age at menarche: a genetically and environmentally controlled sibling study. *Dev Psychol* 2008, 44(5):1409–1420.
38. Ellis BJ, Garber J: Psychosocial antecedents of variation in girls' pubertal timing: maternal depression, stepfather presence, and marital and family stress. *Child Dev* 2000, 71(2):485–501.

39. Bogaert AF: **Age at puberty and father absence in a national probability sample.** *J Adolesc* 2005, **28**(4):541–546. Epub 2005 Jan 20.

40. Mendle J, Turkheimer E, D'Onofrio BM, Lynch SK, Emery RE, Slutske WS, Martin NG: **Family structure and age at menarche: a children-of-twins approach.** *Dev Psychol* 2006, **42**(3):533–542.

41. Bogaert AF: **Menarche and father absence in a national probability sample.** *J Biosoc Sci* 2008, **40**(4):623–636. Epub 2007 Aug 30.

42. Lohr S: *Sampling: Design and Analysis.* Boston: Brooks/Cole; 2010.

43. Kessler RC, Merikangas KR: **The National Comorbidity Survey Replication (NCS-R): background and aims.** *Int J Methods Psychiatr Res* 2004, **13**(2):60–68.

44. Kessler RC, Berglund P, Chiu WT, Demler O, Heeringa S, Hiripi E, Jin R, Pennell BE, Walters EE, Zaslavsky A, Zheng H: **The US National Comorbidity Survey Replication (NCS-R): design and field procedures.** *Int J Methods Psychiatr Res* 2004, **13**(2):69–92X.

45. Breslau N, Novak SP, Kessler RC: **Daily smoking and the subsequent onset of psychiatric disorders.** *Psychol Med* 2004, **34**(2):323–333.

46. Chumlea WC, Schubert CM, Roche AF, Kulin HE, Lee PA, Himes JH, Sun SS: **Age at menarche and racial comparisons in US girls.** *Pediatrics* 2003, **111**(1):110–113.

47. Straus MA, Douglas EM: **A short form of the Revised Conflict Tactics Scales, and typologies for severity and mutuality.** *Violence Vict* 2004, **19**(5):507–520.

48. Molnar BE, Buka SL, Kessler RC: **Child sexual abuse and subsequent psychopathology: results from the National Comorbidity Survey.** *Am J Public Health* 2001, **91**(5):753–760.

49. Courtney ME, Piliavin I, Grogan-Kaylor A, Nesmith A: **Foster youth transitions to adulthood: a longitudinal view of youth leaving care.** *Child Welfare* 2001, **80**(6):685–717.

50. Kendler KS, Silberg JL, Neale MC, Kessler RC, Heath AC, Eaves LJ: **The family history method: whose psychiatric history is measured?** *Am J Psychiatry* 1991, **148**(11):1501–1504.

51. Andreasen NC, Endicott J, Spitzer RL, Winokur G: **The family history method using diagnostic criteria. Reliability and validity.** *Arch Gen Psychiatry* 1977, **34**(10):1229–1235.

52. Herman KM, Craig CL, Gauvin L, Katzmarzyk PT: **Tracking of obesity and physical activity from childhood to adulthood: the Physical Activity Longitudinal Study.** *Int J Pediatr Obes* 2009, **4**(4):281–288.

53. Deshmukh-Taskar P, Nicklas TA, Morales M, Yang SJ, Zakeri I, Berenson GS: **Tracking of overweight status from childhood to young adulthood: the Bogalusa Heart Study.** *Eur J Clin Nutr* 2006, **60**(1):48–57.

54. Research Triangle Institute: *SUDAAN Language Manual, Release 10.0.* Research Triangle Park, NC: Research Triangle Institute; 2008.

55. Draper P, Harpending H: **Father absence and reproductive strategy: An evolutionary perspective.** *J Anthropol Res* 1982, **38**:255–273.

56. Belsky J, Steinberg L, Draper P: **Childhood experience, interpersonal development, and reproductive strategy: and evolutionary theory of socialization.** *Child Dev* 1991, **62**(4):647–670.

57. Jorm AF, Christensen H, Rodgers B, Jacomb PA, Easteal S: **Association of adverse childhood experiences, age of menarche, and adult reproductive behavior: does the androgen receptor gene play a role?** *Am J Med Genet B Neuropsychiatr Genet* 2004, **125B**(1):105–111.

58. Hulanicka B, Gronkiewicz L, Koniarek J: **Effect of familial distress on growth and maturation of girls: a longitudinal study.** *Am J Hum Biol* 2001, **13**(6):771–776.

59. Felitti VJ, Anda RF, Nordenberg D, Williamson DF, Spitz AM, Edwards V, Koss MP, Marks JS: **Relationship of childhood abuse and household dysfunction to many of the leading causes of death in adults. The Adverse Childhood Experiences (ACE) Study.** *Am J Prev Med* 1998, **14**(4):245–258.

60. Damon A, Bajema CJ: **Age at menarche: Accuracy of recall after thirty-nine years.** *Hum Biol* 1974, **46**(3):381–384.

61. Zacharias L, Wurtman RJ, Schatzoff M: **Sexual maturation in contemporary American girls.** *Am J Obstet Gynecol* 1970, **108**(5):833–846.

62. Wang Y, Zhang Q: **Are American children and adolescents of low socioeconomic status at increased risk of obesity? Changes in the** association between overweight and family income between 1971 and 2002. *Am J Clin Nutr* 2006, **84**(4):707–716.

63. Elks CE, Loos RJ, Hardy R, Wills AK, Wong A, Wareham NJ, Kuh D, Ong KK: **Adult obesity susceptibility variants are associated with greater childhood weight gain and a faster tempo of growth: the 1946 British Birth Cohort Study.** *Am J Clin Nutr* 2012, **95**(5):1150–1156.

23

Normative penile anthropometry in term newborns in Kumasi, Ghana: a cross-sectional prospective study

Serwah Bonsu Asafo-Agyei[1*], Emmanuel Ameyaw[1], Jean-Pierre Chanoine[2] and Samuel Blay Nguah[1]

Abstract

Background: Genital measurements are a useful adjunct in the early detection of various endocrine conditions including hypopituitarism and disorders of sexual differentiation. Standards for genital sizes have been published but racial/ethnic differences exist. This study was done to establish norms for genital sizes in term Ghanaian male newborns.

Methods: This was a cross-sectional study of all apparently well full-term newborns of postnatal age < 48 h and birth weight between 2.5 and 4.0 kg delivered at Komfo Anokye Teaching Hospital within the study period. Anthropometric and genital parameters were documented for study subjects as well as parental socio-demographic indices.

Results: A total of 644 male newborns were recruited between May and September 2014. The mean penile length (MPL) was 3.3 ± 0.5 cm and the mean penile width (MPW) was 1.05 ± 0.1 cm. An inverse relationship was found between maternal age and MPL (correlation coefficient −0.062, 95% CI −0.121 to −0.002; $p = 0.04$). MPL was also significantly different ($p = 0.04$) by mode of delivery, with babies delivered by caesarean section having the lowest MPL. MPL correlated positively with both gestational age ($p = 0.04$) and birth length ($p < 0.001$), while MPW correlated proportionally with birth weight and length ($p < 0.001$ for both).

Conclusions: Using the conventional definition of micropenis as stretched penile length (SPL) < 2.5 standard deviation (SD) below the mean and macropenis as an SPL > 2.5 SD, a Ghanaian term newborn may warrant investigation if he has an MPL < 2.1 cm or > 4.4 cm.

Keywords: Penile length, Penile width, Genital size, Ghana, Micropenis, Macropenis

Background

Penile size is a reflection of the adequacy of exposure of the male fetus to androgens, right from hypothalamic/pituitary gonadotropins down to testicular androgens. Normative standards of penile sizes are thus useful for the diagnosis of genital/endocrine abnormalities [1]. Penile length abnormalities consist of micropenis and macropenis ('large penis'). A micropenis is an abnormally small penis with a normal configuration [2]. Conventionally, micropenis has been defined as a stretched penile length (SPL) < 2.5 standard deviation (SD) below the mean for age with normal function and structure. Likewise, an SPL > 2.5 SD is considered as a macropenis [2, 3].

Micropenis is an important sign in neonates, since it may be the only clue to the diagnosis of hypopituitarism, a potentially lethal but treatable condition [4]. It may also raise the clinical suspicion concerning the possibility of associated hypoglycaemia, a life-threatening metabolic emergency associated with hypopituitarism or isolated growth hormone deficiency [5]. Micropenis may also reflect an impairment specific to the hypothalamo-pituitary-gonadal axis, including isolated hypogonadism, poorly functioning, dysgenetic testicular tissue with malignant potential or partial androgen insensitivity [6, 7]. Early diagnosis of micropenis is important, because it

* Correspondence: sbasafoagyei@gmail.com
[1]Department of Child Health, Komfo Anokye Teaching Hospital, Kumasi, Ghana
Full list of author information is available at the end of the article

allows for various treatment options to be implemented early [8].

Conversely, a possibly large penis with hyperpigmentation of the scrotum alerts the physician to the possibility of congenital adrenal hyperplasia (CAH), a condition that can be fatal if not identified [9]. This is especially crucial in resource limited settings where newborn screening for CAH is not routinely done, as newborn males with CAH usually don't have other signs of androgen excess and often die undiagnosed from salt wasting crisis [10]. Macropenis has also been associated with rare syndromes like auriculo-condylar syndrome and caudal dysplasia sequence [11, 12].

Genital anthropometric measurements also help to avoid unwarranted investigations. It is useful in differentiating micropenis from an entirely normal 'inconspicuous' penis (concealed penis) [13].

Normative genital anthropometric data for healthy newborns exist and were mainly derived from Caucasian and Asian infants [3, 6, 14–16]. However, this may not be applicable to African infants. Indeed, previous studies have reported racial/ethnic differences in newborn penile sizes [1, 17, 18]. Some studies have even demonstrated significant differences in the same ethnic group with the passage of time and improvement in national economic conditions [19]. Recent studies from various parts of the world have aimed at establishing genital anthropometric norms representing their own populations [20–24]. No such comparable published data exist for Ghana. Hence, this study aimed at establishing the reference ranges for penile sizes in apparently healthy term newborns in Ghana.

Methods

A cross-sectional prospective study of all apparently well term male newborns delivered at Komfo Anokye Teaching Hospital (KATH) was carried out from May 2014 to September 2014. KATH is a tertiary teaching hospital in Kumasi, the second largest city in Ghana. Kumasi is a metropolitan city but majority of its inhabitants are Akans of the Ashanti tribe.

A nurse attached to the paediatric endocrine unit was trained to assist the principal investigator with the genital and anthropometric measurements. Two research assistants were trained to assist the two examiners with positioning of the babies and data entry. All apparently well male term newborns with a gestational age of 40 ± 2 weeks and birth weight between 2.5 and 4.0 kg were included. An initial clinical assessment guided by a screening form was done to find out which babies were eligible. Newborns with major congenital anomalies/dysmorphism, genital anomalies, breech presentation at birth, maternal pregnancy history of hormonal drug use, maternal signs of virilisation during pregnancy, maternal

pre-eclampsia or diabetes were all excluded. For eligible babies, the study was explained to the parent(s) and written informed consent was sought for. The baby was then enrolled if the parent(s) consented. Recruitment was done within 48 h after delivery. A complete antenatal history was obtained from the mother and from the hospital records, including a history of ingestion of herbal medicine or prescribed medications. The gestational age was determined by using the last menstrual period and early ultrasound results and confirmed if necessary with Dubowitz/Ballard score [25]. The socioeconomic status of the parents was determined using the Oyedeji classification [26]. A complete physical examination of each baby was done and anthropometric measurements taken. All anthropometric measurements were done by a 2-member team, with one person taking the measurements while the other positioned the baby and helped enter the data onto the Case report form.

In a warm environment, the newborns were put in a supine position and the perineum was adequately exposed. The SPL was measured by holding the glans gently between the thumb and forefinger and measuring from the pubic ramus, along the dorsum, to the tip of the glans penis with a disposable wooden spatula. The shaft of the penis was stretched to the point of resistance and the suprapubic fat pad compressed as completely as possible. The foreskin was not included in the measurement. The tip of the glans was marked on the spatula by a pencil. The distance between the tip of the spatula and the marked point was then measured with a measuring tape/ruler. The penile width was determined with a digital Vernier caliper (Resolution 0.01 mm, Accuracy +/–0.02 mm) by measuring the widest diameter along the shaft to the nearest 0.01 mm. All measurements were done twice and the mean value recorded. Majority (72.1%) of the measurements was done by the principal investigator but fortnightly, genital measurements were done on 5 randomly selected babies by both examiners to evaluate for inter-observer variability, which remained insignificant throughout the study. The standard deviations for inter-observer variation were 0.04 cm and 0.13 mm and 95% of paired measurements were within range of 0.09 cm and 0.26 mm for penile length and penile width respectively.

The data was analyzed using R statistical software version 3.1.2. Continuous variables were summarized and presented as means with standard deviation as well as median with their corresponding ranges. Single categorical variables were tabulated and expressed as percentages. The relationships between the genital measurements and the various categorical variables were determined using an analysis of variance, correcting for possible confounders and reporting the respective p-values as appropriate. Relationships between the genital measurement and other continuous variables were however determined using linear regression. These analyses were presented as their regression coefficient with their 95% confidence intervals. To establish the various percentiles for the genital measurements they were each summarized for gestational age to display the; 1st, 3rd, 50th, 97th, and the 99th age specific percentiles with the range. For all analysis a two sided p-value of <0.05 was considered statistically significant.

The study was approved by the Committee on Human Research, Publications and Ethics of KATH/Kwame Nkrumah University of Science and Technology, Kumasi. The Heads of the Department of Child Health and the Obstetrics and Gynaecology department as well as other staff in both departments were briefed about the study. A written Informed Consent Form detailing the study purpose, benefit and possible risk of the study to the children were provided and explained to the parent(s) in a language they could understand. The child was only enrolled if the parent(s) consented.

Results

A total of 644 male infants were studied. A summary data of study subjects is shown in Table 1. The distribution of maternal tribe was Akan 451 (70%), Mole-Dagomba 92 (14.3%), Ewe 20 (3.1%), Ga-Adangbe 7 (1.1%) and 'Others' (including Hausa, Grushie and Wangara tribes) 74 (11.5%). Genital measurements from study subjects were used to construct gestation-specific genital anthropometry percentile charts (Table 2). The mean penile length (MPL) was 3.3 cm and the −2.5 SD

Table 1 Summary data of study subjects

	Mean	SD	Median	Minimum	Maximum
Gestational age *(weeks)*	40.0	1.2	40.1	38.0	42.0
Post-natal age *(hours)*	10.1	8.3	8.0	1	48
Five Minute APGAR score	8.6	0.6	9.0	6	10
Birth weight *(kgs)*	3.2	0.4	3.2	2.5	4.0
Length *(cm)*	48.7	2.1	49.0	39.5	54.0
Head Circumference *(cm)*	34.4	1.3	34.4	30.0	38.2
Penile Length *(cm)*	3.3	0.5	3.2	2.0	4.8
Penile Width*(cm)*	1.05	0.1	1.05	0.69	1.37
Heart Rate *(bpm)*	134	11	136	96	164
Respiratory Rate *(cpm)*	49	11	48	28	90
Temperature *(℃)*	35.9	0.8	36	34.0	37.9
Maternal age *(years)*	28.5	6.2	28.0	15	49
Antenatal Care attendance	7	3	7	0	20
Paternal Age *(years)*	34.7	7.4	34	18	65
Parental socioeconomic score	3.3	1.0	3.5	1	5

Table 2 Percentile chart for penile size by gestational age in male newborns

Gestational age *(weeks)*	Percentiles						
	Min	1st	3rd	50th	97th	99th	Max
Penile Length *(cm)*							
38	2.3	2.3	2.6	3.1	4.2	4.3	4.4
39	2.2	2.2	2.5	3.2	4.1	4.3	4.7
40	2.0	2.2	2.2	3.3	4.4	4.5	4.8
41	2.0	2.2	2.3	3.2	4.0	4.3	4.5
42	2.3	2.5	2.7	3.2	4.0	4.1	4.1
Penile Width *(mm)*							
38	7.6	7.7	8.2	10.3	13.1	13.2	13.2
39	6.9	7.4	8.2	10.6	12.8	13.4	13.7
40	6.9	7.7	8.5	10.5	12.5	12.7	13.5
41	7.8	7.9	8.3	10.5	12.4	12.7	13.2
42	7.3	7.5	8.0	10.9	12.3	13.1	13.7

and +2.5 SD for MPL were 2.1 cm and 4.4 cm respectively.

There was no significant difference in genital size by maternal tribe, parental socioeconomic score or maternal herbal intake. Eighty-three mothers (12.9%) took herbs at varying periods during their pregnancy. There was also no significant difference in genital measurements done in the first 24 h of postnatal life and those done from 24 h up to 48 h. MPL, but not mean penile width (MPW), was negatively correlated with maternal age (Correlation Coefficient −0.062, 95% CI −0.121 to −0.002; $p = 0.04$) but positively correlated with gestational age (Correlation Coefficient 0.33, 95% CI: 0.02–0.64, p-value = 0.04). In an analysis of variance, only MPL was significantly different by mode of delivery. A post hoc analysis found a difference between only the caesarean section (C/S) group and the spontaneous vaginal delivery (SVD) group ($p = 0.038$). Table 3 shows the correlation between genital size and anthropometric parameters.

Discussion

Micropenis result from a heterogenous group of disorders; the most common being fetal testosterone deficiency [18]. In the human male fetus, testosterone synthesis by the fetal Leydig cell during the critical period of male differentiation (8–12weeks) is under the influence of placental human chorionic gonadotrophin. After mid-gestation, fetal pituitary Luteinizing hormone modulates fetal testosterone synthesis by the Leydig cell and, consequently, affects the growth of the differentiated penis [7]. Growth hormone acting in conjunction with insulin-like growth factors may also modulate androgen action [27]. Thus, males with congenital hypopituitarism as well as isolated gonadotropin or growth

Table 3 Association of genital size with anthropometric parameters

	Birth Weight (kgs)		Length (cm)	
	Coeff (95% CI)	P-value	Coeff (95% CI)	P-value
MPL (mm)	0.87 (−0.1–1.85)	0.08	0.34 (0.16–0.51)	**<0.001**
MPW (mm)	0.57 (0.32–0.81)	**<0.001**	0.11 (0.07–0.16)	**<0.001**

Significant p-values are in bold face

hormone deficiency can present with normal male differentiation and micropenis at birth. Rarely micropenis is associated with 5 alpha reductase enzyme deficiency or mild defects in the androgen receptor [7], though patients with 5 alpha reductase enzyme deficiency are more likely to have associated hypospadias than only isolated micropenis [28].

The main purpose of this study was to define normative genital sizes in the Ghanaian male newborn. To the best of our knowledge, this is the first published study of penile size in Ghanaian newborns. The relatively larger sample size allowed for a more precise construction of gestational specific percentile charts than in previously published smaller scale studies. Studies done in different parts of the world have reported varying MPL in newborns ranging from 2.35 to 3.77 cm [3, 14–16, 20, 29, 30]. This study found an MPL of 3.3 ± 0.5 cm. Using the conventional definition of micropenis as SPL < 2.5 SD below the mean and 'macropenis' as an SPL > 2.5 SD, a Ghanaian term newborn may warrant investigation if he has an MPL < 2.1 cm or > 4.4 cm.

Among studies with similar methodology, Akin et al. [21] reported a relatively lower MPL of 3.16 ± 0.39 cm in Turkey and Semiz et al. [30] also reported an even lower MPL of 2.81 ± 0.32 cm in 746 term Turkish newborns. Possible factors accounting for this observed difference are inter-observer variation and differences in the characteristics of the study populations including ethnicity/race [17]. Reports from other parts of Asia have also been relatively lower [23, 31], though not uniformly so [18, 22, 32]. Very low SPL have especially been reported in Indonesian newborns [33, 34]. Faizi et al. [29] for example reported a relatively low MPL of 2.35 ± 0.39 cm in 197 term neonates in Indonesia. Few African studies have been published. Jarrett et al. [24] in Nigeria reported a slightly higher MPL of 3.4 ± 0.48 cm. However, the characteristics of their study population were quite different. The study included preterm, term and post term babies, whilst only term babies were analyzed in the current study. Elsewhere in Africa, Kholy et al. [35] also reported a marginally higher MPL of 3.4 ± 0.37 cm in 150 Egyptian neonates. In Caucasians, Schonfeld et al. [14] published a relatively higher MPL in full-term infant of 3.75 ± 0 cm, while Feldman and Smith [3] and Flatau et al. [16] published an MPL of 3.5 ± 0.7 cm and 3.5 ± 0.4 cm, respectively.

Fewer studies have reported penile width in published literature. This study found an MPW of 1.05 ± 0.1 cm. Semiz et al. [30] reported a comparable MPW of 1.04 ± 0.09 while Akin et al. [21] reported a comparatively higher MPW of 1.21 ± 0.11 cm. The technique for the measurement of penile width was not stated in the former whilst the latter study measured the penile width in the midshaft using a circular scale with measurements being taken to the nearest even 2 mm. Jarrett et al. [24] reported a relatively higher MPW of 1.2 ± 0.14 cm. Here the penile width was measured as the transverse diameter in the middle of the penile shaft using a ruler. This current study measured penile width in its widest diameter along the shaft with a caliper which measures to the nearest 0.01 mm. Differences in measurement techniques and accuracy of the scales employed could play a role in the variation of published MPW values. There have also been reports of a significant association between penile width and other anthropometric parameters as well as maternal age [21, 24, 36]. Consequently, differences in the characteristics of the study population may contribute to the variability seen in reported values of MPW. Elsewhere, Feldman and Smith [3] has reported a comparable MPW of 1.1 ± 0.2 cm in the United States whereas Sutan-Assin et al. [33] reported a relatively low MPW of 0.82 ± 0.33 cm in 336 term babies in Indonesia.

Genital size did not vary significantly by parental socio-economic status, probably as a result of the lack of association between anthropometric parameters and parental socio-economic status. The effect of socioeconomic status on genital sizes is likely an indirect one, through an effect on newborn anthropometric parameters. No study has examined the effect of socioeconomic status on genital sizes per say. However, Lee et al. [19] reported a significant increase in SPL in Korean children when they compared normative data obtained in the year 2011 to that of 1987. They attributed this to a comparative increase in anthropometric indices like weight and length/height from improved economic conditions. Genital size also did not vary significantly with maternal use of herbal medicine during pregnancy. This analysis was done to evaluate for possible hormonal effects of the ingested herbal medicines, since their constituents were largely unknown. MPW was higher (1.15 ± 0.77 cm) in babies of mothers from the Ga-Adangbe tribe but their numbers were too small to compute for statistical significance. There was no significant difference between genital measurements done in the first 24 h and those done afterwards. Contrarily, in 63 Japanese term newborns Matsuo et al. [31] found that penile length measured within 12 h after birth differed significantly (0.3 cm 95% CI 0.22–0.34) from values obtained 1–7 days postnatally by the same examiner. They attributed this to the oedematous prepubic skin hindering sufficient stretching of the penis. However, the sample size was probably too small to establish a definite significance and *p*-values were not given.

There was a weak inverse relationship between maternal age and MPL (Coefficient –0.062, 95% CI –0.121 to –0.002; $p = 0.04$), consistent with what was reported by Romano-Riquer et al. [36]. The association between penile size and maternal age could be related to the finding that older pregnant women tend to have lower testosterone levels [37, 38], and there is a positive correlation between maternal and fetal testosterone levels [39]. Testosterone has a trophic effect on the phallus, as demonstrated by Mohamed et al. [40] who reported a positive correlation between penile length and serum testosterone levels in newborns. Another possibility is that placental aromatase activity, which metabolizes fetal androgens into estriol, may increase with increasing maternal age, thereby resulting in lower fetal testosterone concentrations. Kaijser et al. [41] however found no correlation between maternal age and placental aromatase.

This study found a significant positive correlation between MPL and gestational age ($p = 0.04$). In multivariate analysis, likely because of the small range of gestational ages (only term neonates delivered at 38–42 weeks of gestation were included); this correlation was no longer statistically significant. Other studies have also reported a positive correlation between MPL and gestational age [23, 34]. Jarrett et al. [24] found no correlation between MPL and gestational age. The reasons for these inconsistencies in finding associations are most likely multi-factorial, possibly including differences in study methodology and ethnicity [17]. Similar to Jarrett et al. [24], this study did not find any correlation between MPW and gestational age. In a multiple linear regression analysis with post hoc analysis, babies delivered by SVD had a significantly higher MPL than those delivered by C/S ($p = 0.038$). We performed this analysis to find out whether the inclusion of babies delivered by other means apart from SVD can influence mean genital size. Kutlu [20] in Turkey recruited only babies delivered by SVD, but most other published studies did not state the mode of delivery [17, 21, 22, 24, 30, 32, 42]. The reason for our finding was not clear. More studies need to be done to clarify this. Our study specifically excluded babies with breech presentation because of its known association with hypopituitarism. Debate is ongoing about whether breech presentation is the cause or consequence of hypopituitarism [43]. Hypopituitarism has also been associated with instrumental delivery [5].

In this study, MPL was positively correlated with length ($p < 0.001$) but not with birth weight ($p = 0.08$) while MPW was proportionally correlated with both anthropometric parameters ($p < 0.001$ for all). These observations

closely mirror those of Akin et al. [21]. Likewise, other authors have reported a positive correlation between MPL and birth length [20, 23, 30, 34, 44], although majority also found a positive correlation with birth weight as well, unlike this study [23, 30, 34, 44]. Jarrett et al. [24] and Cheng & Chanoine [17] found no correlation between MPL and birth weight or length. Jarrett et al. [24] also found a positive correlation between MPW and birth weight and length. In contrast, Cheng and Chanoine [17] found no significant correlation between MPW and birth weight or length.

Whether penile length at birth correlates with penile length in adults is unclear. There is to our knowledge no longitudinal study on this topic and no studies directly comparing penile lengths in neonates and adults of diverse origins. Penile length seems to be relatively similar in both neonates and adults from Nigerian and Caucasian descent [14, 24, 45].

Conclusions

In comparing penile size across studies, characteristics of the study population including gestational age, birth weight and length, mode of delivery and maternal age should be taken into consideration. More importantly, over/under-diagnosis of micropenis may occur with its attendant unnecessary investigations and treatment if local normative values for penile size are not established.

Limitations

Measurements were done by two examiners and could have introduced an error due to inter-observer variability. However, an extensive training was done and a subset of study subjects was examined by both 2 examiners to evaluate and control for variability, which remained insignificant throughout the study.

Abbreviations

CI: Confidence interval; Coeff: Correlation coefficient; KATH: Komfo Anokye Teaching Hospital; MPL: Mean penile length; MPW: Mean penile width; SPL: Stretched penile length

Acknowledgements

SBAA, EA and JPC are members of Global Pediatric Endocrinology and Diabetes (GPED, www.globalpedendo.org), which supported the study. The authors will like to acknowledge Prof Margaret Zacharin, the staff of KATH Obstetrics and Gynaecology department and the co-ordinators and fellows of the PETCWA programme.

Funding

This research was jointly funded by Global Paediatric Endocrinology and Diabetes and the European Society for Paediatric Endocrinology.

Authors' contributions

SBAA participated in the study design, data collection and entry and manuscript writing. EA sought for ethical clearance, participated in the study design, data collection and entry and supervision and completion of final manuscript. JPC participated in the study design, supervision and completion of final manuscript. SBN participated in the study design, statistical analysis and completion of final manuscript. All authors read and approved the final manuscript.

Competing interests

The authors declare that they have no competing interests.

Author details

[1]Department of Child Health, Komfo Anokye Teaching Hospital, Kumasi, Ghana. [2]Endocrinology and Diabetes Unit, British Columbia's Children's Hospital, University of British Columbia, Vancouver, BC, Canada.

References

1. Phillip M, De Boer C, Pilpel D, Karplus M, Sofer S. Clitoral and penile sizes of full term newborns in two different ethnic groups. J Pediatr Endocrinol Metab. 1996;9:175–9.
2. Lee P, Mazur T, Danish R, Amrhein J, Blizzard R, Money J, et al. Micropenis I. Criteria, etiologies and classification. Johns Hopkins Med J. 1980;146:156–63.
3. Feldman KW, Smith DW. Fetal phallic growth and penile standards for newborn male infants. J Pediatr. 1975;86:395–8.
4. Salisbury DM, Leonard JV, Dezateux CA, Savage MO. Micropenis: an important early sign of congenital hypopituitarism. Br Med J (Clin Res Ed). 1984;288:621–2.
5. Ameeta Mehta A, Datta MT. Congenital disorders of the hypothalamic–pituitary axis. In: Brook CGD, Clayton PE, Brown RS, editors. Brook's Clinical Pediatric Endocrinology. 5th ed. Oxford: Blackwell Publishing Ltd; 2005. p. 67–89.
6. Tuladhar R, Davis PG, Batch J, Doyle LW. Establishment of a normal range of penile length in preterm infants. J Paediatr Child Health. 1998;34:471–3.
7. Conte FA, Grumbach MM. Disorders of sexual determination and differentiation. In: Gardner DG, Shoback D, editors. Greenspan's Basic & Clinical Endocrinology. 9th ed. New York: The McGraw-Hill Companies; 2011. p. 479–526.
8. Hatipoğlu N, Kurtoğlu S. Micropenis: etiology, diagnosis and treatment approaches. J Clin Res Pediatr Endocrinol. 2013;5:217–23.
9. Kaiser GL. Symptoms and signs in Pediatric surgery. New York: Springer; 2005. p. 565–79.
10. Thorén M. Adrenal disorders, female androgen deficiency, hirsutism, and endocrine hypertension. In: Schenck-Gustafsson K, DeCola PR, Pfaff DW, Pisetsky DS, editors. Handbook of Clinical Gender Medicine. Basel: Karger; 2012. p. 317–26.
11. Kido Y, Gordon CT, Sakazume S, Bdira EB, Dattani M, Wilson LC, et al. Further characterization of atypical features in auriculocondylar syndrome caused by recessive PLCB4 mutations. Am J Med Genet A. 2013;161A:2339–46.
12. Makhoul IR, Aviram-Goldring A, Paperna T, Sujov P, Rienstein S, Smolkin T, et al. Caudal dysplasia sequence with penile enlargement: case report and a potential pathogenic hypothesis. Am J Med Genet. 2001;99:54–8.
13. Praduch DA, Schlegel PN. Male hypogonadism. In: Sarafoglou K, Hoffmann G, Roth KS, Courtney H, editors. Pediatric Endocrinology and Inborn Errors of Metabolism. New York: The McGraw Hill Companies; 2009. p. 575–600.
14. Schonfeld WA, Beebe GW. Normal growth and variation in the male genitalia from birth to maturity. J Urol. 1942;48:759–77.
15. Schonfeld WA. Primary and secondary sexual characteristics: study of their development in males from birth through maturity, with biometric study of penis and testes. Am J Dis Child. 1943;65:535–49.
16. Flatau E, Josefsberg Z, Reisner SH, Bialik O, Laron Z. Letter: Penile size in the newborn infant. J Pediatr. 1975;87:663–4.
17. Cheng PK, Chanoine JP. Should the definition of micropenis vary according to ethnicity? Horm Res. 2001;55:278–81.
18. Lian WB, Lee WR, Ho LY. Penile length of newborns in Singapore. J Pediatr Endocrinol Metab. 2000;13:55–62.
19. Lee JH, Ji YH, Lee SK, Hwang HH, Ryu DS, Kim KS, et al. Change in penile length in children: preliminary study. Korean J Urol. 2012;53:870–4.
20. Kutlu AO. Normative data for penile length in Turkish newborns. J Clin Res Pediatr Endocrinol. 2010;2:107–10.
21. Akın Y, Ercan O, Telatar B, Tarhan F. Penile size in term newborn infants. Turk J Pediatr. 2011;53(3):301–7.
22. Ting TH, Wu LL. Penile length of term newborn infants in multiracial Malaysia. Singapore Med J. 2009;50(8):817–21.
23. Fok TF, Hon KL, So HK, Wong E, Ng PC, Chang A, et al. Normative data of penile length for term Chinese newborns. Biol Neonate. 2005;87:242–5.
24. Jarrett OO, Ayoola OO, Jonsson B, Albertsson-Wikland K, Ritzen EM. Penile size in healthy Nigerian newborns: country-based reference values and international comparisons. Acta Paediatr. 2014;103(4):442–6.
25. Dubowitz LMS, Dubowitz V, Goldberg C. Clinical assessment of gestational age in the newborn infant. J Pediatr. 1970;77:1–10.
26. Oyedeji GA. Socio-economic and cultural background of hospitalized children in Ilesha. Nig J Paediatr. 1985;12:111–7.
27. Laron Z, Klinger B. Effect of insulin-like growth factor-1 treatment on serum androgens and testicular and penile size in males with Laron syndrome (primary growth hormone resistance). Eur J Endocrinol. 1998;138:176–80.
28. Maimoun L, Philibert P, Cammas B, Audran F, Bouchard P, Fenichel P, et al. Phenotypical, biological, and molecular heterogeneity of 5α-reductase deficiency: an extensive international experience of 55 patients. J Clin Endocrinol Metab. 2011;96:297–307.
29. Faizi M, Dyah T, Lita ST, Netty EP. Penile length of newborn infants in Dr. Soetomo Hospital Surabaya. A Preliminary Study. FMI. 2011;47:64–7.
30. Semiz S, Küçüktaşçi K, Zencir M, Sevinç O. One-year follow-up of penis and testis sizes of healthy Turkish male newborns. Turk J Pediatr. 2011;53(6):661–5.
31. Matsuo N, Ishii T, Takayama J, Miwa M, Hasegawa T. Reference standard of penile size and prevalence of buried penis in Japanese newborn male infants. Endocr J. 2014;61(9):894–53.
32. Al-Herbish AS. Standard penile size for normal full term newborns in the Saudi population. Saudi Med J. 2002;23:314–6.
33. Sutan-Assin M, Rukman J, Dahlan A. Penile dimensions of newborn infants. Paediatr Indones. 1989;29(7–8):146–50.
34. Moelyo AG, Widyastuti M. Penile length of newborns and children in Surakarta, Indonesia. Paediatr Indones. 2013;53:65–9.
35. Kholy ME, Hamza RT, Saleh M, Elsedfy H. Penile length and genital anomalies in Egyptian male newborns: epidemiology and influence of endocrine disruptors. JPEM. 2013;26:509–13.
36. Romano-Riquer SP, Hernandez-Avila M, Gladen BC, Cupul-Uicab LA, Longnecker MP. Reliability and determinants of anogenital distance and penis dimensions in male newborns from Chiapas, Mexico. Paediatr Perinat Epidemiol. 2007;21:219–28.
37. Carlsen SM, Jacobsen G, Bjerve KS. Androgen levels in pregnant women decrease with increasing maternal age. Scand J Clin Lab Invest. 2003;63:23–6.
38. Troisi R, Potischman N, Roberts J, Siiteri P, Daftary A, Sims C, et al. Associations of maternal and umbilical cord hormone concentrations with maternal, gestational and neonatal factors (United States). Cancer Causes Control. 2003;14:347–55.
39. Gitau R, Adams D, Fisk NM, Glover V. Fetal plasma testosterone correlates positively with cortisol. Arch Dis Child Fetal Neonatal Ed. 2005;90:F166–9.
40. Mohamed MH, Abdoua RM, Hamzab MT, Husseina MMS. Penile length and cord total and free testosterone in full term male Egyptian neonates. Gaz Egypt Paediatr Assoc. 2015;63:58–62.
41. Kaijser M, Jacobsen G, Granath F, Cnattingius S, Ekbom A. Maternal age, anthropometrics and pregnancy oestriol. Paediatr Perinat Epidemiol. 2002;16:149–53.
42. Alaee E, Gharib MJ, Fouladinejad M. Penile length and anogenital distance in male newborns from different Iranian ethnicities in Golestan province. Iran Red Crescent Med J. 2014;16:1–4.
43. Backeljauw PF, Dattani MT, Cohen P, Rosenfeld RG. Disorders of growth hormone/insulin-like growth factor secretion and action. In: Sperling MA, editor. Pediatric Endocrinology. 4th ed. Philadelphia: Elsevier; 2014. p. 338.
44. Çamurdan AD, Öz MO, Ilhan MN, Çamurdan OM, Sahin F, Beyazova U. Current stretched penile length: cross-sectional study of 1040 healthy Turkish children aged 0 to 5 years. Urology. 2007;70:572–5.

24

An audit of the management of childhood-onset growth hormone deficiency during young adulthood in Scotland

M. Ahmid[1], V. Fisher[1], A. J. Graveling[2], S. McGeoch[2], E. McNeil[1], J. Roach[3], J. S. Bevan[2], L. Bath[3], M. Donaldson[1], G. Leese[4], A. Mason[1], C. G. Perry[5], N. N. Zammitt[6], S. F. Ahmed[1] and M. G. Shaikh[1]*

Abstract

Background: Adolescents with childhood onset growth hormone deficiency (CO-GHD) require re-evaluation of their growth hormone (GH) axis on attainment of final height to determine eligibility for adult GH therapy (rhGH).

Aim: Retrospective multicentre review of management of young adults with CO-GHD in four paediatric centres in Scotland during transition.

Patients: Medical records of 130 eligible CO-GHD adolescents (78 males), who attained final height between 2005 and 2013 were reviewed. Median (range) age at initial diagnosis of CO-GHD was 10.7 years (0.1–16.4) with a stimulated GH peak of 2.3 μg/l (0.1–6.5). Median age at initiation of rhGH was 10.8 years (0.4–17.0).

Results: Of the 130 CO-GHD adolescents, 74/130(57 %) had GH axis re-evaluation by stimulation tests /IGF-1 measurements. Of those, 61/74 (82 %) remained GHD with 51/74 (69 %) restarting adult rhGH. Predictors of persistent GHD included an organic hypothalamic-pituitary disorder and multiple pituitary hormone deficiencies (MPHD). Of the remaining 56/130 (43 %) patients who were not re-tested, 34/56 (61 %) were transferred to adult services on rhGH without biochemical retesting and 32/34 of these had MPHD. The proportion of adults who were offered rhGH without biochemical re-testing in the four centres ranged between 10 and 50 % of their total cohort.

Conclusions: A substantial proportion of adults with CO-GHD remain GHD, particularly those with MPHD and most opt for treatment with rhGH. Despite clinical guidelines, there is significant variation in the management of CO-GHD in young adulthood across Scotland.

Keywords: Childhood onset growth hormone deficiency, Retesting, Re-evaluation, Transition, Adolescence

Background

The transition of care from childhood to adulthood for many chronic disorders requires a careful coordinated approach and this is particularly important in growth hormone deficiency (GHD). Traditionally, children with childhood onset GHD (CO-GHD) discontinue recombinant human GH therapy (rhGH) after attaining final height. However, adults with CO-GHD may have increased fat mass, decreased muscle mass and low bone mineral density, as well as reduced cardiac performance, altered lipid status, reduced physical performance, impaired cognitive function and reduced well-being [1, 2]. Reports suggest that these adults may benefit from rhGH [3, 4]. A number of studies have shown that a high proportion of CO-GHD patients remain GH deficient as adults especially those with multiple pituitary hormone deficiencies (MPHD) and/or structural abnormalities, whereas the majority of those with idiopathic or isolated GHD no longer have GHD in adulthood [5–7]. Therefore, after childhood treatment it is necessary to review GH status in order to assess appropriateness of adult rhGH replacement [8]. However, the extent of benefit from this therapy may be variable and the decision to reinstitute rhGH needs to be undertaken carefully.

* Correspondence: guftar.shaikh@nhs.net
[1]Developmental Endocrinology Research Group, Royal Hospital for Children, School of Medicine, University of Glasgow, 1345 Govan Road, Glasgow G51 4TF, UK
Full list of author information is available at the end of the article

In this context, clinical practice guidelines have been issued on the subject of transition of care of young adults with CO-GHD [9–12]. However, the practicalities of these guidelines as well as the extent to which these guidelines have been implemented in clinical practice are unclear. The purpose of this multicentre study was to understand the variation that may exist in the management of young adults with CO-GHD after attainment of final height.

Methods

We reviewed databases from the four specialist endocrine centres in Scotland and identified young adults who had been diagnosed as having CO-GHD and who had been treated with GH during childhood and had subsequently reached final height between 2005 and 2013. Study entry criteria were: CO-GHD (low GH peak response on stimulation test <6.6 µg/l), GH treatment during childhood, attainment of final height between 2005 and 2013 (height velocity <1 cm/year as defined in all centres), and evaluation of GH- axis by stimulation tests and/or IGF-1 levels after withdrawal of GH for at least one month. Exclusion criteria included: untreated CO-GHD, GH-treated patients with CO-GHD who have not yet attained final height. Baseline demographic data included: aetiology of CO-GHD, age at diagnosis of CO-GHD, duration of GH treatment, presence of multiple pituitary hormone deficiencies (MPHD), re-evaluation of GH axis, and whether adult GH treatment was recommenced or not. The persistent GHD after retesting for four centers was defined as cutoff <5 µg/L GH peak response for dynamic stimulation testes and/or low serum IGF-1 levels (<2 SD for age and sex) [9]. IGF-1 level measurement for centres A, B, and D were done using IDS iSys and centre C measured IGF-1 levels by immunoassay on the Siemens Immulite. All IGF-1 levels were corrected for age and sex accordingly.

Statistical analysis

Data were analyzed using Minitab software (Version 16) with a significance level of <0.05 and are described as median, ranges and percentage. Additionally, the Mann–Whitney U–test was used for calculation of significance of differences between median values. Association with clinical factors was assessed by Spearman's rank coefficient and a positive predictive value (PPV) was calculated for the identified predictors of persistent GHD.

Results
General characteristics

A total of 142 patients were screened, 130 of whom met inclusion criteria. The 130 patients (78 male) comprised of: 70 from centre A, 32 from B, 18 from C and 10 from D. Table 1 displays the aetiology of CO-GHD. Median age at diagnosis of CO-GHD was 10.7 years (0.1–16.4) with an initial stimulated GH peak of 2.3 µg/l (0.1–6.5), and basal IGF-1 was 74 µg/l (4.0–410.0). Median age at initiation of rhGH was 10.8 years (0.4–17.0). GH peak at diagnosis was lower in those with MPHD compared to IGHD (1.9 µg/l (<0.1–6.4) vs 3.0 µg/l (0.3–6.5) respectively: $p < 0.01$).

Re-evaluation of GH axis

A total of 74/130 (57 %) patients with CO-GHD (IGHD = 31 (42 %): MPHD = 43(58 %)) were biochemically retested at a median age of 18.2 years (14.5–21.3) (with one outlier patient who was retested at the age of 27.5 years), rhGH treatment was discontinued at the median age of 16.4 years (10.8–21.0). Biochemical retesting was performed after a median period of 0.5 years (0.1–5.6) off rhGH (21/74 (28 %) were retested over period of (0.1–0.3 years) and 34/74(46 %) over a period of (0.4–5.7 years), with incomplete data on timing of re-testing in 20/74 (27 %). Median duration of childhood treatment was 5.3 years (0.4–16.8). At retesting, the median GH peak was 1.6 µg/l (0.1–23.7) and IGF-1 was 88.0 µg/l (15.0–631.0). Of those retested, 61/74 (82 %) (32 males) remained GHD and were eligible for adult rhGH, with 51/61 (84 %) re-starting adult rhGH and 10/61 (16 %) declining therapy although it is possible that they may have restarted at a later stage. The remaining 13/74 (18 %)(10 males) who were no longer GH deficient consisted of eight with idiopathic IGHD, two brothers with central hypothyroidism and normal pituitary MRI, one with an ectopic pituitary, one with hypogonadism and Coeliac disease and one with a history of cranial irradiation. Of the 56 of 130 (43 %) cases of CO-GHD who were not retested 34 (61 %) were transferred from paediatric to adult services without biochemical retesting during transition, 12 (21 %) stopped treatment without biochemical re-evaluation and 10 (18 %) were lost to follow up whilst on treatment (Fig. 1).

Dynamic function stimulation tests were performed in 40/74 (54 %) patients who were retested, with 35/40 (88 %) of subjects having a low GH peak response <5 µg/l, with 27/35 of them having severe GHD with a GH peak response <3 µg/l. Of the remaining 34/74 (46 %) patients who were retested, IGF-1 levels alone were available and low enough to confirm GHD (≤ -2 SD for age and gender) in 19/34 (56 %) of which 15 had MPHD and 4 had IGHD (organic causes and abnormal pituitary MRI). Two patients (MPHD) had IGF-1 levels within normal range on initial retesting (>2 SD for age and gender), but were confirmed to have GHD following GH stimulation tests.

Reconfirmation of GHD and initiation of adult GH replacement therapy

Of the 130 with CO-GHD, 34 (26 %) patients continued adult rhGH without temporary cessation of therapy or

Table 1 The categories of patients with CO-GHD according to aetiology and centres distribution is shown as (A, B, C, D)

	Total number of cases 130	IGHD 48/130 (37 %)	MPHD* 82/130 (63 %)
Congenital n (%) (A,B,C,D)	38/130 (29 %)	12 (8,1,2,1)	26 (14,3,4,5)
-Pituitary axial structural abnormalities (A,B,C,D)	24	9 (6,1,1,1)	15 (6,3,1,5)
-Midline axial structure defects (SOD) (A,B,C,D)	14	3 (2,0,1,0)	11 (8,0,3,0)
Oncology/cranial irradiation n (%) (A,B,C,D)	51/130 (40 %)	8 (5,3,0,0)	43 (18,19,4,2)
- Craniopharyngioma (A,B,C,D)	15	–	15 (6,7,1,1)
- Hematologic malignancies (A,B,C,D)	12	4 (4,0,0,0)	8 (6,0,1,1)
- Medulloblastoma (A,B,C,D)	6	1 (0,1,0,0)	5 (1,4,0,0)
- Other CNS tumors (A,B,C,D)	18	3 (1,2,0,0)	15 (5,8,2,0)
Idiopathic[a] n (%) (A,B,C,D)	15/130 (11 %)	13 (7,1,5,0)	2 (1,1,0,0)
Others[b] n (%) (A,B,C,D)	26/130 (20 %)	15 (12,1,1,1)	11 (5,3,2,1)
-Crohn's disease (A,B,C,D)	4	4 (3,0,0,1)	–
-Coeliac disease (A,B,C,D)	2	–	2 (0,1,1,0)
-Haematological diseases[c] (A,B,C,D)	2	1 (1,0,0,0)	1 (1,0,0,0)
-Other diseases[d] (A,B,C,D)	11	8 (6,1,1,0)	3 (0,2,1,0)
-Syndromes[e](A,B,C,D)	6	2 (2,0,0,0)	4 (3,0,0,1)
-Acquired brain injury (A,B,C,D)	1	–	1 (1,0,0,0)

Data are presented as the numbers of patients and percentages are given in *parentheses*

*33/82 patients with one additional pituitary hormone deficiency, 17/82 with two additional deficiencies, 19/82 with three and 13/82 with four additional deficiencies 'panhypopituitarism'

IGHD, isolated growth hormone deficiency; MPHD, multiple-pituitary hormone deficiencies; SOD, Septo-optic dysplasia

[a]Normal pituitary MRI, GHD is not associated with other conditions

[b]Normal pituitary MRI (or no MRI report), but GHD is associated with other conditions

[c](Thalassemia, X-linked Sideroblastic Anaemia)

[d](Microephaly with learning disability, history of intrauterine growth retardation, gastrochisis with history of small for gestational age, Asthma, joint hypermobility syndrome, pesudohypoparathyrodism)

[e](Charge syndrome, Noonan syndrome, Kallman Syndrome, trisomy 22, Klinefelter's syndrome, Turner's syndrome with GHD)

formal retesting. Of these 34, nine had structural abnormalities on MRI, 22 were related to late effects of cancer therapy and three had unexplained GHD. Of those 34, 31 (91 %) had MPHD (17/32 of them had three or more additional pituitary hormone deficiencies (PHDs)); and 3/34 (9 %) had IGHD (two with pituitary structural abnormalities on MRI and one with tumour related GHD).

These patients were advised to continue rhGH until their mid-20s.

For patients who were re-tested, GH cut offs for considering rhGH varied between centres. Not all patients found to have persistent GHD restarted adult GH therapy despite low peak GH levels at re-testing. There were four patients who were found not to have severe GHD with GH peaks

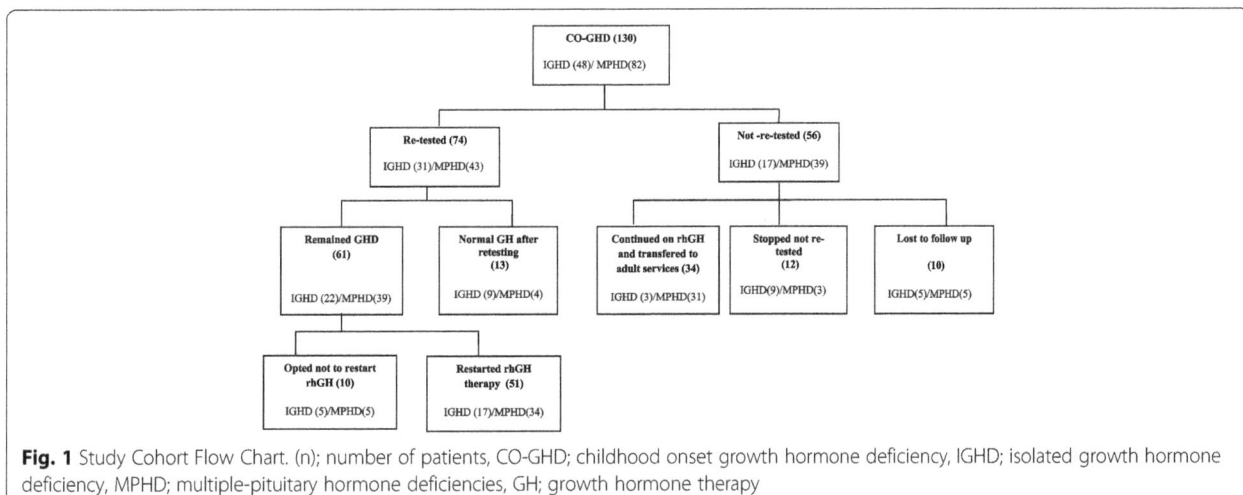

Fig. 1 Study Cohort Flow Chart. (n); number of patients, CO-GHD; childhood onset growth hormone deficiency, IGHD; isolated growth hormone deficiency, MPHD; multiple-pituitary hormone deficiencies, GH; growth hormone therapy

4-5 µg/l (three patients from centre B, one from centre A) and were not offered rhGH as they did not meet adult criteria for replacement. However, among those who were offered rhGH after retesting, one patient with IGHD (centre C) had a GH peak >5 µg/l (5.5 µg/l).

Variation in the management between centres

There were substantial variations in the management of CO-GHD between Scottish centres. Re-testing with stimulation testes and/or IGF-1 levels was found to be the highest in centre A (68 %), while centre C had the lowest percentage of retested patients (28 %), although this did include all IGHD patients from centre C. Centre B did not retest those with a high likelihood of permanent GHD (especially those with three or more additional PHDs) and had the highest percentage of adults on rhGH without biochemical re-evaluation (Table 2). A total of 32/130 patients in the cohort had three or more additional PHDs (Table 3). Of these 32, 14 (44 %) were retested using their IGF-1 levels alone and all were confirmed to have adult GHD, 17 (53 %) continued on rhGH without biochemical retesting and one was lost to follow up whilst on treatment.

Predictors of persistent GHD on re-evaluation

Patients with persistent GHD were diagnosed at an earlier age ((8.4 years (0.3–16.0) vs 11.6 years (7.1–15.5)) and reached final height with re-evaluation of their GH axis in earlier adolescence ((17.9 years (14.2–21.2) vs 19.3 years (17.3–21.3)) than those who were no longer GH deficient on retesting. No significant differences in the other parameters between persistent GHD and non-persistent GHD were identified at time of diagnosis or re-evaluation. In this population the peak GH level on retesting was positively related with the GH peak level at childhood ($r = 0.4$, $P = 0.02$). The number of additional PHDs was a predictor of a low peak GH on retesting as all patients with two or more additional PHDs had a lower GH response (<5 µg/l) at reassessment with a PPV (93 %). The presence of hypothalamic–pituitary structural abnormalities has a high PPV (96 %) of persistent

GHD, as of the 25 who were retested, 24 were reconfirmed with persistent GHD. Similarly, CO-GHD with a history of cranial irradiation predicted persistent GHD in adulthood (96 %).

Discussion

Our data confirm that a high proportion (82 %) of the retested patients with CO-GHD continue to have GHD as adults. The majority (80 %) of those who remain GH deficient opted to resume adult GH treatment, however it is unknown whether they complied with therapy and for how long they continued with the treatment. It may also be the case that those adults who were GHD initially declined to restart rhGH during transition, but later reconsidered GH therapy. Factors influencing this decision would be an important area for future studies.

Previous published studies have reported variable estimates of persistent GHD in adulthood ranging from 12.5–90 % [13, 14] but the high incidence of ongoing GHD in adulthood in our cohort may be attributed to the large proportion of patients with organic causes for their GHD. Some of our subjects with MPHD who had no structural abnormalities on MRI continued to have GHD, raising the possibility of an underlying genetic disorder. Similarly, the majority of idiopathic IGHD who were re-evaluated were GH deficient which may also indicate an underlying genetic predisposition. These findings suggest the importance of follow up and regular assessment of pituitary function in those with a low probability of persistent GHD, as they may develop other pituitary hormone deficiencies as previously demonstrated [15, 16]. On the other hand, some patients who would be considered as having a moderate to high probability of persistent GHD (IGHD with structural abnormalities, patients with MPHD or those with a history of cranial irradiation) were no longer GH deficient. These findings demonstrate the limitations in using "at risk" groups to determine who require re-evaluation of their GH axis and those who do not.

Our data confirm that while there are no unequivocal auxological or clinical signs that predict the transiency

Table 2 Management of patients with CO-GHD according to each Scottish centre

	All centres	A	B	C	D
Total number of patients (n)	130	70	32	18	10
Total number of patients re-tested n (%)	74/130 (57)	48/70 (69)	16/32 (50)	5/18 (28)	5/10 (50)
Persistent GHD n (%)	61/74 (82)	43/48 (90)	12/16 (75)	1/5 (20)	5/5 (100)
Those with persistent GHD who restarted rhGH n (%)	51/61 (83)	35/43 (81)	11/12 (92)	1/1 (100)	4/5 (80)
Total number of patients not-retested n (%)	56/130 (43)	22/70 (31)	16/32 (50)	13/18 (72)	5/10 (50)
Continued adult rhGH therapy without re-testing n (%)	34/56 (61)	7/22 (32)	16/16 (100)	7/13 (54)	4/5 (80)
Lost to follow up whilst on treatment n (%)	10/56 (18)	9/22 (41)	0	0	1/5 (20)
Stopped GH, no re-testing required n (%)	12/56 (21)	6/22 (27)	0	6/13 (46)	0

Data are presented as the numbers of patients and percentages are given in *parentheses*

Table 3 Variation in the management of patients with CO-GHD between the four Scottish centres according to GHD categories

Centres	A		B		C		D	
	IGHD	MPHD	IGHD	MPHD	IGHD	MPHD	IGHD	MPHD
Total CO-GHD n = 130 [32]	32	38[16]	6	26[10]	8	10[3]	2	8[3]
Retested n = 74 [14]	21	27[13]	4	12[0]	4	1 [0]	2	3[1]
With structural abnormalities[a]	8	13[5]	–	2	1	–	–	–
Tumour related[b]	3	13[8]	2	7	–	1	–	1
Idiopathic/unexplained[c]	10	1	2	3	3	–	2	2[1]
Re-confirmed GHD	16	27[13]	3	9[0]	1	0	2	3[1]
Not retested (*but on adult rhGH*) n = 34 [17]	0	7[2]	2	14[10]	1	6 [3]	–	4[2]
With structural abnormalities[a]	–	–	2	1	1	3 [3]	–	1
Tumour related[b]	–	5[2]	–	12[10]	–	3	–	1[1]
Idiopathic/unexplained[c]	–	2	–	1	–	–	–	2[1]

Data are presented as number of patients with CO-GHD and [number of patients who have three and more additional pituitary hormones deficiencies

[a]MRI imaging reported hypothalamic-pituitary axial structural abnormalities

[b]Cranial irradiation

[c]Normal pituitary MRI/Congenital GHD unexplained (no MRI report)/and/or associated with chronic disease

or the persistence of GHD, a history of organic disease, the presence of two or more additional PHDs [17, 18], presence of hypothalamic-pituitary structural abnormalities and tumour related organic GHD are strong indicators of persistence GHD [19–22].

In terms of timing of retesting, the current guidelines suggest that a period from one to three months off rhGH is sufficient for retesting [9]. Our data show a variable interval between stopping treatment and reassessment, with only 28 % of patients off rhGH for less than 3 months. It is not clear for those who were off rhGH for longer duration before reassessment whether their stopping rhGH was for reasons other than re-testing. However, this prolonged period off rhGH may be associated with detrimental effects on somatic bone and body composition development during transition [23, 24], with recommendations for prompt resumption of rhGH in individuals with clinical evidence of persistent GHD [25]. Furthermore, a longer interval off rhGH may increase the risk of being lost to follow up in these already vulnerable patients and continued follow up around this time is essential [26]. We recommend that in patients who are under the care of paediatric services, the evaluation of GHD in transition should be undertaken by the paediatric clinic, ideally in the context of a joint transition service to improve the follow up and smooth transfer of adolescents with chronic endocrine conditions to the adult services as previously suggested [27].

The principle of offering rhGH during transition for those who have ongoing severe deficiency was variable between centres as the cut-offs chosen are variable, though the majority were in keeping with the guidance suggesting a GH peak <5 µg/l constituting severe GHD in transition [9, 10]. Few patients in our cohort declined restarting adult rhGH, they may be asymptomatic and therefore reluctant to restart rhGH therapy. Approximately one third of our subjects were considered to be very likely to have permanent GHD and therefore continued rhGH uninterrupted, apart from adjustment to an adult GH dose. This is in line with current guidelines which recommend that patients with severe congenital or acquired panhypopituitarism with three or more pituitary hormone deficiencies or identified genetic mutations may not require re-evaluation of their GH status; otherwise all patients with CO-GHD require biochemical re-evaluation and reconfirmation of GHD during transition before reinstituting adult GH replacement therapy [9, 12]. However, of the 34 patients who continued adult rhGH without formal retesting, nine had structural abnormalities on MRI probably were at high risk of ongoing GHD, but three had unexplained GHD and probably should have been retested. Furthermore, some centres still retested those with a high likelihood of permanent GHD, by checking their IGF1 levels, although all were reconfirmed GHD and resumed rhGH. On these grounds, it seems that no clear consensus has been reached as to whether or not to withdraw treatment and retest those at high risk of permanent GHD. It is also unclear whether those who continued rhGH without biochemical re-testing were re-evaluated at a later stage. For those who restarted rhGH, according to the current guidelines, at completion of somatic growth (approximately 25–30 years old) further re-evaluation should be undertaken with the offer of adult GH replacement therapy and monitoring in accordance with National Institute for Health and Care Excellence guidance (NICE) (TA 64 August 2003).

Conclusion

In conclusion, this study not only provided a snapshot of the differences in management of CO-GHD during transition across Scotland, but it has also enabled us to identify areas of uncertainty despite there being clinical practice recommendations. Our data showed a substantial proportion of patients with CO-GHD remain GH deficient and most opt for rhGH as adults, although not all patients may require re-evaluation of their GH axis. This study also raises concerns about follow up of those who no longer have GHD and patients with GHD who opted not to resume adult rhGH. The optimal management of adolescents with CO-GHD requires continuous follow up during transition and effective communication between paediatric and adult services.

Abbreviations
CO-GHD: childhood onset growth hormone deficiency; GH: growth hormone; GHD: growth hormone deficiency; IGF-1: insulin-like growth factor 1; IGHD: isolated growth hormone deficiency; MPHD: multiple pituitary hormone deficiencies; MRI: magnetic resonance imaging; PPV: positive predictive value; SDS: standard deviation score.

Competing interests
The authors declare that they have no competing interests.

Authors' contributions
MA and MGS designed, performed data collection, performed the main part of statistical analysis, and wrote the initial draft of the manuscript. SFA conceived of the study and participated in its design and coordination as well as drafting the manuscript. AJG, SM, GL, JSB contributed in data collection and interpretations. All authors made substantial contributions read, edited and approved the final manuscript.

Acknowledgements
MA is currently supported by the Government of Libya.

Author details
[1]Developmental Endocrinology Research Group, Royal Hospital for Children, School of Medicine, University of Glasgow, 1345 Govan Road, Glasgow G51 4TF, UK. [2]JJR Macleod Centre for Diabetes, Endocrinology & Metabolism, Aberdeen Royal Infirmary, Aberdeen, UK. [3]Department of Endocrinology, Royal Hospital for Sick Children, Edinburgh, UK. [4]Ninewells Hospital and Medical School in Dundee, Dundee, UK. [5]Department of Endocrinology, Queen Elizabeth University Hospitals, Glasgow, UK. [6]Royal Infirmary of Edinburgh, Edinburgh, UK.

References
1. deBoer H, vanderVeen EA. Why retest young adults with childhood-onset growth hormone deficiency? J Clin Endocrinol Metab. 1997;82(7):2032–6.
2. Moller N, Jorgensen JO. Effects of growth hormone on glucose, lipid, and protein metabolism in human subjects. Endocr Rev. 2009;30(2):152–77.
3. Carroll PV, Christ ER, Bengtsson BA, Carlsson L, Christiansen JS, Clemmons D, et al. Growth hormone deficiency in adulthood and the effects of growth hormone replacement: a review. Growth Hormone Research Society Scientific Committee. J Clin Endocrinol Metab. 1998;83(2):382–95.
4. Clayton P, Gleeson H, Monson J, Popovic V, Shalet SM, Christiansen JS. Growth hormone replacement throughout life: insights into age-related responses to treatment. Growth Horm IGF Res. 2007;17(5):369–82.
5. Geffner ME. Growth hormone replacement therapy: transition from adolescence to adulthood. J Clin Res Pediatr Endocrinol. 2009;1(5):205–8.
6. Tauber M, Moulin P, Pienkowski C, Jouret B, Rochiccioli P. Growth hormone (GH) retesting and auxological data in 131 GH-deficient patients after completion of treatment. J Clin Endocrinol Metab. 1997;82(2):352–6.
7. Loche S, Bizzarri C, Maghnie M, Faedda A, Tzialla C, Autelli M, et al. Results of early reevaluation of growth hormone secretion in short children with apparent growth hormone deficiency. J Pediatr. 2002;140(4):445–9.
8. Koltowska-Haggstrom M, Geffner ME, Jonsson P, Monson JP, Abs R, Hana V, et al. Discontinuation of growth hormone (GH) treatment during the transition phase is an important factor determining the phenotype of young adults with nonidiopathic childhood-onset GH deficiency. J Clin Endocrinol Metab. 2010;95(6):2646–54.
9. Clayton PE, Cuneo RC, Juul A, Monson JP, Shalet SM, Tauber M, et al. Consensus statement on the management of the GH-treated adolescent in the transition to adult care. Eur J Endocrinol. 2005;152(2):165–70.
10. Radovick S, DiVall S. Approach to the growth hormone-deficient child during transition to adulthood. J Clin Endocrinol Metab. 2007;92(4):1195–200.
11. Ho KK. Consensus guidelines for the diagnosis and treatment of adults with GH deficiency II: a statement of the GH Research Society in association with the European Society for Pediatric Endocrinology, Lawson Wilkins Society, European Society of Endocrinology, Japan Endocrine Society, and Endocrine Society of Australia. Eur J Endocrinol. 2007;157(6):695–700.
12. Cook DM, Rose SR. A review of guidelines for use of growth hormone in pediatric and transition patients. Pituitary. 2012;15(3):301–10.
13. Maghnie M, Strigazzi C, Tinelli C, Autelli M, Cisternino M, Loche S, et al. Growth hormone (GH) deficiency (GHD) of childhood onset: reassessment of GH status and evaluation of the predictive criteria for permanent GHD in young adults. J Clin Endocrinol Metab. 1999;84(4):1324–8.
14. Attanasio AF, Howell S, Bates PC, Blum WF, Frewer P, Quigley C, et al. Confirmation of severe GH deficiency after final height in patients diagnosed as GH deficient during childhood. Clin Endocrinol (Oxf). 2002;56(4):503–7.
15. Lange M, Feldt-Rasmussen U, Svendsen OL, Kastrup KW, Juul A, Muller J. High risk of adrenal insufficiency in adults previously treated for idiopathic childhood onset growth hormone deficiency. J Clin Endocrinol Metab. 2003;88(12):5784–9.
16. Blum WF, Deal C, Zimmermann AG, Shavrikova EP, Child CJ, Quigley CA, et al. Development of additional pituitary hormone deficiencies in pediatric patients originally diagnosed with idiopathic isolated GH deficiency. Eur J Endocrinol. 2014;170(1):13–21.
17. Juul A, Holm K, Kastrup KW, Pedersen SA, Michaelsen KF, Scheike T, et al. Free insulin-like growth factor I serum levels in 1430 healthy children and adults, and its diagnostic value in patients suspected of growth hormone deficiency. J Clin Endocrinol Metab. 1997;82(8):2497–502.
18. Hartman ML, Crowe BJ, Biller BM, Ho KK, Clemmons DR, Chipman JJ, et al. Which patients do not require a GH stimulation test for the diagnosis of adult GH deficiency? J Clin Endocrinol Metab. 2002;87(2):477–85.
19. Tillmann V, Tang VW, Price DA, Hughes DG, Wright NB, Clayton PE. Magnetic resonance imaging of the hypothalamic-pituitary axis in the diagnosis of growth hormone deficiency. J Pediatr Endocrinol Metab. 2000;13(9):1577–83.
20. Kalina MA, Kalina-Faska B, Gruszczynska K, Baron J, Malecka-Tendera E. Usefulness of magnetic resonance findings of the hypothalamic-pituitary region in the management of short children with growth hormone deficiency: evidence from a longitudinal study. Childs Nerv Syst. 2012;28(1):121–7.
21. Bonfig W, Bechtold S, Bachmann S, Putzker S, Fuchs O, Pagel P, et al. Reassessment of the optimal growth hormone cut-off level in insulin tolerance testing for growth hormone secretion in patients with childhood-onset growth hormone deficiency during transition to adulthood. J Pediatr Endocrinol Metab. 2008;21(11):1049–56.
22. Quigley CA, Zagar AJ, Liu CC, Brown DM, Huseman C, Levitsky L, et al. United States multicenter study of factors predicting the persistence of GH deficiency during the transition period between childhood and adulthood. Int J Pediatr Endocrinol. 2013;2013(1):6. doi:10.1186/1687-9856-2013-6.
23. Carroll PV, Drake WM, Maher KT, Metcalfe K, Shaw NJ, Dunger DB, et al. Comparison of continuation or cessation of growth hormone (GH) therapy on body composition and metabolic status in adolescents with severe GH deficiency at completion of linear growth. J Clin Endocrinol Metab. 2004;89(8):3890–5.
24. Tritos NA, Hamrahian AH, King D, Greenspan SL, Cook DM, Jonsson PJ, et al. A longer interval without GH replacement and female gender are associated with lower bone mineral density in adults with childhood-onset GH deficiency: a KIMS database analysis. Eur J Endocrinol. 2012;167(3):343–51.
25. Nguyen VT, Misra M. Transitioning of children with GH deficiency to adult dosing: changes in body composition. Pituitary. 2009;12(2):125–35.
26. Courtillot C, Baudoin R, Du Souich T, Saatdjian L, Tejedor I, Pinto G, et al. Monocentric study of 112 consecutive patients with childhood onset GH deficiency around and after transition. Eur J Endocrinol. 2013;169(5):587–96.
27. Downing J, Gleeson HK, Clayton PE, Davis JR, Wales JK, Callery P. Transition in endocrinology: the challenge of maintaining continuity. Clin Endocrinol (Oxf). 2013;78(1):29–35.

25

Change in BMI after radioactive iodine ablation for graves disease

Melinda Chen[1*], Matthew Lash[2], Todd Nebesio[1] and Erica Eugster[1]

Abstract

Background: We aimed to determine the extent of post-treatment weight gain that occurs in pediatric patients in the first year following radioactive iodine (RAI) therapy for Graves disease (GD) and its relationship to clinical characteristics.

Methods: A retrospective chart review of patients receiving RAI therapy for GD between 1998–2015 was performed. Change in BMI SDS (ΔBMI SDS) from baseline to one year after treatment was determined. We also investigated whether individual clinical and/or biochemical factors were associated with the weight trajectory in these patients.

Results: One hundred fifty seven patients aged 12.7 ± 3 years (80% girls) were included in the analysis. Average ΔBMI SDS was 0.70 ± 0.71 ($p < 0.001$) at 1 year. Patients with weight loss at presentation had a greater ΔBMI SDS than those without (0.92 vs 0.56, $p = 0.005$), whereas no association was seen with gender, pubertal status, use of antithyroid drugs, history of ADHD, or Down syndrome. Baseline BMI SDS was negatively correlated with ΔBMI SDS, with a stronger correlation in males. From baseline to 1 year, the proportion of overweight and obese patients increased from 9.6% to 18.5% and from 6.4% to 21%, respectively. In a subset of 81 patients, a positive correlation was noted between time to euthyroidism and ΔBMI SDS, particularly in boys.

Conclusions: The number of our patients in the overweight category doubled and the number in the obese category more than tripled in the first year following RAI treatment for GD. Anticipatory guidance regarding this important issue is badly needed.

Keywords: RAI, Obesity, Graves disease

Background

Graves disease (GD), characterized by autoimmune over-stimulation of the thyroid gland, is the most common cause of hyperthyroidism in children and adolescents [1–4]. The overall incidence within the pediatric population is approximately 1 in 10,000 [5] with the highest prevalence seen in adolescent girls [2]. Although the hypermetabolic state in GD typically results in weight loss, stable weight or even weight gain due to increased caloric intake can be seen [5].

Therapeutic modalities for the treatment of GD include surgery, radioactive iodine (RAI) ablation and anti-thyroid drugs (ATDs). Surgery and RAI are considered definitive therapy and result in permanent hypothyroidism. Patients receiving definitive therapy often become hypothyroid for a period of time before appropriate levothyroxine replacement and biochemical euthyroidism is achieved. Weight gain following treatment of GD has been reported in both children and adults. Proposed explanations include continued increased caloric consumption with resolution of the prior hypermetabolic state [5], a return to or exaggeration of premorbid weight [6], or a result of post-treatment hypothyroidism [7]. Previous studies reporting change in weight following treatment of GD in children have focused primarily on patients treated with ATDs as first-line therapy. In contrast, the change in BMI after RAI treatment has not been systematically studied. It is unknown whether the treatment modality itself affects the degree of weight gain or whether there are clinical or

* Correspondence: chenmeli@iupui.edu
[1]Department of Pediatrics, Section of Pediatric Endocrinology, Riley Hospital for Children, Indiana University School of Medicine, 705 Riley Hospital Drive, Room # 5960, Indianapolis, IN 46202, USA
Full list of author information is available at the end of the article

biochemical factors that might modulate the degree of weight gain in these patients [7–9].

Thus, the goal of our study was to investigate the degree of weight gain in the first year following RAI therapy for GD. We also sought to explore whether individual characteristics were associated with differences in weight gain among our patients.

Methods

Following ethical review and approval of Protocol #1412088318 by the Indiana University Institutional Review Board, a retrospective chart review was performed of pediatric patients receiving RAI ablation for GD at Riley Hospital for Children between 1998 and 2015. All patients with a documented height and weight within four months before RAI treatment and a follow up visit with documented height and weight between 6 and 18 months after RAI date were included. Regardless of whether patients had been treated for GD prior to evaluation at our institution, all patients were hyperthyroid at the time of RAI. If a second dose of RAI was needed, the dose leading to successful ablation (i.e. the second dose) was used as the event of interest to determine pre- and post-treatment height and weight.

Medical records were searched for variables of interest, which included age, gender, pubertal status, history of weight loss, DS (Down Syndrome), use of medications for ADHD, ATD use for ≥ one month prior to RAI, start date of levothyroxine replacement, and the date of documented euthyroidism. Weight and height were collected at baseline (last appointment prior to RAI) and at the one-year follow up appointment. BMI was calculated using the formula {BMI = weight in kilograms/height in meters^2}. Pubertal status was classified as either prepubertal (Tanner I) or pubertal (Tanner II-V). Euthyroidism was considered to be a TSH and free T4 or total T4 within the performing laboratory's reference range, or (in a small subset of cases), documented interpretation of lab tests as "normal" by the primary endocrinologist.

All BMIs were categorized according to Centers for Disease Control (CDC) standards as underweight (<5th percentile), normal weight (5- < 85th percentile), overweight (85- < 95th percentile) or obese (≥95th percentile) [10]. Time to euthyroidism (TTE) was calculated by determining the time in weeks between the date of starting levothyroxine replacement and the date of documented euthyroidism.

Statistics

Analyses were performed using SPSS statistical software (version 24; IBM Corp.). All variables of interest were evaluated for normality to determine appropriateness of statistical methods and found to be normally distributed. Descriptive statistics were used to report anthropometric data and time intervals. Chi-square tests and Fisher's exact tests were used to analyze differences in weight status category distribution before and after RAI. Paired t-tests were used to assess differences in BMI before and after treatment. Unpaired t-tests were used to analyze the effect of clinical risk factors on weight gain. Linear regression was used to describe strength of association between change (Δ) in BMI SDS over time and contributing factors. The level of significance was α = 0.05, with all p-values lower than 0.05 considered statistically significant. Results are expressed as mean ± SD in the text, with medians and ranges also provided in Table 1.

Results

Of 247 patients receiving RAI for GD, 157 (79.6% female) had complete data and were included in the analysis. Mean baseline age was 12.7 ± 3.0 years and mean baseline BMI SDS was 0.003 ± 1.18 kg/m^2. Ten patients (6.4%) had DS (Down Syndrome) and 33 (21.0%) had received ATDs before RAI ablation. Of 135 patients with documented pubertal status, 88 (65.2%) were ≥ Tanner stage II at the baseline evaluation. Post-treatment BMI data were obtained at 50.65 ± 11.32 weeks after RAI.

Average ΔBMI SDS from baseline to one year was 0.70 ± 0.71 ($p < 0.001$), with no difference noted by gender, pubertal status, history of ATDs, use of stimulant medications for ADHD, or presence of DS (Down Syndrome). In contrast, BMI SDS increased more in those with a history of weight loss (ΔBMI SDS 0.92 vs 0.56, $p = 0.005$). These results are shown in Table 1. On regression analysis, baseline BMI SDS was negatively correlated with ΔBMI SDS ($p < 0.001$, R = –0.529), with a stronger correlation in males ($p < 0.001$, R = –0.696).

From baseline to follow-up, the proportion of underweight patients in the study decreased from 10.2% to 0.6% ($p ≤ 0.001$), while those in the overweight and obese categories increased from 9.6% to 18.5% ($p ≤ 0.001$) and from 6.4% to 21% ($p ≤ 0.001$), respectively, as shown in Fig. 1. Of 157 patients, 2 (0.1%) moved into a lower weight category, while 62 (39.5%) moved into a higher weight category. Notably, nearly one third of our patients (31.2%) moved into the overweight or obese category from a lower weight category.

A sub-analysis was performed on 81 patients (85.2% female) with evidence of good compliance in whom the exact TTE was available. Within this group, TTE was 24.16 ± 13.28 weeks and ΔBMI SDS at one year was not different from the group as a whole. Unlike what was seen for the entire cohort, a history of weight loss had no impact on ΔBMI SDS by 1 year, (0.77 ± 0.62 vs. 0.55 ± 0.56, $p = 0.12$), whereas prepubertal patients were found to have greater ΔBMI SDS than pubertal patients at 1 year (0.90 ± .71 vs 0.57 ± .58, $p = 0.037$). In males, a longer TTE was

Table 1 Potential factors associated with weight gain in patients following RAI treatment of GD

Variable – Mean ± SD Median (range)	Whole population ($n = 157$)		p-value	Sub-analysis ($n = 81$)		p-value
Age	12.68 ± 3.00 y 12.86 (5.34-17.89) y			12.79 ± 3.02 y 12.77 (5.34-17.83) y		
	ΔBMI SDS			ΔBMI SDS		
Gender	Female (%) 0.71 ± 0.66 (79.6)	Male (%) 0.71 ± 0.92 (20.4)	0.99	Female (%) 0.69 ± 0.65 (85.2)	Male (%) 0.35 ± 0.47 (14.8)	0.09
	0.61 (−0.4-2.97)	0.41 (−0.55-3.85)		0.69 (−0.4-2.68)	0.24 (−0.55-1.24)	
	Yes (%)	No (%)		Yes (%)	No (%)	
ATD use	0.64 ± 0.68 (21)	0.73 ± 0.73 (79)	0.55	0.67 ± 0.77 (18.5)	0.63 ± 0.60 (81.5)	0.81
	0.46 (−0.37-2.68)	0.54 (−0.55-3.85)		0.55 (−0.25-2.68)	0.66 (−0.55-2.04)	
Down syndrome	0.85 ± 0.86 (6.4)	0.70 ± 0.71 (93.6)	0.53	1.04 ± 0.90 (7.4)	0.61 ± 0.60 (92.6)	0.10
	0.88 (0.0-2.68)	0.53 (−0.55-3.85)		0.88 (0.17-2.68)	0.59 (−0.55-2.04)	
ADHD treatment	0.97 ± 1.08 (7.6)	0.69 ± 0.68 (92.4)	0.40	0.98 ± 0.79 (4.9)	0.62 ± 0.62 (95.1)	0.26
	0.44 (0.08-3.85)	0.55 (−0.55-2.97)		0.97 (0.08-1.92)	0.59 (−0.55-2.68)	
History of weight loss	0.92 ± 0.84 (38.2)	0.56 ± 0.57 (49)	0.005*	0.77 ± 0.62 (39.5)	0.55 ± 0.56 (50.6)	0.12
	0.74 (−0.55-3.85)	0.45 (−0.4-2.47)		0.74 (−0.55-2.00)	0.57 (−0.4-2.04)	
Pubertal	0.67 ± 0.63 (56.1)	0.91 ± 0.90 (29.9)	0.10	0.57 ± 0.58 (56.8)	0.90 ± 0.71 (29.6)	0.04*
	0.49 (−0.4-2.71)	0.75 (−0.37-3.85)		0.50 (−0.4-2.04)	0.82 (−0.35-2.68)	

Significant findings ($p < 0.05$) are marked with an asterisk (*). Mean ± SD are on line 1 and median, range on line 2 for all variables. Not all percentages add to 100% due to missing patient information. BMI = body mass index; ATD = anti-thyroid drug; ADHD = attention deficit-hyperactivity disorder

correlated with greater increase in BMI z-score (R = 0.63, $p = 0.029$) (Fig. 2), while a similar, though weaker, association was seen in females (R = 0.59, $p ≤ 0.001$).

Discussion

Weight gain after treatment for GD is well recognized in adults, but only two previous studies have been published in pediatric patients to our knowledge [5, 11]. These studies included patients who were almost exclusively treated with ATDs as first-line therapy, and did not closely examine as many potential modifying factors. We observed a ΔBMI SDS of 0.70 ± 0.71 over the first year in our population receiving RAI therapy as definitive treatment for GD. One previous study followed children for up to 3 years and observed a similar

increase in BMI z-score after treatment from −0.02 ± 1.05 to 0.79 ± 0.81 with subsequent stabilization of weight, with most weight gain seen within the first 6 months of treatment [5]. A second study comparing changes in weight following treatment of both hypothyroidism and hyperthyroidism also reported weight gain after treatment for GD early in follow up, though the exact time frame was not specified [11].

Unsurprisingly, a history of weight loss before RAI was associated with greater weight gain at follow up in our population, though this relationship was not present in the sub-analysis. However, prepubertal patients in our sub-analysis did have a greater ΔBMI SDS. This is in line with another study that observed greater increases in

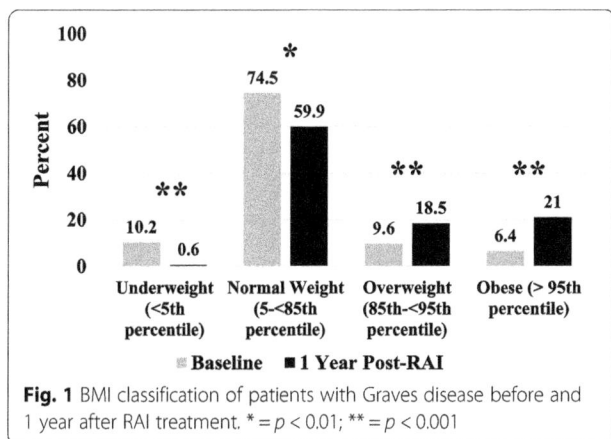

Fig. 1 BMI classification of patients with Graves disease before and 1 year after RAI treatment. * = $p < 0.01$; ** = $p < 0.001$

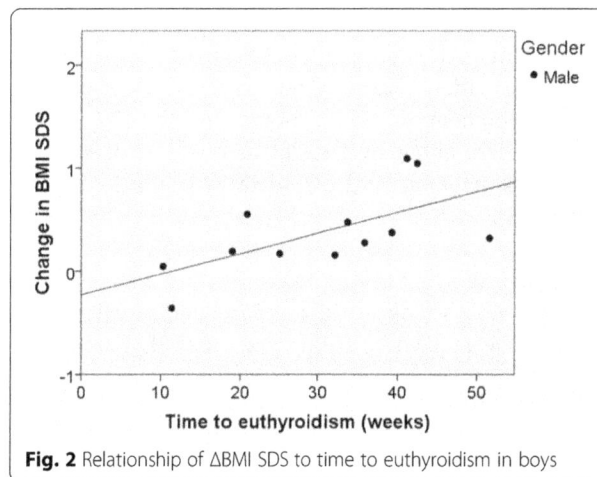

Fig. 2 Relationship of ΔBMI SDS to time to euthyroidism in boys

BMI after treatment for GD in children under 11 years compared with older children [5]. It is unknown whether this relationship is a result of age or of the metabolic changes that occur during puberty. No other factors were found to clearly define higher-risk groups for weight gain in our population. All patients receiving RAI for GD should be considered at high risk for weight gain and counseled accordingly.

Although our study was focused on the effects of RAI therapy, 21% of patients had previously received ATDs and experienced no difference in ΔBMI SDS at one year compared with those who had not. Most patients treated with ATDs were not seen at our institution at their initial presentation with GD, and thus their pre-treatment BMIs were not available. However, previous research has suggested that the use of sequential treatment modalities in adults can result in continued weight gain compared with definitive treatment as a first line approach [8]. This question would be interesting to investigate in pediatric patients as well. If corroborated, this may be further reason to advocate for earlier definitive treatment rather than pursuing medical therapy which only rarely results in permanent remission in children and adolescents and carries the potential for rare but serious side effects [12].

While TTE was negatively correlated with ΔBMI SDS in our subanalysis, the weakness of this association suggests that other factors should also be considered. Though some studies in adults show differences in BMI outcome by treatment modality [8, 9], this has not been demonstrated consistently, and it is unknown whether these expectations can be extended to children. We found similar outcomes in our population when compared to reports from other centers [5].

To our knowledge, our study represents the largest cohort of pediatric patients in whom weight gain following treatment for GD is investigated, and the only one in which all patients were treated with RAI. Limitations include its retrospective nature as well as the fact that data documenting the precise TTE was only available in 81 of our patients. An additional weakness is that we did not have information regarding our patients' BMIs prior to the development of GD. However, nearly 40% of our patients were either overweight or obese at one year, a rate above national BMI SDS data in youth 2–19 years of age [13].

Conclusions

In conclusion, we observed a striking and nearly universal increase in BMI SDS one year after RAI treatment for GD resulting in a doubling in the number of overweight and a tripling in the number of obese patients, placing them at higher risk for adverse health consequences over time. Future studies should focus on targeted interventions aimed at attenuating the rate of weight gain in children and adolescents undergoing treatment for GD.

Abbreviations
ΔBMI SDS: Change in BMI standard deviation score; ATDs: Anti-thyroid drugs; DS: Down syndrome; GD: Graves Disease; RAI: Radioactive iodine; TTE: Time to euthyroidism

Acknowledgements
Dr. Chen was supported by NIH 2 T32DK065549.

Funding
Dr. Chen was supported by NIH 2 T32DK065549.

Authors' contributions
MC collected data, carried out the initial analyses, drafted the initial manuscript, reviewed and revised the manuscript, and approved the final manuscript as submitted. ML designed the study, obtained regulatory approval, collected data, and approved the final manuscript as submitted. TN conceptualized the study, reviewed and revised the manuscript, and approved the final manuscript as submitted. EE conceptualized the study, provided supervision of the research, critically reviewed the manuscript, and approved the final manuscript as submitted

Competing interests
The authors declare that they have no competing interests.

Author details
[1]Department of Pediatrics, Section of Pediatric Endocrinology, Riley Hospital for Children, Indiana University School of Medicine, 705 Riley Hospital Drive, Room # 5960, Indianapolis, IN 46202, USA. [2]Department of Pediatrics, Naval Medical Center, 34800 Bob Wilson Dr, San Diego, CA 92134, USA.

References
1. Rivkees SA. Pediatric Graves' disease: controversies in management. Horm Res Paediatr. 2010;74(5):305–11. doi:10.1159/000320028.
2. Leger J, Carel JC. Hyperthyroidism in childhood: causes, when and how to treat. J Clin Res Pediatr Endocrinol. 2013;5 Suppl 1:50–6. doi:10.4274/jcrpe.854.
3. Kaguelidou F, Alberti C, Castanet M, Guitteny MA, Czernichow P, Leger J, et al. Predictors of autoimmune hyperthyroidism relapse in children after discontinuation of antithyroid drug treatment. J Clin Endocrinol Metab. 2008;93(10):3817–26. doi:10.1210/jc.2008-0842.
4. Pinto T, Cummings EA, Barnes D, Salisbury S. Clinical Course of Pediatric and Adolescent Graves' Disease Treated with Radioactive Iodine. Journal of Pediatric Endocrinology and Metabolism. 2007;20(9). doi:10.1515/jpem.2007.20.9.973.
5. van Veenendaal NR, Rivkees SA. Treatment of pediatric Graves' disease is associated with excessive weight gain. J Clin Endocrinol Metab. 2011;96(10):3257–63. doi:10.1210/jc.2011-1601.

6. Jansson S, Berg G, Lindstedt G, Michanek A, Nystrom E. Overweight–a common problem among women treated for hyperthyroidism. Postgrad Med J. 1993;69(808):107–11. doi:10.1136/pgmj.69.808.107.

7. Tigas S, Idiculla J, Beckett G, Toft A. Is excessive weight gain after ablative treatment of hyperthyroidism due to inadequate thyroid hormone therapy? Thyroid. 2000;10(12):1107–11. doi:10.1089/thy.2000.10.1107.

8. Schneider DF, Nookala R, Jaraczewski TJ, Chen H, Solorzano CC, Sippel RS. Thyroidectomy as primary treatment optimizes body mass index in patients with hyperthyroidism. Ann Surg Oncol. 2014;21(7):2303–9. doi:10.1245/s10434-014-3542-8.

9. Dale J, Daykin J, Holder R, Sheppard MC, Franklyn JA. Weight gain following treatment of hyperthyroidism. Clin Endocrinol. 2001;55(2):233–9. doi:10.1046/j.1365-2265.2001.01329.x.

10. Defining Childhood Obesity. In: Overweight and Obesity. Centers of Disease Control and Prevention. https://www.cdc.gov/obesity/childhood/defining.html.

11. Crocker MK, Kaplowitz P. Treatment of paediatric hyperthyroidism but not hypothyroidism has a significant effect on weight. Clin Endocrinol. 2010;73(6):752–9. doi:10.1111/j.1365-2265.2010.03877.x.

12. Rivkees SA, Szarfman A. Dissimilar hepatotoxicity profiles of propylthiouracil and methimazole in children. J Clin Endocrinol Metab. 2010;95(7):3260–7. doi:10.1210/jc.2009-2546.

13. Ogden CL, Carroll MD, Kit BK, Flegal KM. Prevalence of childhood and adult obesity in the United States, 2011–2012. JAMA. 2014;311(8):806–14. doi:10.1001/jama.2014.732.

26

Peak cortisol response to corticotropin-releasing hormone is associated with age and body size in children referred for clinical testing: a retrospective review

Mary Ellen Vajravelu[1], Jared Tobolski[1], Evanette Burrows[2], Marianne Chilutti[2], Rui Xiao[3], Vaneeta Bamba[1], Steven Willi[1], Andrew Palladino[4], Jon M. Burnham[5] and Shana E. McCormack[1*]

Abstract

Background: Corticotropin-Releasing Hormone (CRH) testing is used to evaluate suspected adrenocorticotropic hormone (ACTH) deficiency, but the clinical characteristics that affect response in young children are incompletely understood. Our objective was to determine the effect of age and body size on cortisol response to CRH in children at risk for ACTH deficiency referred for clinical testing.

Methods: Retrospective, observational study of 297 children, ages 30 days – 18 years, undergoing initial, clinically indicated outpatient CRH stimulation testing at a tertiary referral center. All subjects received 1mcg/kg corticorelin per institutional protocol. Serial, timed ACTH and cortisol measurements were obtained. Patient demographic and clinical factors were abstracted from the medical record. Patients without full recorded anthropometric data, pubertal assessment, ACTH measurements, or clear indication for testing were excluded (number remaining = 222). Outcomes of interest were maximum cortisol after stimulation (peak) and cortisol rise from baseline (delta). Bivariable and multivariable linear regression analyses were used to assess the effects of age and size (weight, height, body mass index (BMI), body surface area (BSA), BMI z-score, and height z-score) on cortisol response while accounting for clinical covariates including sex, race/ethnicity, pubertal status, indication for testing, and time of testing.

Results: Subjects were 27 % female, with mean age of 8.9 years (SD 4.5); 75 % were pre-pubertal. Mean peak cortisol was 609.2 nmol/L (SD 213.0); mean delta cortisol was 404.2 nmol/L (SD 200.2). In separate multivariable models, weight, height, BSA and height z-score each remained independently negatively associated ($p < 0.05$) with peak and delta cortisol, controlling for indication of testing, baseline cortisol, and peak or delta ACTH, respectively. Age was negatively associated with peak but not delta cortisol in multivariable analysis.

Conclusions: Despite the use of a weight-based dosing protocol, both peak and delta cortisol response to CRH are negatively associated with several measures of body size in children referred for clinical testing, raising the question of whether alternate CRH dosing strategies or age- or size-based thresholds for adequate cortisol response should be considered in pediatric patients, or, alternatively, whether this finding reflects practice patterns followed when referring children for clinical testing.

Keywords: Adrenal insufficiency, Corticotropin-releasing hormone (CRH) stimulation test, Exogenous glucocorticoid exposure, Adrenal stimulation testing, Cortisol

* Correspondence: mccormacks1@email.chop.edu
[1]Division of Endocrinology and Diabetes, The Children's Hospital of Philadelphia, 3401 Civic Center Blvd, Suite 11NW, Philadelphia, USA
Full list of author information is available at the end of the article

Background

Undiagnosed adrenal insufficiency can be life-threatening [1–3]. Children exposed to prolonged courses of exogenous glucocorticoids or with congenital or acquired forms of hypopituitarism are at increased risk for adrenocorticotropic hormone (ACTH) deficiency, or central adrenal insufficiency [1, 4]. Despite considerable clinical experience, the diagnosis of ACTH deficiency remains complex [5], and the "optimal" method to reliably diagnose ACTH deficiency remains unclear [6], particularly in children. While the insulin tolerance test (ITT) is often considered a "gold standard," its use is limited due to the potential for severe hypoglycemia and its contraindication in patients with a history of seizures or cardiovascular disease [7, 8]. Although frequently used, the low-dose ACTH stimulation test does not allow for direct measurement of pituitary response, and concerns have been raised about the difficulty of reliably diluting the low dose of medication with precision [9]. The standard-dose ACTH stimulation test may be used to assess for primary adrenal insufficiency, but the large dose of 250 mcg produces supra-physiologic ACTH levels, which may lead to falsely reassuring cortisol responses in patients who may truly have inadequate responses to stress under more physiologic conditions [9].

Stimulation of the pituitary with corticotropin-releasing hormone (CRH), or corticorelin, can be used to test for both primary and secondary adrenal insufficiency through its stimulation of the release of ACTH from the pituitary [10–12]. The CRH stimulation test has been suggested as a useful and safe alternative to the ITT, as the cortisol response to CRH has been found to be significantly correlated with cortisol response to insulin-induced hypoglycemia [13, 14]. However, distinguishing between "healthy" and "inadequate" cortisol responses to this test remains a challenge, in part because there is not a clear consensus from previous studies on the patient-specific clinical factors that determine peak cortisol, particularly in children. Indeed, although some pediatric studies suggest that cortisol response after stimulation with CRH remains constant with increasing age [12, 15, 16], in other investigations, cortisol response after stimulation using other strategies, including low- [4] or standard-dose [17] ACTH, was negatively associated with age in children. The current recommended dosing for CRH is weight-based, which assumes a comparable pituitary and adrenal response to this medication across all ages and sizes. Previously published studies have not systematically focused on the relationship of body size to CRH response, particularly in children younger than six years [12, 15, 16]. Children under six years of age, in particular, may differ in clearance rates of medications due to incomplete maturation of physiologic and enzymatic processes [18]. Thus, the objective of the present study was to determine the effect of both age and body size on cortisol response, as measured by peak cortisol and cortisol rise from baseline (delta) to a standard CRH test in a cohort of nearly 300 children referred to a tertiary care center for suspicion of ACTH deficiency.

Methods

Design

This is a retrospective electronic medical record review of all children and adolescents referred for outpatient adrenal stimulation testing with CRH between January 2007 and April 2013 at The Children's Hospital of Philadelphia Day Medicine Unit.

Subjects

Subjects were less than 18 years of age at the time of testing; neonates (<30 days), most of whom receive clinically indicated adrenal stimulation testing as inpatients, were excluded. For subjects who underwent multiple stimulation tests, only the first was used for this analysis. All subjects underwent stimulation with 1 mcg/kg corticorelin (CRH) intravenously, prepared as a solution of 50 mcg corticorelin/mL by our institution's main pharmacy. Per standard protocol at our institution, cortisol and ACTH were measured at baseline and 15, 30, 60, and 90 min after CRH administration. This study was reviewed, approved, and granted a waiver of consent by the Institutional Review Board of The Children's Hospital of Philadelphia.

Anthropometric and pubertal data

Height and weight were abstracted from electronic medical record as measured on the day of stimulation testing. If unavailable from the day of the test, heights were abstracted from the closest Endocrinology clinic visit that occurred no more than 3 months before or after stimulation. BSA was calculated using the Mosteller formula [19]. The following additional elements of the physical examination from the closest Endocrinology clinic visit within 3 months of stimulation testing were also abstracted: breast Tanner stage (girls only), testicular volume and Tanner stage (boys only), and Tanner stage for pubic hair (both girls and boys). Subjects without either height or weight data or without pubertal exam were excluded from further analysis; this was 54 out of 297 subjects initially identified to have completed testing.

Laboratory assessment of ACTH and cortisol values

The main hospital laboratory at the Children's Hospital of Philadelphia performed all laboratory testing. Cortisol and ACTH were measured by chemiluminescence. The lower limit of detection for cortisol was 1.0 mcg/dL (30 nmol/L) and for ACTH was 5 pg/mL (1 pmol/L). For the hospital's main laboratory, the coefficient of variation for the cortisol assay was approximately 3–4 % and for ACTH was 5 %. (Personal communication with Tracey G. Polsky, MD, PhD, assistant director of the Clinical Chemistry Laboratory, The Children's Hospital of Philadelphia, February 20, 2015) Subjects without available ACTH values were excluded from further analysis ($n = 11$).

Indication for testing

All outpatient Endocrinology clinic visits within 3 months before or after stimulation testing were reviewed to determine the indication for referral for adrenal stimulation testing. A step-wise hierarchical approach was applied in order to assign a single, primary indication for each subject for the purpose of these analyses, even though patients could have more than one indication for testing. This is described here and illustrated graphically in Fig. 1. This categorization approach was developed based on a comprehensive review of pediatric adrenal insufficiency [1]. First, all subjects with exogenous glucocorticoid exposure noted as an indication for testing were assigned "exogenous glucocorticoid exposure" as their primary indication for testing. For remaining subjects, if short stature was listed as an indication for testing, they were categorized as either "concern for isolated growth hormone deficiency," or "concern for multiple pituitary abnormalities (excluding neoplasm)," depending on whether the medical history or imaging suggested a possibility of multiple pituitary abnormalities. Many of these patients underwent CRH stimulation testing as well as growth hormone (GH) stimulation testing. Subjects who subsequently had a likely inadequate response to growth hormone stimulation testing (GH <10 mcg/L) [20] were classified into "possible growth hormone insufficiency." Those with GH peak ≥ 10 mcg/L were considered to have "growth hormone sufficient short stature;" these subjects

had apparently intact pituitary GH axis and no other indication of abnormal pituitary function aside from short stature. Next, the remaining subjects who did not have short stature listed as an indication for testing were categorized into one of the following groups: "neoplastic process with condition or therapy placing patient at risk for pituitary injury" or "known multiple pituitary abnormality." No subjects were suspected of having primary adrenal insufficiency. Subjects without documentation of concern for central adrenal insufficiency as the indication for testing were excluded from further analysis ($n = 10$), for a final subject total of 222.

Statistical analysis

"Peak cortisol" was defined as the maximum observed cortisol value measured following CRH administration. Change in cortisol, or "Δ cortisol," was defined as the difference between the baseline and peak cortisol. Cortisol values below the detection limit of 1 mcg/dL were recorded as 1 mcg/dL for the purpose of data analysis. Units were converted to SI using the standard conversions of 27.59 nmol/L per 1.0 mcg/dL cortisol and 0.22 pg/mL per 1.0 pmol/L ACTH. Descriptive variables were summarized by mean ± standard deviation (SD), and outcome variables by mean ± standard error of the mean (SEM) unless otherwise stated. Categorical variables, including pubertal stage, were assessed across groups and sex using the chi-square test. Peak cortisol was assessed across weight and age quartiles using one-way ANOVA. Baseline, delta, and peak cortisol and ACTH were assessed across indication for testing using one-way ANOVA. Rate of peak cortisol < 500 nmol/L was compared across indications and age category (six years or younger vs older than six years) using the chi-square test. Two-sample t-test was used to compare the groups with suspected GH deficiency (those found to be likely GH sufficient and those likely to

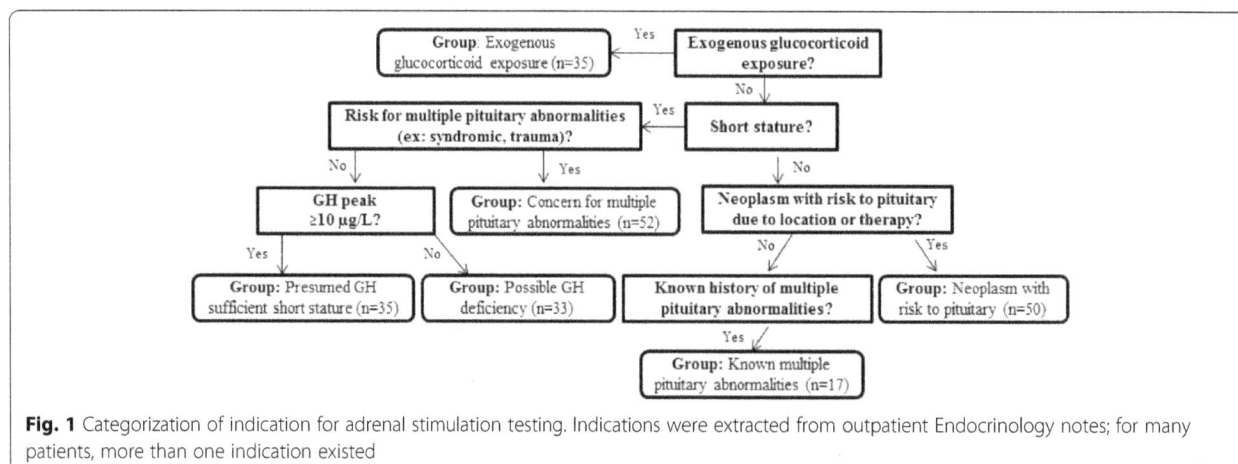

Fig. 1 Categorization of indication for adrenal stimulation testing. Indications were extracted from outpatient Endocrinology notes; for many patients, more than one indication existed

have GHD) and to compare cortisol response of subjects categorized by age younger than six years or older. Z-scores for height and BMI were calculated using CDC 2000 growth standards for children 2 years and older and WHO 2006 growth standards for children younger than 2 years, as recommended by the CDC [21]. To assess any potential confounding effect on the outcomes of interest (laboratory parameters of the CRH stimulation test, including peak cortisol, baseline cortisol, and Δ cortisol), bivariable linear regression analysis was first performed for covariates of interest, including: age, size (as measured by weight, height, BMI, BSA, BMI z-score, and height z-score), indication for testing, baseline cortisol, pubertal status, race/ethnicity, and time of day (AM or PM). Factors with p-value of <0.2 were included in multivariable linear regression models for peak and delta cortisol. Next, backward elimination using $p < 0.1$ was used to determine final multivariable models for peak and delta cortisol. Each model included only one "size factor" (i.e., weight, height, BMI, or BSA) or age due to the strong positive correlation ($p < 0.0005$) between age and each of weight, height, BMI, and BSA. BMI z-score and height z-score were also included in separate models because z-scores were determined using both age and absolute height or BMI. Thus, to avoid the collinearity problem, only one of each of age or "size factors" was included per model. Of note, weight, height, BMI, BSA are absolute size factors, while BMI z-score and height z-score are calculated based on reference values for age and sex, and thus are relative size factors.

Data analysis was performed with Stata, Release 13.0 (College Station, TX) and R version 3.0.0. A two-sided p value of <0.05 was considered statistically significant.

Results

Subjects

Table 1 shows subject characteristics, summarized by indication for testing. The 222 subjects (27 % female) who met inclusion criteria had a mean age of 8.9 years (SD 4.5, range 0.4–17.8 years). Seventy-five percent were pre-pubertal (Tanner I), 22 % were peri-pubertal (Tanner II-IV), and 4 % were post-pubertal (Tanner V). These proportions were not significantly different between boys and girls ($p = 0.07$). Seventy-nine percent of subjects did not have pubic hair at time of stimulation testing. By body mass index (BMI) z-score, 26 % of subjects were overweight or obese (BMI z-score ≥1.04) [21]. As expected in a population including glucocorticoid-treated children, as well as those with known pituitary abnormalities and/or clinically referred for short stature, subjects were relatively short (mean height z-score −1.96, range −6.07 to 3.2). Subjects with known multiple pituitary abnormalities tended to be older and weighed more than those who were undergoing initial evaluation for pituitary abnormalities ($p < 0.0005$ for both; see Table 1). Additionally, for each group, the majority of subjects were male. This was most notable for the group with neoplasms with risk to the pituitary. The two groups of subjects screened for growth hormone deficiency (GHD) were similar in age, weight, height, and gender distribution ($p > 0.05$), and 49 % of those tested for GHD had peak growth hormone of < 10 mcg/L.

Cortisol and ACTH response to stimulation

Mean peak cortisol for all subjects was 609.2 nmol/L (SD 213.0, range 27.59–1404.3). Mean Δ cortisol was

Table 1 Subject characteristics by indication for testing

Indication for testing	Presumed GH sufficient short stature (GH ≥ 10 µg/L)	Possible GHD (GH < 10 µg/L)	Concern for multiple pituitary abnormalities	Neoplasm with risk to pituitary	Exogenous glucocorticoid exposure	Known multiple pituitary abnormalities	p-value[a]
n	35	33	52	50	35	17	-
Sex (% female)	34 %	27 %	29 %	16 %	34 %	29 %	0.4
Age (years)	9.1 (4.6)	8.4 (4.1)	7.3 (5.0)	10.1 (3.0)	8.1 (4.9)	12.6 4.2)	0.0002
Tanner stage (Breast/Genital)							
I	28 (80 %)	29 (88 %)	44 (85 %)	33 (66 %)	25 (71 %)	7 (41 %)	<0.0005
II–IV	7 (20 %)	4 (12 %)	7 (13 %)	17 (34 %)	6 (17 %)	7 (41 %)	
V	0	0	1 (2 %)	0	4 (11 %)	3 (18 %)	
Presence of pubic hair							
No	29 (83 %)	32 (97 %)	47 (90 %)	32 (64 %)	27 (77 %)	8 (47 %)	<0.0005
Yes	6 (17 %)	1 (3 %)	5 (10 %)	18 (36 %)	8 (23 %)	9 (53 %)	
Weight (kg)	23.6 (11.1)	24.5 (14.2)	25.9 (17.4)	31.8 (13.1)	31.0 (22.9)	47.5 (22.4)	<0.0005
BMI z-score	−0.50 (0.98)	−0.04 (1.25)	0.55 (1.12)	0.27 (1.05)	0.45 (1.36)	0.57 (1.53)	0.0009
Height z-score	−2.8 (0.8)	−2.6 (0.9)	−1.8 (1.6)	−1.6 (1.4)	−1.4 (1.3)	−1.6 (1.5)	<0.0005

Data are presented as mean (SD)

[a] As determined by ANOVA across indication for testing

404.2 nmol/L (SD 200.2, range 0–905.0). Using cortisol of 500 nmol/L, a commonly used threshold to define "failure" to achieve reassuring cortisol response to CRH stimulation [6, 22], failure rate varied significantly by indication for testing ($p = 0.0066$ by ANOVA). Forty-eight (22 %) of all subjects had peak cortisol less than 500 nmol/L. The greatest failure rate occurred in the group tested due to exogenous glucocorticoid exposure; this group had 63 % (22/35) of subjects with peak cortisol < 500 nmol/L.

Mean peak ACTH for all subjects was 20.2 pmol/L (SD 18.7, range 1.1–197.8). Mean baseline ACTH was 4.1 pmol/L (SD 3.6, range 1.1–30.4); mean delta ACTH was 16.1 pmol/L (SD 18.2, range 0–192.5). Mean peak ACTH for subjects with peak cortisol less than 500 nmol/L was 11.4 pmol/L (SD 9.0, range 1.1–36.3), compared to mean peak ACTH of 22.6 pmol/L (SD 19.9, range 3.6–197.8) for subjects with peak cortisol of 500 nmol/L or greater. This difference was statistically significant ($p = 0.0002$ by two-sample t-test).

Relationship between cortisol response, body size, age, and other clinical covariates

Table 2 displays results of bivariable analysis of factors predicted to have a potential effect on peak or delta cortisol. In bivariable analysis, peak cortisol was significantly negatively associated with age, weight, height, BMI, BSA, and height z-score ($p < 0.05$ for each). Negative associations between body size factors and delta cortisol were also found but were less robust, with only height z-score reaching a similar level of statistical significance ($p < 0.05$). For purposes of further investigation of the relationship between outcomes with the predictive factors, factors with p-value < 0.2 were included in multivariable analysis and noted in Table 2, as described in Methods; for delta cortisol, these factors included weight, height, and BSA. Unlike for peak cortisol, age was not correlated with delta cortisol ($p > 0.2$). Baseline cortisol was significantly positively correlated with peak cortisol and negatively correlated with delta cortisol ($p < 0.0005$ for each). Baseline ACTH ($p = 0.007$), delta ACTH ($p < 0.0005$), and peak ACTH ($p < 0.0005$) were significantly positively correlated with peak cortisol. Delta and peak ACTH were also significantly positively correlated with delta cortisol ($p < 0.0005$ for each) (Table 2). To assess for bias conferred by subjects considered to have central cortisol deficiency, sensitivity analysis was performed. In bivariable analysis excluding subjects with peak cortisol < 500 nmol/L, age and size variables of interest (weight, height, BSA, and height z-score) remained significantly negatively associated with peak cortisol ($p < 0.05$). BMI also remained negatively associated with peak cortisol ($p = 0.13$) (data not shown).

Table 2 Bivariable analysis of peak and delta cortisol

	Peak cortisol (nmol/L)		Delta cortisol (nmol/L)	
	Coefficient	p-value	Coefficient	p-value
Age (years)	−7.6	0.02*		NS
Weight (kg)	−2.5	0.002 **	−1.4	0.06#
Weight inverse (1/kg)	1153.9	0.004 **		NS
Height (m)	−174.1	0.001 **	−85.9	0.08#
BMI (kg/m²)	−6.5	0.04*		NS
BSA (m²)	−123.8	0.001 **	−67.4	0.05#
BMI z-score	−14.6	NS		NS
Height z-score	−41.7	<0.0005**	−33.4	<0.005**
Sex (vs female)	−42.8	0.18#	−19.1	NS
Race		NS		NS
Ethnicity (Hispanic/Latino vs Non-Hispanic/Latino)		NS	−94.3	0.09#
Pubertal status (vs Tanner I)		0.21		0.09#
Tanner II-IV		NS		NS
Tanner V	−115.2	0.14#	−154.7	0.03*
Pubic hair development (yes vs no)		NS		NS
Indication for testing (vs GH sufficient short stature)		<0.0005**		<0.0005**
GHD		NS		NS
Concern for multi-pituitary abnormalities	−65	0.11#	−55.1	0.16
Neoplasm with risk to pituitary		NS		NS
Exogenous glucocorticoid exposure	−312.7	<0.0005**	−239.0	<0.0005**
Known multi-pituitary abnormalities	−133.7	0.02*	−105.3	0.05
Time of testing (PM vs AM)	−40.1	0.17#	−62.2	0.02*
Baseline cortisol (nmol/L)	0.72	<0.0005**	−0.35	<0.0005**
Baseline ACTH (pmol/L)	10.6	0.01*	−5.9	0.11#
Delta ACTH (pmol/L)	3.4	<0.0005**	4.0	<0.0005**
Peak ACTH (pmol/L)	3.6	<0.0005**	3.6	<0.0005**

#p-value <0.2 (for use in multivariate analysis); *p-value;<0.05, **p-value < 0.005

Other factors with marginal significance ($p < 0.2$) in bivariable analysis of peak cortisol were sex (male vs female, $p = 0.182$) and time of testing (after vs before 12:00 PM, $p = 0.17$); both factors were negatively associated with peak cortisol. For delta cortisol, ethnicity (Hispanic/Latino vs non-Hispanic/Latino, $p = 0.09$) and time of testing (after vs before 12:00 PM, $p = 0.023$) were significantly negatively correlated. Pubertal status (post-pubertal vs pre-pubertal: $p = 0.003$) was significantly negatively correlated with delta cortisol but not peak cortisol. These factors were included in initial multivariable models for peak and delta cortisol.

For peak and delta cortisol, indication for testing was associated with cortisol response ($p < 0.0005$). To account for this in multivariable linear regression, interaction terms between indication for testing and the size variable of interest were created and included in each model.

Multivariable model for peak cortisol response to stimulation

Multivariable linear regression analysis was used to determine factors that were independently associated with cortisol response to CRH stimulation. Table 3 displays final multivariable linear regression models obtained after backward elimination of non-significant ($p > 0.1$) variables that were initially included from bivariable analysis. Baseline cortisol and peak ACTH remained significantly

positively associated with peak cortisol. Sex was marginally associated with peak cortisol in each multivariable model, with p-values ranging from 0.048 for the model including age to 0.057 for the model including height z-score. Each model also included interaction terms between indication for testing and either age or the size factor of interest. Because age and size are highly associated, only one of these was included in each model to avoid collinearity, as described in Methods.

Models for weight, height z-score, and BSA included significant interaction terms between indication for testing and size. For these models, an interaction between size and exogenous glucocorticoid administration was detected ($p < 0.05$); within glucocorticoid-exposed children, the smallest children seemed to have the lowest peak cortisol, as described in more detail below. Multivariable linear regression analysis was repeated separately for the group with exogenous glucocorticoid exposure (Additional file 1: Table S1). In this analysis, the exogenous glucocorticoid group did not have an independent association between peak cortisol and weight or BSA ($p > 0.05$), but did have a significant positive

Table 3 Multivariable models for peak cortisol

	Age (years)		Weight (kg)		Height (m)		BSA (m²)		Height z-score	
	Coefficient	p-value	Coefficient	p-value	Coefficient	p-value	Coefficient	p-value	Coefficient	p-value
Age or size factor	−6.6	0.01*	−5.9	0.01*	−135.3	0.001**	−221.3	0.01*	−70.8	0.02*
Sex (vs female)	−46.4	0.05*	−45.7	0.05	−45.1	0.05	−45.2	0.06		
Indication for testing (vs GH sufficient short stature)										
GHD		NS		NS		NS		NS		NS
Concern for multi-pituitary abnormalities	−67	0.05*	−137	0.06	−63	0.06	−173	0.07		NS
Neoplasm with risk to pituitary		NS		NS		NS		NS		NS
Exogenous glucocorticoid exposure	−249	<0.0005**	−398	<0.0005**	−242	<0.0005**	−425	<0.0005**		NS
Known multi-pituitary abnormalities	−104	0.02*	−244.0	0.03*	−94	0.04*		NS		NS
Interaction variables (vs GH sufficient group*age or size factor)										
GHD*(age or size factor)				NS				NS		NS
Concern for multi-pituitary*(age or size factor)				NS				NS		NS
Neoplasm*(age or size factor)				NS				NS		NS
Exogenous glucocorticoids*(age or size factor)			6.4	0.02*			212	0.05*	129.3	<0.0005**
Known multi-pituitary*(age or size factor)				NS				NS		NS
Baseline cortisol (nmol/L)	0.59	<0.0005**	0.60	<0.0005**	0.58	<0.0005**	0.60	<0.0005**	0.65	<0.0005**
Peak ACTH (pmol/L)	2.56	<0.0005**	2.49	<0.0005**	2.47	<0.0005**	2.49	<0.0005**	2.20	<0.0005**
R², n	0.5092, 222		0.5201, 222		0.5182, 222		0.5196, 222		0.5481, 222	

*p-value <0.05, **p-value < 0.005 by multivariate linear regression association between peak cortisol and height z-score (beta = 58.6, $p = 0.015$), opposite the direction of the negative association between size and peak cortisol over all other subjects.

Multivariable model for delta cortisol

Table 4 displays final multivariable linear regression models obtained after backward elimination of non-significant ($p > 0.1$) variables that were initially included from bivariable analysis with delta cortisol. In the final multivariable models, pubertal status, ethnicity, and time of stimulation testing were no longer significantly independently associated with delta cortisol. Baseline cortisol remained significantly negatively and delta ACTH significantly positively associated with delta cortisol.

Similar to the models for peak cortisol, each model of delta cortisol included interaction terms between indication for testing and the size factor of interest, as described above. Models for weight, BSA, and height z-score included significant interaction terms between indication for testing and size. Again, for these models, the association between delta cortisol and size (weight, BSA, or height z-score) among subjects tested due to exogenous glucocorticoids was positive, opposite that of overall subjects. Similar to the findings for peak cortisol, when analysis of delta cortisol was repeated by indication for testing, a significant positive association ($p = 0.003$) between height z-score (but not weight or BSA) and delta cortisol was found for subjects with exogenous glucocorticoid exposure (data shown in Additional 2: Table S2).

Relationship between weight, age and peak cortisol response

Figure 2 displays peak cortisol response by quartiles of absolute weight. As shown, subjects in the highest weight quartile tended to have the lowest peak cortisol, consistent with the negative correlation found on multivariable regression. By one-way ANOVA, peak cortisol differed significantly across weight quartiles ($p = 0.0076$). In the highest weight quartile, 36 % (20/55) of subjects failed to achieve a peak cortisol of 500 nmol/L, as opposed to 17 % (28/167) of subjects in quartiles 1–3 ($p = 0.002$ by chi-square test). To better understand the interaction between weight, age, and cortisol response, this analysis was repeated by age quartile, and no significant difference in peak cortisol across age quartiles was noted ($p > 0.05$, data not shown).

Relationship between peak and baseline cortisol and time of testing

Although mean baseline cortisol drawn between 8:00 and 9:00 AM tended to be higher than those drawn after 9:00 AM (226.2 nmol/L, SD 88.0 for 12 subjects vs 200.2 nmol/L, SD 148.2 for 206 subjects), this did not reach statistical significance ($p = 0.5$). Peak cortisol also did not differ significantly between these groups (mean peak 562.8 nmol/L, SD 171.4 vs 610.0 nmol/L, SD 216.6,

Table 4 Multivariable models for delta cortisol

	Weight		Height		BSA (m²)		Height z-score	
	Coefficient	p-value	Coefficient	p-value	Coefficient	p-value	Coefficient	p-value
Size factor	−5.8	0.02*	−128.3	0.003 **	−216.8	0.02	−71.5	0.02*
Indication for testing (vs GH sufficient short stature)								
GHD		NS		NS		NS		NS
Concern for multi-pituitary abnormalities		NS		NS		NS		NS
Neoplasm with risk to pituitary		NS		NS		NS		NS
Exogenous glucocorticoid exposure	−429	<0.0005**	−256	<0.0005**	−472	<0.0005**		NS
Known multi-pituitary abnormalities	−230.0	0.05*	−96	0.05*		NS		NS
Interaction variables (vs GH sufficient group*size factor)								
GHD*(size factor)		NS				NS		NS
Concern for multi-pituitary*(size factor)		NS				NS		NS
Neoplasm*(size factor)		NS				NS		NS
Exogenous glucocorticoids*(size factor)	7.0	0.01*			245.5	0.03*	159	<0.0005**
Known multi-pituitary*(size factor)		NS				NS		NS
Baseline cortisol (nmol/L)	−0.44	<0.0005**	−0.46	<0.0005**	−0.44	<0.0005**	−0.40	<0.0005**
Delta ACTH (pmol/L)	2.47	<0.0005	2.49	<0.0005**	2.49	<0.0005**	2.22	<0.0005**
R², n	0.3956, 222		0.3875, 22		0.3947, 222		0.4621, 222	

*p-value <0.05, **p-value < 0.005 by multivariate linear regression

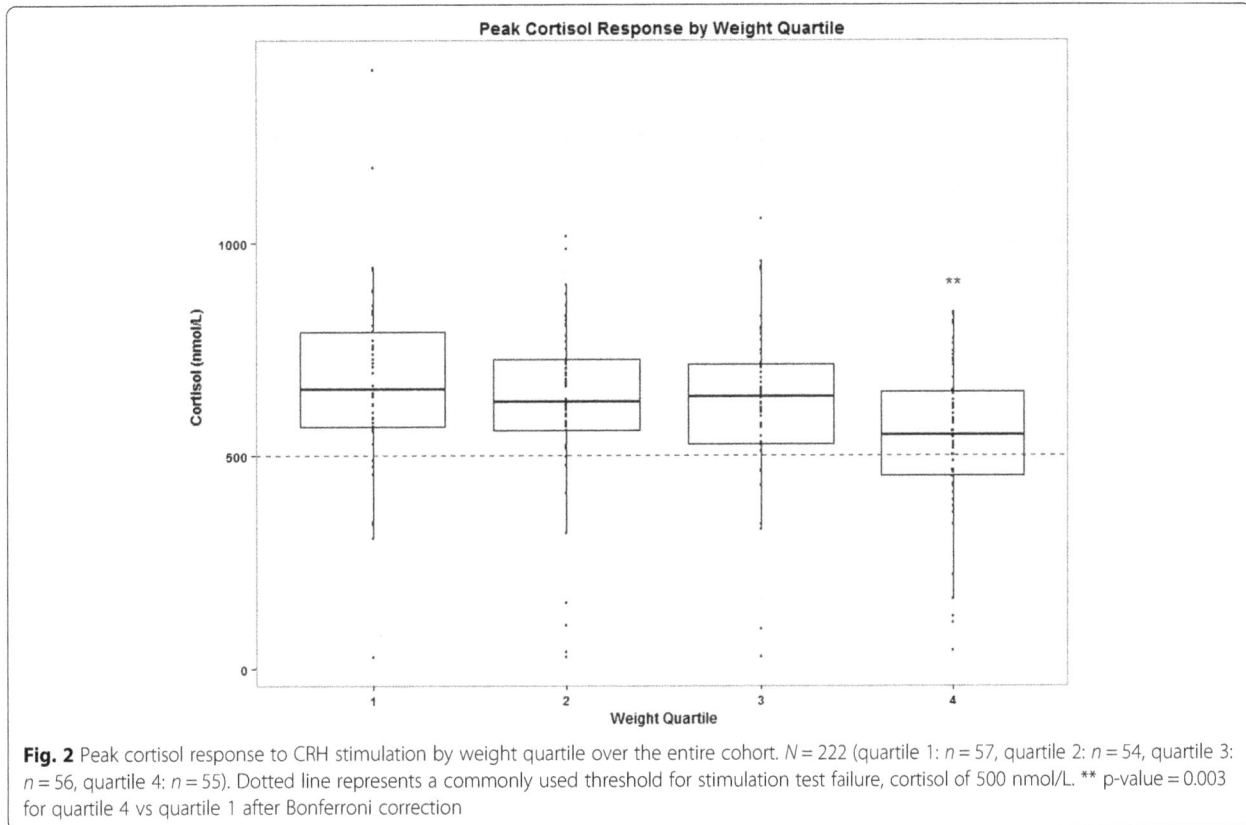

Fig. 2 Peak cortisol response to CRH stimulation by weight quartile over the entire cohort. $N = 222$ (quartile 1: $n = 57$, quartile 2: $n = 54$, quartile 3: $n = 56$, quartile 4: $n = 55$). Dotted line represents a commonly used threshold for stimulation test failure, cortisol of 500 nmol/L. ** p-value $= 0.003$ for quartile 4 vs quartile 1 after Bonferroni correction

$p = 0.5$). Similarly, when divided into subjects tested before and after noon, baseline cortisol did not differ significantly (192.0 nmol/L, SD 106.6 for 117 subjects vs 212.9 nmol/L, SD 180.3 for 101 subjects, $p = 0.3$).

Baseline and peak cortisol response in children six years or younger

We sought to characterize cortisol response in children 6 years and younger, as limited data is available for children of this age referred for clinical testing. Baseline cortisol was significantly higher in children 6 years or younger (239.4 nmol/L, SD 172.0 for 57 subjects vs 188.7 nmol/L, SD 132.5 for 165 subjects, $p = 0.0223$ by two-sample t-test). Peak cortisol, however, did not significantly differ between these groups (652.1 nmol/L, SD 221.8 for 57 subjects vs 594.4 nmol/L, SD 208.5 for 165 subjects, $p = 0.08$). Rate of peak cortisol response less than 500 nmol/L also did not differ significantly between these groups (11/57 (19 %) vs 37/165 (22 %), $p = 0.6$ by chi-square).

Relationship between weight, indication for testing, and peak cortisol

To better understand the interaction between weight and indication for testing in the multivariable model for peak cortisol, subjects who "failed" (peak cortisol < 500 nmol/L) CRH stimulation were compared across

weight quartiles and indication for testing, as shown in Fig. 3. As shown, the group with exogenous glucocorticoid exposure had significantly higher rates of failure, particularly for the middle two weight quartiles. A summary of failure rates for all groups is shown in black; this demonstrates the trend across groups toward higher failure rates among the highest weight quartile. Overall failure rates for each indication for testing are summarized in Table 5.

Finally, to minimize effects of indication of testing on cortisol response, bivariable analysis was repeated for the two groups with the most similar subjects: those tested due to concern for GHD and subsequently found to be either likely GH sufficient or deficient. These groups had similar weight and age distributions ($p = 0.79$ and $p = 0.50$ by two-sample t test). In this analysis, the negative association between weight and peak cortisol ($p = 0.008$) and age and peak cortisol ($p = 0.021$) persisted, suggesting that the differences among subjects due to indication for testing cannot solely explain the negative correlation between body size or age and cortisol response.

Discussion

In both bivariable and multivariable analyses, peak cortisol after CRH stimulation testing was significantly negatively associated with age and multiple measures of body

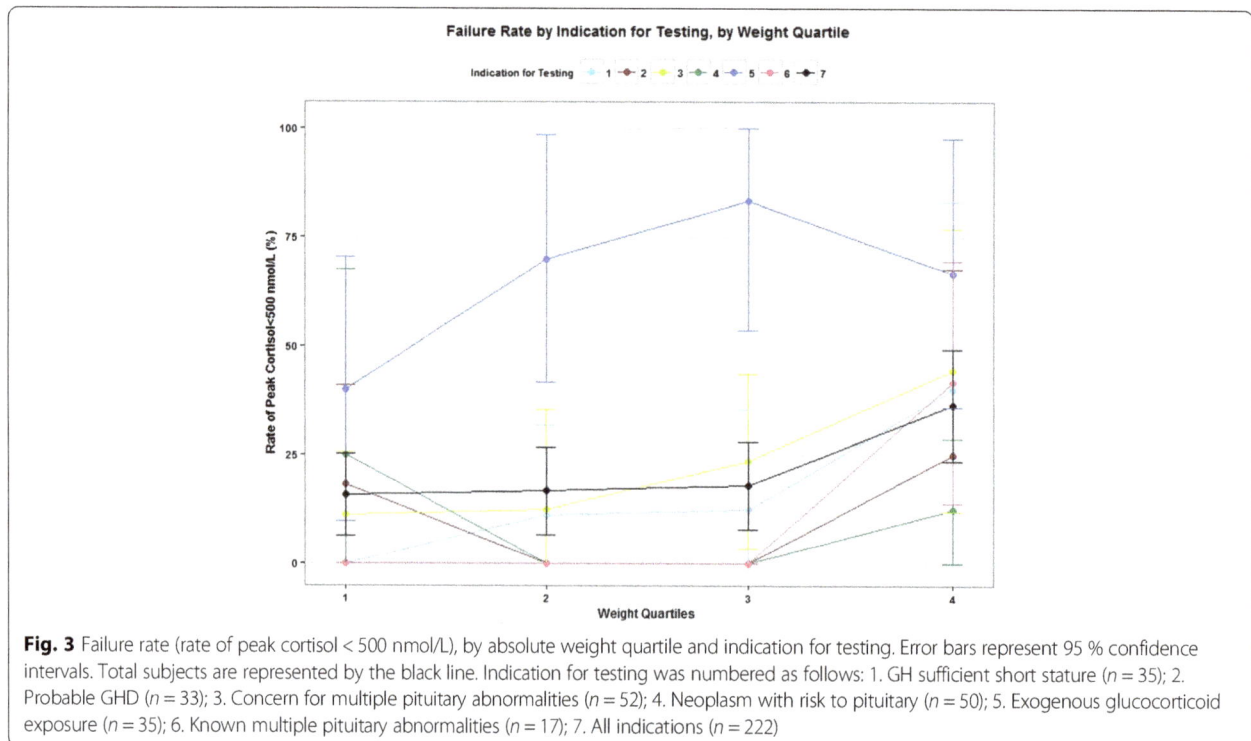

Fig. 3 Failure rate (rate of peak cortisol < 500 nmol/L), by absolute weight quartile and indication for testing. Error bars represent 95 % confidence intervals. Total subjects are represented by the black line. Indication for testing was numbered as follows: 1. GH sufficient short stature (n = 35); 2. Probable GHD (n = 33); 3. Concern for multiple pituitary abnormalities (n = 52); 4. Neoplasm with risk to pituitary (n = 50); 5. Exogenous glucocorticoid exposure (n = 35); 6. Known multiple pituitary abnormalities (n = 17); 7. All indications (n = 222)

size, including weight, height, height z-score, and BSA in our study of over 200 children referred for clinical testing. Delta cortisol, another measure of cortisol response to stimulation, was similarly negatively associated with weight, height, height z-score, and BSA, but was not significantly associated with age.

These findings may be interpreted in several ways. First, due to the retrospective nature of our study, referral bias may have played a role. For example, the high failure rate among glucocorticoid-exposed subjects may be due to referral of the most severely affected individuals, raising the pre-test probability of failure. Additionally, younger (and smaller) subjects may have been referred more readily despite their relatively healthy clinical status, making these subjects more likely to pass their stimulation test. Another possibility is the changing nature of indication for testing across age and size. For example, older and larger subjects may have been tested for indications that also increased their pre-test probability of failure, independent of their size and age. To account for these possibilities, we performed several sensitivity analyses. As explained above in Results, when bivariable analysis was repeated only for subjects tested due to concern for isolated growth hormone deficiency, the negative association between peak cortisol and weight or age persisted. Therefore, another important

Table 5 Cortisol and ACTH response by indication for testing

Indication for testing	Presumed GH sufficient short stature (GH ≥ 10 μg/L)	Possible GHD (GH < 10 μg/L)	Concern for multiple pituitary abnormalities	Neoplasm with risk to pituitary	Exogenous glucocorticoid exposure	Known multiple pituitary abnormalities	p-value[a]
n	35	33	52	50	35	17	
Baseline cortisol (nmol/L)	231.0 (124.3)	203.3 (136.6)	221.1 (182.0)	199.1 (119.4)	145.7 (139.8)	202.2 (139.6)	0.18
Delta cortisol (nmol/L)	454.9 (168.1)	485.2 (139.7)	399.8 (160.4)	470.2 (189.2)	215.9 (218.4)	349.6 (219.5)	<0.0005
Peak cortisol (nmol/L)	685.9 (161.8)	688 .5 (179.8)	620.9 (178.6)	675.8 (138.5)	373.2 (246.1)	552.2 (227.0)	<0.0005
Baseline ACTH (pmol/L)	3.2 (1.8)	5.9 (6.6)	4.2 (2.6)	3.6 (1.9)	3.7 (4.1)	4.7 (2.8)	0.036
Delta ACTH (pmol/L)	14.9 (9.3)	23.0 (18.5)	13.2 (11.6)	21.4 (26.6)	6.3 (4.9)	18.3 (25.6)	0.0007
Peak ACTH (pmol/L)	18.1 (9.6)	28.9 (17.9)	17.4 (11.5)	25.0 (27.0)	10.1 (7.5)	23.0 (26.3)	0.0003
Failure Rate (peak cortisol < 500 nmol/L)	11.4 %	9.1 %	21.2 %	6.0 %	62.9 %	29.4 %	<0.0005

Data are presented as mean (SD)
[a]As determined by ANOVA across indication for testing for cortisol and ACTH values; by Chi-square for Failure Rate

possible explanation to explore is that true physiologic differences in adrenal response to CRH exist, despite weight-based dosing, across the wide range of body sizes and ages of children included in the present study.

An important previous study in healthy children did not find age- or size-based differences in pharmacokinetic or pharmacodynamic parameters in the response to CRH, but the sample size was relatively small ($n = 21$, girls and boys ages 6–15 years), and these investigators themselves noted the lack of data for children under 6 years of age [16]. However, in investigations using other techniques to assess hypothalamic-pituitary-adrenal axis function (low- and standard-dose ACTH), peak cortisol response in healthy children [17] and in children exposed to exogenous glucocorticoids [4] did decrease with age, consistent with our findings using CRH stimulation testing over all subjects. As noted previously, the subjects in our study with glucocorticoid exposure did not demonstrate a similar negative relationship between peak or delta cortisol and height z-score (Additional file 1: Table S1 and Additional file 2: Table S2). This may reflect the higher likelihood of adrenal suppression in subjects who had glucocorticoid exposure great enough to negatively affect height growth, as even inhaled corticosteroids have been associated with decreased height growth, particularly in prepubertal children [23].

Other studies have also found associations between cortisol levels and age in healthy children, but the direction of effect has differed between studies depending on statistical approaches, highlighting how the simultaneous effects of age and size are challenging to disentangle [24–27]. For example, in one of these investigations, salivary cortisol concentration was initially found to increase with age, but after statistical adjustment for BSA, the relationship with age seemed reversed [25]. The authors posit that this finding could reflect a lower production rate or higher rate of clearance of cortisol with age [25]. A separate study focused on this question found that daily cortisol production remained constant with age, again after adjustment for body surface area [28]. Taken together, these studies illustrate the important challenge in pediatrics of scaling for size when interpreting experimental results across a wide range of subject ages [29], particularly in the youngest children, in whom there is the additional complexity of incomplete maturation of kidney and liver function, which also affects drug metabolism [30].

To our knowledge, an independent, negative relationship between cortisol response to CRH and body size has not been demonstrated previously. As discussed above, due to the high correlation between age and body size, discerning the relative effects on cortisol response of each of these is a challenging undertaking, particularly due to differences in indication for testing across age

and weight. For example, the association between peak cortisol response and age/size may be due to maturational differences in the responsiveness of the adrenal gland to ACTH and/or clearance of cortisol, differences that cannot be fully adjusted by the current weight-based dosing regimen of CRH.

Differences in adrenal gland size may also partly explain differences in responsiveness across the ages and body sizes tested. The adrenal gland does not grow at the same pace as the rest of the body; instead, it decreases in size from birth to around one year of age, then gains mass, but more slowly than the body as a whole [31]. If circulating cortisol concentration were to remain constant or even increase with age as has been described by several authors [24–26], these relatively smaller adrenal glands would need to produce proportionally more cortisol to distribute across relatively larger blood volumes, assuming constant clearance. Although these relatively smaller adrenal glands would thus produce larger amounts of cortisol relative to body size on a constant basis, they may not produce as robust a response to acute stimulation, as they may already be operating at a "higher capacity." This "lower reserve" could explain the lower peak cortisol response to stimulation in subjects with larger body surface area and relatively smaller adrenal glands.

Alternatively, age may be the driving force in the negative association, through mechanisms not primarily driven by body size. We looked for but did not find an effect of puberty and/or presumed adrenarche (pubic hair development alone) on cortisol response, but the sample was enriched in young, pre-pubertal children, so these effects may have been more difficult to detect. Indeed, at least one previous study has suggested increased volume of distribution and more rapid clearance of cortisol with the onset of puberty [32]. Sampling beyond the usual prescribed time range for CRH stimulation testing would be required to estimate these parameters. Additional careful pharmacokinetic and pharmacodynamics studies in children could help answer these questions.

Strengths and limitations

The strengths of the present study include its large size and wide range of ages studied, including 57 children age six years and younger, the largest study to our knowledge of children in this age range who have undergone stimulation with CRH. As mentioned above, our study has limitations related to its retrospective nature. One potential limitation was the health status of our subjects, who had a wide range of diagnoses and exposures to medications and therapies. Although this limits our ability to generalize to healthy children, our subjects are representative of the patients who most often undergo adrenal stimulation testing. As noted above, however, 89 % of subjects with presumed growth hormone sufficient short stature reached a cortisol peak of 500 nmol/L, consistent with our belief that this group was representative of subjects with a likely intact HPA axis, regardless of their short stature. In addition, we considered the possibility that age- or size-related differences in indication for testing could introduce bias into our results. We observed the negative association between peak cortisol and age or size even in multivariable regression analyses including testing indication and interaction terms between testing indication and age/size (Table 3). However, it would be optimal to reproduce these results in additional cohorts prospectively grouped by age and indication for testing and to consider studies in healthy children as well. Additionally, referral patterns may be valuable to study, as one interpretation of our results may be that younger/smaller children with intact adrenal function may be more likely to undergo testing to exclude ACTH deficiency as part of an initial evaluation. This may explain our finding that smaller, shorter children tended to have higher peak cortisol, opposite of what one would expect if these children were short due to underlying pathology associated with ACTH deficiency. Finally, an additional limitation is that cumulative glucocorticoid exposure was unavailable for analysis; although this was not the primary focus of our study, it may have allowed for a better understanding of the cortisol response among this group of subjects.

The present study, the largest collection to date of pediatric CRH stimulation testing results to our knowledge, demonstrates that cortisol response to CRH stimulation is negatively associated with both age and size, as reflected by weight, height, BSA, and height z-score, in children referred for clinical testing, even after accounting for important clinical covariates. Additional careful pharmacokinetic and pharmacodynamic studies, including serial measurements of CRH, ACTH, and cortisol, could help clarify the etiology of these differences. That is, the volume of distribution of CRH, and/or the clearance of cortisol are at least two potential sources of age- or size-related variation.

Conclusions

Our results suggest that to better interpret peak cortisol response across a wide range of ages and sizes in the pediatric population, it may be helpful to consider the possibility of greater cortisol responses in the youngest and smallest patients. Specifically, for patients with "borderline" peak cortisol response, it may be helpful to consider the patient-specific characteristics of age and size when determining whether the patient has "passed" or "failed" the stimulation test. Our study was limited to a

population referred for clinical testing, but the potential for generalizability of these findings make future prospective studies focused on size and age very important. Optimally, prospective development of age- or size-dependent thresholds for cortisol response might increase the clinical utility of this provocative test, particularly in the youngest at-risk patients.

Abbreviations
CRH: Corticotropin-releasing hormone, corticorelin; ACTH: Adrenocorticotropic hormone; BSA: Body surface area; ITT: Insulin tolerance test; GH: Growth hormone; GHD: Growth hormone deficiency; BMI: Body mass index; HPA: Hypothalamic-pituitary-adrenal.

Competing interests
Since the initial submission of this manuscript to the International Journal of Pediatric Endocrinology, AP has become an employer of Pfizer. All other authors deny competing financial or non-financial interests.

Authors' contributions
MEV wrote the initial draft of this manuscript. All authors contributed significantly to this work; MEV and SEM were primary authors. Data collection and analysis assistance was provided by JT, MC, EB, and RX. VB, AP, JMB, and SW edited the manuscript. All authors read and approved the final manuscript.

Acknowledgements
Grants or fellowships that supported this project include: 5K12DK94723-2 (SEM, PI: SW) and 228950000-RESD5 CTSA (CHOP Center for Biomedical Informatics).

Author details
[1]Division of Endocrinology and Diabetes, The Children's Hospital of Philadelphia, 3401 Civic Center Blvd, Suite 11NW, Philadelphia, USA. [2]Center for Biomedical Informatics, The Children's Hospital of Philadelphia, 3535 Market St, Philadelphia, PA 19104, USA. [3]Department of Biostatistics and Epidemiology, University of Pennsylvania, 635 Blockley Hall, 423 Guardian Drive, Philadelphia, PA 19104-6021, USA. [4]Global Innovative Pharma, Pfizer, Inc, 500 Arcola Road, Collegeville, PA 19426, USA. [5]The Children's Hospital of Philadelphia, Division of Rheumatology, 10103 Colket Building, 34th & Civic Center Blvd, Philadelphia, PA 19104, USA.

References
1. Shulman DI, Palmert MR, Kemp SF. Adrenal insufficiency: still a cause of morbidity and death in childhood. Pediatrics. 2007;119:e484–94.
2. Buchanan CR, Preece MA, Milner RD. Mortality, neoplasia, and Creutzfeldt-Jakob disease in patients treated with human pituitary growth hormone in the United Kingdom. BMJ. 1991;302:824–8.
3. Taback SP, Dean HJ. Mortality in Canadian children with growth hormone (GH) deficiency receiving GH therapy 1967–1992. The Canadian Growth Hormone Advisory Committee. J Clin Endocrinol Metab. 1996;81:1693–6.

Peak cortisol response to corticotropin-releasing hormone is associated with age and body...

189

4.	Wildi-Runge S, Deladoëy J, Bélanger C, Deal CL, Van Vliet G, Alos N, et al. A search for variables predicting cortisol response to low-dose corticotropin stimulation following supraphysiological doses of glucocorticoids. J Pediatr. 2013;163:484–8.

5.	Crowley RK, Argese N, Tomlinson JW, Stewart PM. Central hypoadrenalism. J Clin Endocrinol Metab. 2014;99:4027–36.

6.	Maghnie M, Uga E, Temporini F, Di Iorgi N, Secco A, Tinelli C, et al. Evaluation of adrenal function in patients with growth hormone deficiency and hypothalamic-pituitary disorders: comparison between insulin-induced hypoglycemia, low-dose ACTH, standard ACTH and CRH stimulation tests. Eur J Endocrinol. 2005;152:735–41.

7.	Shah A, Stanhope R, Matthew D. Hazards of pharmacological tests of growth hormone secretion in childhood. BMJ. 1992;304(6820):173–4.

8.	Gonzálbez J, Villabona C, Ramón J, Navarro MA, Giménez O, Ricart W, et al. Establishment of reference values for standard dose short synacthen test (250 microgram), low dose short synacthen test (1 microgram) and insulin tolerance test for assessment of the hypothalamo-pituitary-adrenal axis in normal subjects. Clin Endocrinol (Oxf). 2000;53:199–204.

9.	Magnotti M, Shimshi M. Diagnosing adrenal insufficiency: Which test is best—The 1-μg or the 250-μg Cosyntropin stimulation test? Endocr Pract. 2008;14:233–8.

10.	Orth DN, Jackson RV, Decherney GS, Debold CR, Alexander AN, Island DP, et al. Effect of synthetic ovine corticotropin-releasing factor: dose response of plasma adrenocorticotropin and cortisol. J Clin Invest. 1983;71:587–95.

11.	DeBold C, Orth D. Corticotropin-releasing hormone: stimulation of ACTH secretion in normal man. Horm Metab Res. 1986;16:8–16.

12.	Attanasio A, Rosskamp R, Bernasconi S, Terzi C, Ranke MB, Giovanelli G, et al. Plasma adrenocorticotropin, cortisol, and dehydroepiandrosterone response to corticotropin-releasing factor in normal children during pubertal development. Pediatr Res. 1987;22:41–4.

13.	Goji K. The corticotropin-releasing hormone test in normal short children: comparison of plasma adrenocorticotropin and cortisol responses to human corticotropin-releasing hormone and insulin-induced hypoglycemia. Acta Endocrinol (Copenh). 1989;120:390–4.

14.	Schlaghecke R, Kornely E. The effect of long-term glucocorticoid therapy on pituitary–adrenal responses to exogenous corticotropin-releasing hormone. N Engl J Med. 1992;326:226–30.

15.	Dahl RE, Siegel SF, Williamson DE, Lee PA, Perel J, Birmaher B, et al. Corticotropin releasing hormone stimulation test and nocturnal cortisol levels in normal children. Pediatr Res. 1992;32:64–8.

16.	Ross JL, Schulte HM, Galucci WT, Cutler GB, Loriaux DL, Chrousos GP. Ovine corticotropin-releasing hormone stimulation test in normal children. J Clin Endocrinol Metab. 1986;62:390–2.

17.	Lashansky G, Saenger P, Fishman K, Gautier T, Mayes D, Berg J, et al. Normative data for adrenal steroidogenesis in a healthy pediatric population: age- and sex-related changes after adrenocorticotropin stimulation. J Clin Endocrinol Metab. 1991;73:674–86.

18.	Edginton AN, Shah B, Sevestre M, Momper JD. The integration of allometry and virtual populations to predict clearance and clearance variability in pediatric populations over the age of 6 years. Clin Pharmacokinet. 2013;52:693–703.

19.	Mosteller R. Simplified calculation of body-surface area. N Engl J Med. 1987;317:1098.

20.	Reiter E, Martha Jr PM. Pharmacological testing of growth hormone secretion. Horm Res Paediatr. 1990;33:121–6.

21.	Centers for Disease Control and Prevention. CDC growth charts: United States. Percentile data files with LMS values. 2005.

22.	Maguire AM, Biesheuvel CJ, Ambler GR, Moore B, McLean M, Cowell CT. Evaluation of adrenal function using the human corticotrophin-releasing hormone test, low dose Synacthen test and 9 am cortisol level in children and adolescents with central adrenal insufficiency. Clin Endocrinol (Oxf). 2008;68:683–91.

23.	Kelly H, Sternberg A. Effect of inhaled glucocorticoids in childhood on adult height. N Engl J Med. 2012;367:904–12.

24.	Bailey D, Colantonio D, Kyriakopoulou L, Cohen AH, Chan MK, Armbruster D, et al. Marked biological variance in endocrine and biochemical markers in childhood: establishment of pediatric reference intervals using healthy community children from the CALIPER cohort. Clin Chem. 2013;59:1393–405.

25.	Kiess W, Meidert A, Dressendörfer R. Salivary cortisol levels throughout childhood and adolescence: relation with age, pubertal stage, and weight. Pediatr Res. 1995;37:502–6.

26.	Knutsson U, Dahlgren J, Marcus C, Rosberg S, Brönnegård M, Stierna P, et al. Circadian cortisol rhythms in healthy boys and girls: relationship with age, growth, body composition, and pubertal development. J Clin Endocrinol Metab. 1997;82:536–40.

27.	Soldin SJ, Murthy JN, Agarwalla PK, Ojeifo O, Chea J. Pediatric reference ranges for creatine kinase, CKMB, troponin i, iron, and cortisol. Clin Biochem. 1999;32:77–80.

28.	Kenny F, Preeyasombat C, Migeon C. Cortisol production rate II. Normal infants, children, and adults. Pediatrics. 1966;37:34–42.

29.	Abernethy DR, Burckart GJ. Pediatric dose selection. Clin Pharmacol Ther. 2010;87:270–1.

30.	Momper JD, Mulugeta Y, Green DJ, Karesh A, Krudys KM, Sachs HC, et al. Adolescent dosing and labeling since the food and drug Administration amendments act of 2007. JAMA Pediatr. 2013;167:926–32.

31.	Basic anatomical and physiological data for use in radiological protection reference values. ICRP Publication 89. ICRP. 2002;32:3–4.

32.	Charmandari E. Congenital adrenal hyperplasia due to 21-hydroxylase deficiency: alterations in cortisol pharmacokinetics at puberty. J Clin Endocrinol Metab. 2001;86:2701–8.

27

Effects of fiber supplementation on glycemic excursions and incidence of hypoglycemia in children with type 1 diabetes

Nicole Nader[1], Amy Weaver[2], Susan Eckert[3] and Aida Lteif[1*]

Abstract

Background: Nutritional therapy is an important component of diabetes management. There is data to suggest that fiber content of foods may affect glycemic response.

Materials and methods: 10 children, diagnosed with type 1 diabetes, participated. In the first phase of the study, children followed their usual meal plan. In the second phase, subjects followed the same meal plan except that fiber was added to the diet using a powder supplement (wheat dextrin). Data was collected using a continuous glucose monitoring device. The blood glucose excursion level following each meal was compared between the two phases of the study by fitting a repeated measures regression model. The incidence of hypoglycemia was also compared by fitting a logistic regression model.

Results: There was no difference in the mean blood glucose excursion after meals or the incidence of hypoglycemia between the two phases. There was a strong negative correlation between the amount of fiber supplemented and the mean maximum post-prandial blood sugar after the lunch and breakfast meals (Spearman rank correlation coefficient = −0.86 lunch and −0.76 breakfast).

Conclusion: Our study did not show an overall decrease in glucose excursion or incidence of hypoglycemia with fiber supplementation. We did find a strong negative correlation between the amount of fiber added during the supplemental phase and the mean maximum post-prandial blood sugar after the lunch and breakfast meals. We speculate that different types of fiber may have different effects on blood glucose with wheat dextrin having a greater dampening effect.

Introduction

Nutritional therapy is an important component of diabetes management. The American Diabetes Association currently recommends that patients with type 1 diabetes monitor their carbohydrate intake either by carbohydrate counting or by the use of exchange diets and match prandial insulin to carbohydrate intake [1]. This method implies that equal portions of carbohydrate have equivalent effects on blood sugar levels. However, there is data to suggest that other factors such as the molecular structure of the carbohydrate and its fiber content result in differential blood glucose responses [2]. High fiber foods as a preferred source of carbohydrate and higher amount of fiber per day are currently recommended [3,4].

Fibers are known to slow down the absorption of carbohydrates after a meal [5].

Despite the fact that children with type 1 diabetes are known to have sub-optimal fiber intake [6,7] and have a tendency towards greater glycemic excursions, there is limited data looking at the effects of a fiber on metabolic control in children. In a cross over study of 23 patients who consumed either a low glycemic diet or a standard diet for two days, it was shown that the low glycemic diet contained more fiber than the standard diet and resulted in lower mean daytime blood glucose values [8]. Rami et al. demonstrated that giving a high-fiber bedtime snack to children with type 1 diabetes flattened the blood glucose curve until midnight [9].

* Correspondence: lteif.aida@mayo.edu
[1]Division of Pediatric Endocrinology, Mayo Clinic, 200 1st St SW, Rochester, MN 55905, USA
Full list of author information is available at the end of the article

It currently remains unclear what effects a diet rich in fiber would have on diabetes control and glycemic excursions in children with type 1 diabetes. The aim of this study was to determine whether the addition of a fiber supplement to the diet of pediatric patients with type 1 diabetes has an effect on the magnitude of glucose excursions and or the incidence of hypoglycemia. We hypothesized that children with type 1 diabetes receiving a high fiber diet will have lower glucose excursions and a lower incidence of hypoglycemia.

Research design and methods

Recruitment

Ten children with type 1 diabetes were recruited from a pediatric endocrinology clinic in Rochester, MN between September 2008 and March 2010. Study staff approached potential participants during their routine diabetes clinic visit and invited them to participate. Inclusion criteria were: diagnosis of type 1 diabetes for at least two years prior to enrollment in the study and 4–16 years of age. Exclusion criteria were: any other associated medical conditions that could potentially affect absorption of nutrients such as celiac disease or inflammatory bowel disease and intercurrent illness during the study period. The study protocol was approved by the Mayo Clinic Institutional Review Board. Study subjects signed assent or consent forms (depending on their age) and both parents signed consent forms prior to participation.

Study procedure

The study was a prospective interventional observation study with a within-subject cross over design. During the study period the subjects were asked to maintain their usual level of activity. All subjects were asked to present to the outpatient diabetes clinic for an initial study visit. They first met with a dietitian who worked with them on a 3 day meal plan which was representative of their typical daily intake. The subjects were asked to follow that meal plan very closely. They then met with a physician who performed a brief physical exam including an Ears/Nose/Throat, heart, lung, and abdominal exam. Subjects were also asked about the presence of the following signs and symptoms in the preceding 3 days: upper respiratory infection symptoms, vomiting, diarrhea, and fever. If subjects had any signs or symptoms of an infection, upon presentation or during the study period, they were excluded from the study. Subjects were then connected to a continuous blood glucose monitoring device (Medtronic CGMD gold system). Subjects were instructed to continue using their own reflectance meters to check their blood sugars at least four times per day. They were also asked to keep a detailed food diary. Three days later, subjects returned to the clinic and the monitoring device was removed. The study dietitian analyzed the food diary to determine daily caloric intake and fiber intake using the Nutritionist Pro program. Subjects were instructed to contact the study team if they developed any symptoms or signs of infection at any time during the study period.

During the washout period, subjects were asked to lower their insulin dose for unexplained hypoglycemia and increase it for a pattern of hyperglycemia that lasts for three days.

For the second phase of the study which was conducted on similar days of the week, the subjects again returned to the outpatient diabetes clinic and met with a dietitian. There was a two to four week washout period between the study phases. The same meal plan was given except fiber was added to the diet using a powder supplement (Benefiber, fiber supplement, sugar free) in an amount to total 20 grams/1000Kcal/day of fiber. The Benefiber was mixed with beverages and soft foods. The needed total daily amount was divided equally between breakfast, lunch and supper. Subjects again met with a physician, had a brief physical exam performed, and were asked about the presence of symptoms of infection. If subjects had any signs or symptoms of infection, they were excluded from continuing the study. Subjects were then connected to the continuous monitoring device, and given the same instructions as during the first phase of the study. Subjects returned to clinic in three days, at which time the monitoring device was removed.

Data was collected on plasma glucose concentrations using the continuous blood glucose device. The CGMS System Gold provides up to 288 glucose measurements every 24 hours. This data is stored in a Holter-style monitor and can be downloaded into a computer. The system does not display glucose values to the subjects. For each meal, the blood glucose excursion level was determined as the difference between the glucose at the start of the meal and the maximum post prandial glucose within two hours after the meal, but prior to the start of the subsequent meal. Hypoglycemia was defined as a glucose measurement < 70 mg/dL.

Data analysis

The blood glucose excursion levels following each meal were compared between the two phases (non-fiber and fiber-supplemented) by fitting repeated measures regression models using the MIXED procedure in SAS (version 8.2; SAS Institute, Inc.; Cary, NC). The models were fit after applying the square root transformation to the excursion levels to obtain a more normally distributed outcome. Since each subject had multiple meals over each 3-day phase, the excursion levels were not independent of each other and therefore the appropriate statistical model needed to take into account the correlated nature of the data. To accommodate for this issue and the issue that the multiple meals for each subject were not equally spaced over time, a spatial covariance structure (SP(POW)) was specified. This structure also assumes that measurements closer together are more correlated than measurements obtained further apart in time.

The incidence of hypoglycemia was compared between the two phases (non-fiber and fiber-supplemented) by fitting a logistic regression model using general estimating equation (GEE) methodology available in the GENMOD procedure in SAS. In this model the unit of analysis was an individual glucose measurement. An autoregressive covariance structure was specified to model the correlation between the repeated glucose measurements (i.e. every 5 minutes) over time per subject. This structure assumes that measurements closer together are more correlated than measurements obtained further apart in time.

Results

A total of 10 subjects (7 females and 3 males) participated in the study. Median age was 11.1 years (range, 8.3-14.2 years). Median duration of diabetes was 4.0 years (range, 2.0-7.3 years). Half of the subjects (5/10) were following a multiple daily injection insulin program and the other half (5/10) were following a continuous subcutaneous insulin infusion program. The amount of fiber added to each subject's meal plan in order to total 20 grams/1000 kilocalories/day varied from 9–27 (median, 18) grams daily. During the non-fiber-supplemented and fiber-supplemented phases of the study, the subjects recorded a mean of 14.5 and 13.7 meals or snacks, respectively.

The overall median glucose value was determined for each subject during each 3-day phase. During the non-fiber-supplemented phase the overall median glucose level ranged from 89 to 236 mg/dL for the 10 subjects. For 2 of the subjects, the overall median glucose was lower during the fiber-supplemented phase (117 vs 81 mg/dL; 236 vs. 123 mg/dL). However, for the 8 remaining subjects, the overall median glucose level was between 1.5 and 59.3 mg/dL higher during the fiber-supplemented phase.

Glucose excursions

The mean blood glucose excursion (maximum post prandial glucose - glucose at the time of meal) after meals was not significantly different between the non-fiber-supplemented phase of the study and the fiber-supplemented phase (p = 0.17). The results were similar using a model adjusted for the subject's glucose at the start of each phase (p = 0.18).

The mean (SD) glucose excursion after breakfast during the non-fiber-supplemented phase was 114.7 (71.3) vs. 121.2 (49.6) mg/dL during the fiber supplementation phase. For lunch, the mean (SD) glucose excursion during the non- fiber supplemented phase was 47.9 (45) vs. 56.5

(59.8) mg/dL during the fiber supplementation phase (Figure 1A and B). For the evening meal, the mean (SD) glucose excursion during the non-fiber-supplemented phase was 44.7 (34.5) vs. 62.9 (40.2) mg/dL during the fiber supplementation phase.

To determine if there was a relationship between the amount of fiber supplemented and glucose excursion, the amount of fiber supplemented per subject was compared with their mean peak blood glucose after the each meal during the fiber supplemented phase. There was not a correlation between the amount of fiber supplemented and the mean maximum blood glucose after the evening meal (Spearman rank correlation coefficient = –0.17). However, there was a strong negative correlation between the amount of fiber added and the mean maximum post-prandial blood sugar after the lunch and breakfast meals, respectively (Spearman rank correlation coefficient = –0.86 for lunch and –0.76 for breakfast, Figure 2).

Hypoglycemia

During the non-fiber-supplemented phase, the subjects had a total of 8123 glucose measurements, of which 767 (9.4%) were <70 mg/dL. During the fiber phase, the subjects had a total of 8099 glucose measurements, of which 975 (12.4%) were <70 mg/dL. There was no statistical difference in the incidence of hypoglycemia during the two phases of the study (p = 0.55). Half the subjects (5/10) tended to have more hypoglycemia episodes during the non-fiber-supplemented phase (compared to the fiber phase) and the other half tended to have more hypoglycemia episodes during the fiber supplemented phase (Table 1).

The results were also analyzed separately for daytime (8:00 am-7:59 pm) and nighttime (8:00 pm-7:59 am). During the day, 8.5% of blood sugar readings were < 70 mg/dL during the non-fiber supplemented phase vs. 7.5% of measurements during the fiber supplemented phase (p = 0.44). At night, 10.3% of blood glucose measurements were in the hypoglycemic range during the non-fiber supplemented phase vs. 16.3% of measurements during the fiber supplemented phase (p = 0.60).

Hyperglycemia

During the non-fiber-supplemented phase, the percent of glucose measurements in the hyperglycemic range, defined as blood glucose greater than 180, was 28.0%. During the fiber phase, it was 39%.

Conclusions

Although our study did not show an overall decrease in glucose excursion or incidence of hypoglycemia with fiber supplementation, we did find a strong negative correlation between the amount of fiber added during the supplemented phase and the mean maximum post-prandial blood sugar after the lunch and breakfast meals.

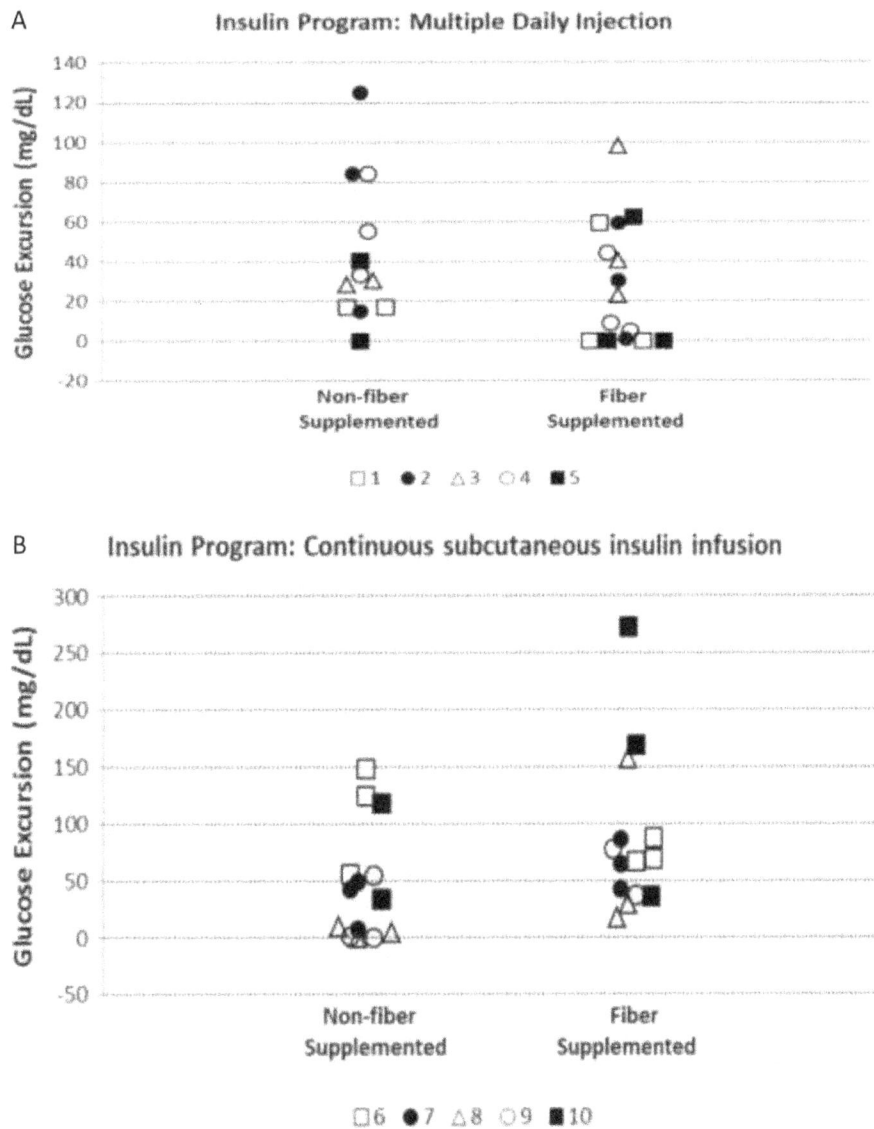

Figure 1 Blood glucose excursion (maximum post prandial glucose - glucose at the start of the meal) following lunch, separately for the 2 study phases. During each phase, each such had 2 or 3 lunch meals. **A**. Data for the 5 subjects who followed a multiple daily injection insulin program. **B**. Data of the 5 subjects who followed a continuous subcutaneous insulin infusion program.

Dietary sources of fiber vary in composition and include different types of soluble and insoluble fibers. In contrast, the fiber in Benefiber is exclusively wheat dextrin. Wheat dextrin is a soluble fiber that has low viscosity and that is slowly fermented in the large intestine to form short chain fatty acids (SCFAs). A previous study has shown that different types of fibers have differential effects on post prandial blood sugar responses, with pectin administration inhibiting post-prandial glucose rise, but fiber from barley and citrus (Dumovital) having no such effect [10]. Through the production of SCFAs, soluble fibers such as wheat dextrin, can stimulate pancreatic insulin release and may interfere with glycogen breakdown. As a result, blood sugar levels may decrease. Dextrin has been shown

to reduce post prandial blood sugars in healthy subjects and reduce fasting blood sugars in type 2 diabetics [11]. We may speculate that wheat dextrin has a greater dampening effect on blood sugar excursion as compared to other types of dietary fiber, so those who added the most wheat dextrin to their diet saw the greatest effects. The effects were only seen after the breakfast and lunch meals. In our patients, breakfast and lunch had higher carbohydrate content. It has been shown that the effect of fibers is most evident in diabetics with more than 55% of their caloric intake coming from carbohydrates [11].

Other studies have shown more significant effects of fiber supplementation on glucose excursion and hypoglycemia. When 60 adult patients with type 1

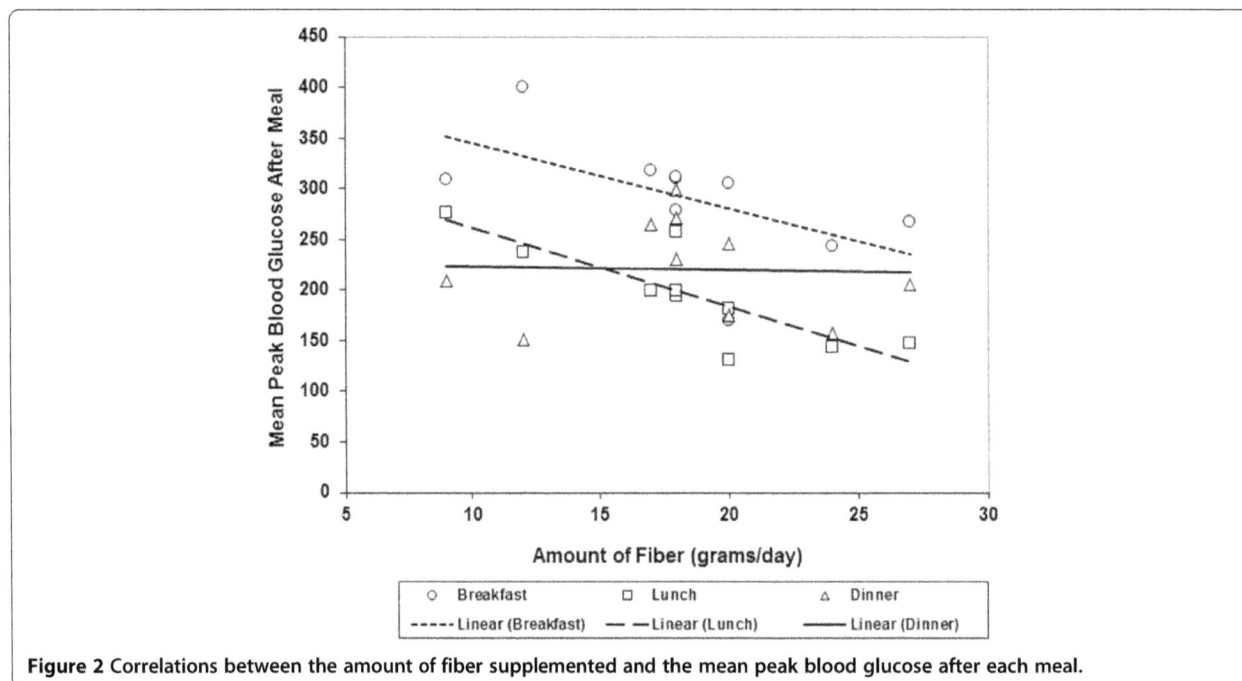

Figure 2 Correlations between the amount of fiber supplemented and the mean peak blood glucose after each meal.

diabetes were randomized to either a high fiber or low fiber diet for 24 weeks, those in the high fiber diet group had decreased mean daily blood glucose concentrations and fewer hypoglycemic events. Patients who were compliant with the high fiber diet also showed a reduction

Table 1 Incidence of hypoglycemia during the two study phases for each of the 10 subjects

Subject	Amount of fiber added (grams)	% of glucose measurements < 70 mg/dL	
		During the non-supplemented phase	During the fiber supplemented phase
1	27	24.9%	8.2%
2	18	15.5%	11.1%
3	20	8.2%	41.7%
4	18	3.3%	12.3%
5	12	0%	7.6%
6	18	12.0%	8.6%
7	20	6.0%	4.5%
8	17	18.4%	3.1%
9	24	1.8%	3.2%
10	9	2.4%	17.0%
Overall		9.4%	12.4%

in hemoglobin A1c [12]. Perhaps, we did not see similar results in our study because the duration of fiber supplementation was significantly shorter. The fermentation of wheat dextrin occurs slowly over 24 hours. Part of the effect of fiber supplements is mediated through the production of

SCFAs. We might have seen greater effects if the subjects wore the sensors for greater than 72 hours and if data was analyzed after the first 24 hours. On the other hand, the effect of fiber supplementation has been seen even during very short studies. Monnier et al. showed that the addition of fiber to an oral glucose load improves the pattern of the oral glucose tolerance test by blunting the peak blood glucose, prolonging the time interval to reach the peak blood glucose, and decreasing the rate of blood glucose rise [13].

There are a variety of other factors that influence glucose excursion. These factors include the carbohydrate, fat, and protein contents of the meal, the glycemic index of the food consumed, as well as the cooking methods, processing methods, and the form of foods. Additionally, an individual's degree of insulin resistance, rate of gastric emptying, and level of physical activity affect blood glucose excursions. Although we asked patients to eat the same types of foods during both phases of the study and we asked them to maintain the same level of physical activity, it is certainly possible that they did not do so and this may have impacted the results. We did review all food records. 6 of 10 participants consumed exactly the same diet at each meal during both study phases. 4 had minor dietary variations but carbohydrate, fat and protein proportions were followed as the subjects were on an exchange type diet with fixed amounts of the different food groups for each meal. A separate analysis was performed. The percent glucose measurement in the hyperglycemic and hypoglycemic range was not significantly different between patients who followed the same exact diet (6/10) and those who did not (4/10).

The strength of this study is the use of the continuous glucose monitoring system, which allowed us to look at data that would otherwise be unavailable using intermittent self-monitoring of blood sugars. However, the limitations include the small sample size and the fact that the meals were not standardized and we relied on patient's self reported intake. The variability of the insulin doses is also an inherent limitation to the study design. Subjects who were following an exchange type diet received overall a similar insulin dose with each meal. However, and if they had an unexplained low during the washout period, they were asked to decrease their dose. If they had a pattern of three highs, the dose was increased. Subjects using insulin to carbohydrate ratio also adjusted the ratio for unexplained hypoglycemia and a pattern of three high blood sugars. The standardized dose adjustment protocol was outlined by the treating physician. Adjusting the insulin dose for unexplained hypoglycemia was deemed necessary from a safety standpoint.

Based on the results of the current study, there is not enough evidence to recommend fiber supplementation to patients with type 1 diabetes in order to improve glycemic excursions the incidence of hypoglycemia. Future studies, in which all factors including diet, exercise and insulin dose are kept constant, are warranted. Further research in a larger sample size is required. However, all patients should strive to meet dietetic guidelines for the intake of fiber since this level of intake results in very few side effects and may have other benefits.

Article summary
Article focus

- It currently remains unclear what effects a diet rich in fiber would have on diabetes control and glycemic excursions in children with type 1 diabetes.
- The aim of this study was to determine whether the addition of a fiber supplement to the diet of pediatric patients with type 1 diabetes has an effect on the magnitude of glucose excursions and or the incidence of hypoglycemia.
- We hypothesized that children with type 1 diabetes receiving a high fiber diet will have lower glucose excursions and a lower incidence of hypoglycemia.

Key messages

- There is no overall decrease in glucose excursion or incidence of hypoglycemia with fiber supplementation in children with type 1 diabetes
- There is a negative correlation between the amount of wheat dextrin supplemented and the mean maximum post-prandial blood sugar after the lunch and breakfast meals

Strengths and limitations

- The strength of this study is the use of the continuous glucose monitoring system, which allowed us to look at data that would otherwise be unavailable using intermittent self-monitoring of blood sugars.
- However, the limitations include the small sample size and the fact that the meals were not standardized and we relied on patient's self reported intake.

Competing interests
The authors declare that they have no competing interests.

Authors' contributions
NN designed research, conducted research, and wrote manuscript. SE conducted research. AW performed statistical analysis. AL designed research, wrote manuscript, and had primary responsibility for the final content. All authors read and approved the final manuscript.

Funding
Mayo Clinic Department of Pediatrics.

Author details
[1]Division of Pediatric Endocrinology, Mayo Clinic, 200 1st St SW, Rochester, MN 55905, USA. [2]Biomedical Statistics and Informatics, Mayo Clinic, Rochester, MN 55905, USA. [3]Division of Endocrinology, Mayo Clinic, Rochester, MN 55905, USA.

References
1. American Diabetes Association: **Standards of medical care in diabetes.** *Diabetes Care* 2010, **34**(Supplement 1):S11–S61.
2. Mann J, De Leeuw I, Hermansen K, Karamanos B, Karlström B, Katsilambros N, Riccardi G, Rivellese AA, Rizkalla S, Slama G, Toeller M, Uusitupa M, Vessby B, On behalf of the Diabetes and Nutrition Study Group of the European Association for the Study of Diabetes: **Evidence based approaches to the treatment and prevention of diabetes mellitus.** *Nutr Metab Cardiovasc Dis* 2004, **14**:373–394.
3. Clinical Practice Consensus Guidelines 2009 Compendium ISPAD: **Nutritional management in children and adolescents with diabetes.** *Pediatr Diabetes* 2009, **10**(Suppl. 12):100–117.
4. Diabetes and Nutrition Study Group of the EASD: **Recommendations for the nutritional management of patients with diabetes mellitus.** *Diabetes Nutr Metab* 1995, **8**:1–4.
5. Anderson JW, Chen WL: **Plant fiber. Carbohydrate and lipid metabolism.** *Am J Clin Nutr* 1979, **32**(2):346–363.
6. Randecker GA, Smiciklas-Wright H, McKenzie JM, Shannon BM, Mitchell DC, Becker DJ, Kieselhorst K: **The dietary intake of children with IDDM.** *Diabetes Care* 1996, **12**:1370–1374.
7. Overby NC, Flaaten V, Veierod MB, Bergstad I, Margeirsdottir HD, Dahl-Jorgensen K, Andersen LF: **Children and adolescents with type 1 diabetes eat a more atherosclerosis prone diet than healthy control subjects.** *Diabetologia* 2007, **50**:307–316.
8. Rovner AJ, Nansel TR, Gellar L: **The effect of a low glycemic diet vs standard diet on blood glucose levels and macronutrient intake in children with type 1 diabetes.** *J Am Diet Assoc* 2009, **109**(2):303–307.

9.   Rami B, Zidek T, Schober E: Influence of beta-glucan-enriched bedtime snack on nocturnal blood glucose levels in diabetic children. *J Pediatr Gastroenterol Nutr* 2001, **32**(1):34–36.

10. Vaaler S, Hanssen KF, Aagenaes O: Effect of different kinds of fibre on post-prandial blood glucose in insulin-dependent diabetics. *Acta Med Scand* 1980, **208**(5):389–391.

11. Slavin JL, Savarino V, Paredes Diaz A: A Review of the role of soluble fiber in health with specific reference to wheat dextrin. *J Int Med Res* 2009, **37**:1–17.

12. Giacco R, Parillo M, Rivellese AA, Lasorella G, Giacco A, D'Episcopo L, Riccardi G: Long term dietary treatment with increased amounts of fiber rich low glycemic index natural foods improves blood glucose control and reduces the number of hypoglycemic events in type 1 diabetic patients. *Diabetes Care* 2000, **10**:1461–1466.

13. Monnier L, Pham TC, Aguirre L, Orsetti A, Mirgjze I: Influence of indigestible fibers on glucose tolerance. *Diabetes Care* 1978, **1**(2):83–88.

28

Clitoral size in term newborns in Kumasi, Ghana

Serwah Bonsu Asafo-Agyei[1*], Emmanuel Ameyaw[1], Jean-Pierre Chanoine[2], Margaret Zacharin[3] and Samuel Blay Nguah[1]

Abstract

Background: Data on normative clitoral sizes in newborns is relatively sparse and racial/ethnic differences have also been reported. This study was performed to establish norms for clitoral size in term Ghanaian female newborns.

Methods: This was a cross-sectional study of all apparently well full-term newborns of postnatal age < 48 h and birth weight between 2.5 and 4.0 kg delivered at Komfo Anokye Teaching Hospital between May and September, 2014. Anthropometric and genital parameters were documented for study subjects as well as parental socio-demographic indices.

Results: In 612 newborn females studied, the mean (±SD) clitoral length (MCL) and the mean (±SD) clitoral width (MCW) were 4.13 ± 1.6 mm and 4.21 ± 1.1 mm, respectively. MCL was inversely related to birth weight ($r = -0.62$; $p < 0.001$) while MCW was inversely related to both gestational age ($r = -0.1$; $p = 0.02$) and birth weight ($r = -0.54$; $p < 0.001$). Babies with a clitoris that was completely covered by the labia majora had relatively lower clitoral sizes ($p < 0.001$) than those who had a partially covered or prominent clitoris. Neither MCL nor MCW differed significantly by birth length or maternal tribe.

Conclusions: Clitoral size varies with birth weight and gestational age. Babies with a completely covered clitoris are unlikely to warrant detailed clitoral measurements for clitoromegaly.

Keywords: Clitoral length, Clitoral width, Clitoral size, Ghana, Newborns, Clitoromegaly

Background

Early detection of genital anomalies in the female infant is crucial. Significant clitoromegaly at birth usually reflects virilization and suggests that the female foetus has been exposed to androgens during the intrauterine period [1]. Congenital adrenal hyperplasia (CAH) is the most common cause of virilization of a female foetus. Failure to identify and treat this disorder results in potentially fatal adrenal crisis, an avoidable outcome if the endocrine emergency is correctly diagnosed and treated [2]. Since the technique of analyzing 17-hydroxyprogesterone (17-OHP) in filter paper blood samples was developed by Pang et al. [3] in 1977, the utility of newborn screening for CAH has been amply demonstrated and several developed countries have established a newborn screening

programme [4–7]. Unfortunately, newborn screening is still not available in most developing countries including Ghana. Thus, until routine newborn CAH screening is commenced, comprehensive clinical assessment including genital examination remains the simplest and most cost-effective option of circumventing the challenges imposed by financial and diagnostic restraints in resource limited settings.

Propitiously, females with classical CAH usually have ambiguous genitalia or clitoromegaly which may be readily detected by genital examination [2]. Hospital statistics at the study site indicate that about 9000 - 12,000 babies are delivered annually in the hospital, with about 16 - 18% of these being preterms. Newborn screening for congenital adrenal adrenal hyperplasia is not carried out in the hospital but between May 2014 and April 2015 we diagnosed 4 females with CAH in a cohort of 9255 neonates through systematic newborn examination (unpublished data). Although it has been reported that clinical examination may

* Correspondence: sbasafoagyei@gmail.com
[1]Department of Child Health, Komfo Anokye Teaching Hospital, Kumasi, Ghana
Full list of author information is available at the end of the article

miss some cases of non-classical and even classical CAH [5, 8, 9], detailed genital examination still has distinct benefits over a cursory look at the genitalia and may even help prevent extremely virilized females from being labelled as "males".

Conversely, the clitoris may seem prominent in some healthy newborns, leading to many unnecessary investigations [10]. Clitoral size measurements permit accurate clitoral assessment and avoid over- or misdiagnosis of abnormalities based on clinical impression alone, thus minimizing unnecessary cost and psychological trauma to the parents [11].

Normative clitoral anthropometric data for healthy newborns has been reported but is sparse and mainly derived from Caucasian and Asian infants. However, racial/ethnic differences in newborn clitoral sizes have been reported [12, 13] and existing data may therefore not be applicable to our population in Ghana, for which no published data exist.

Aim: To establish reference ranges for clitoral sizes in apparently healthy term newborns in Ghana.

Methods

This cross-sectional study was conducted in Komfo Anokye Teaching Hospital (KATH) between May 2014 and September 2014. KATH is a tertiary care teaching hospital in Kumasi, the second largest city in Ghana. It serves as a referral centre for the Kumasi Metropolis and the whole northern half of Ghana.

A complete antenatal history was obtained from the mother and from the hospital records, including a history of ingestion of herbal medicine or prescribed medications. The gestational age was determined by using the last menstrual period and early ultrasound results and confirmed if necessary with Dubowitz/Ballard score [14]. Physical examination of both mother and newborn was done. All apparently well female term newborns with a gestational age of 40 ± 2 weeks and birth weight between 2.5 and 4.0 kg were considered for recruitment into the study. Exclusion criteria for newborns included major congenital anomalies/dysmorphism, apparent disorders of sexual development, breech presentation and twins of different gender. Maternal exclusion criteria were pregnancy history of hormonal drug intake, signs of virilization during pregnancy, pre-eclampsia and diabetes mellitus.

Anthropometric measurements of newborns were taken within 48 h after delivery. A nurse attached to the paediatric endocrine unit was trained to assist the principal investigator with the genital and anthropometric measurements. Two research assistants were also trained to assist the two examiners with positioning of the newborns and with data entry. In a warm environment, the newborns were put in the supine position and the perineum was adequately exposed. It was noted on inspection whether the clitoris was visible or completely covered by the labia majora. The baby was then placed in a frog-like position and the position secured by an assistant. The labia majora were separated and the prepuce of the clitoris gently retracted. Clitoral size was measured as described by Verkauf et al. [15], with clitoral length measured as the distance from the crura insertion at the pubis symphysis to the tip of the glans and clitoral width measured in the greatest transverse diameter (Fig. 1). Both the clitoral length and width were measured twice using digital Vernier calipers (Resolution 0.01 mm, Accuracy +/−0.02 mm) and their respective means were recorded. The weight was measured to the nearest 10 g with a Salter scale (Model 180, Salter Brecknell, England) and the length was measured to the nearest centimetre with an infantometer (Seca 416 Mobile infantometer, Seca GmbH & Co. KG, Germany). All anthropometric measurements were done by a 2-member team, with one person taking the measurements while the other positioned the baby and helped enter the data onto the Case report form. Majority (72.1%) of the measurements were done by the principal investigator. Inter-observer variability for genital measurements was checked on a 2-weekly basis throughout the study on 5 randomly selected newborns and it remained insignificant. The standard deviations for inter-observer variation were 0.05 mm and 0.09 mm and 95% of paired measurements were within range of 0.09 mm and 0.03 mm for clitoral length and clitoral width respectively.

The data was analyzed using R statistical software version 3.1.2. Continuous variables were presented as means with standard deviation as well as median with their corresponding ranges. Single categorical variables were tabulated and expressed as percentages. The relationships between genital measurements and various categorical variables were determined using an analysis of variance, correcting for possible confounders and reporting the

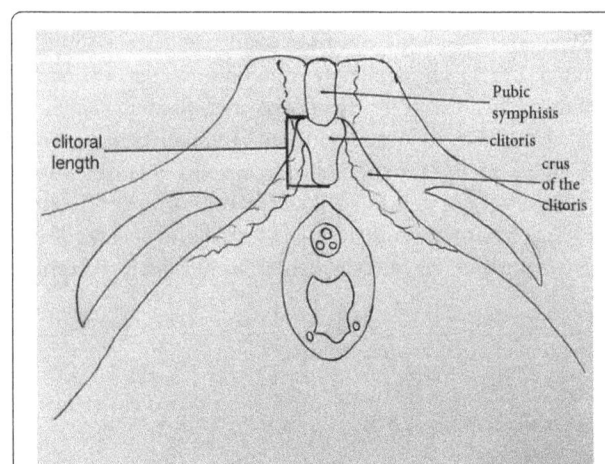

Fig. 1 Schematic diagram of clitoris and surrounding structures showing the anatomic landmarks utilized for clitoral length measurement

respective *p*-values as appropriate. Relationships between genital measurement and other continuous variables were determined using linear regression. These analyses were presented as their regression coefficient (r) with their 95% confidence intervals. For all analysis a two sided *p*-value of <0.05 was considered statistically significant. This study was approved by the Committee on Human Research, Publications and Ethics of KATH/Kwame Nkrumah University of Science and Technology, Kumasi. Written informed consent was received from the parents prior to enrollment.

Results

A total of 612 female infants were studied including one set of identical twins. One mother/baby pair was excluded because of maternal virilization. A descriptive data of study subjects is shown in Table 1. The distribution of maternal tribe is shown in Fig. 2. Genital measurements from study subjects were used to construct clitoral size percentile charts (Table 2). The mean (±SD) clitoral length [MCL] was 4.13 ± 1.6 mm and the mean (±SD) clitoral width [MCW] was 4.21 ± 1.1 mm. There were 3/612 females (0.49%) with a clitoral length ≥ 1 cm and 31/612 female newborns (5.1%) with a clitoral width greater than 6 mm. Using the 97th percentile, a newborn will be considered to have clitoromegaly if clitoral length is greater than 7.5 mm and/or clitoral width is greater than 6.2 mm.

No correlation was seen between genital size and maternal herbal intake or mode of delivery. Seventy-nine (12.9%) mothers took herbs at varying periods during their pregnancy. There was also no significant difference in genital measurements done in the first 24 h of postnatal life and those done from 24 h up to 48 h. After correcting for confounders, there was no significant difference in MCL or MCW by tribe. Table 3 shows the correlation between clitoral size and gestational age, birth weight and birth length. There was a strong negative correlation between clitoral size and birth weight.

Both clitoral length and width varied significantly with appearance of the clitoris (Table 4). A completely covered clitoris was significantly smaller than a partially covered one, which was in turn smaller than a prominent clitoris.

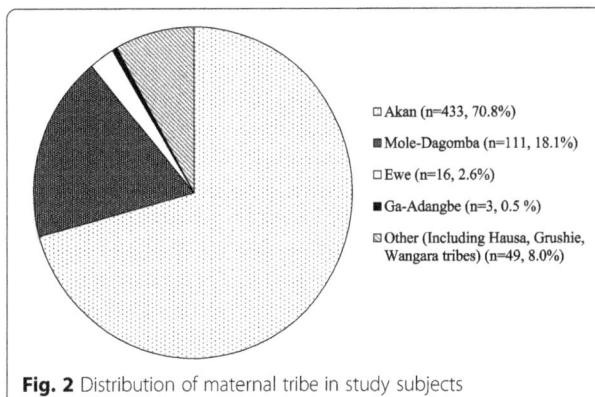

Fig. 2 Distribution of maternal tribe in study subjects

□ Akan (n=433, 70.8%)
■ Mole-Dagomba (n=111, 18.1%)
□ Ewe (n=16, 2.6%)
■ Ga-Adangbe (n=3, 0.5 %)
▨ Other (Including Hausa, Grushie, Wangara tribes) (n=49, 8.0%)

Discussion

This is the first description of the characteristics and size of the clitoris in Ghana and the largest cohort of newborn clitoral sizes in published literature. Traditionally, normal clitoral length is accepted as < 1.0 cm, although rare variations exist [16]. In our study, only 3/612 females (0.49%) had a clitoral length ≥ 1 cm. These patients were followed up for a year and their clitoral size did not increase with time, nor did they develop any clinical features suggestive of CAH. Studies in newborns from different parts of the world have reported MCL ranging from 3.1–7.7 mm [10, 13, 17–21]. Most published studies done in newborns did not elaborate on how the clitoral measurements were done. Amongst studies with similar inclusion criteria, our MCL of 4.13 ± 1.60 mm was comparable to the 4.0 ± 1.24 mm reported by Oberfield et al. [17] in United States and the 4.93 ± 1.61 mm reported by Kutlu et al. [10] in Turkey. Our MCL was also similar to that of other studies that involved preterms, including the 3.66 ± 0.13 mm reported by Riley and Rosenbloom [13] in black term and preterm newborns in United States. Mondal et al. [20] also reported a comparable albeit slightly lower MCL of 3.1 ± 1.54 mm in India and Jarrett et al. [19] reported a relatively higher MCL of 7.7 ± 1.37 mm in 244 term and preterm newborns in Nigeria.

A clitoral width > 6 mm has been said to suggest virilization [22], probably based on earlier studies by

Table 1 Descriptive characteristics of study subjects

	Mean	SD	Median	Minimum	Maximum
Gestational age (weeks)	40.0	1.1	40.0	38.0	42.0
[a]Post-natal age (hours)	10.1	7.8	8.0	1	47
Birth weight (kgs)	3.1	0.4	3.1	2.5	4.0
Length (cm)	48.1	2.1	48.2	37.6	53.6
Clitoral Length (mm)	4.1	1.6	3.7	1.1	10.8
Clitoral Width (mm)	4.2	1.1	4.3	1.3	8.8

[a]Age in hours at which anthropometric measurements were done

Table 2 Clitoral size percentiles

Percentile	Clitoral Length (mm)	Clitoral Width (mm)
3	1.6	2.2
10	2.3	2.8
50	3.9	4.3
90	6.3	5.6
97	7.5	6.2
99	8.6	6.8

Table 3 Association of clitoral size with gestational age, birth weight and birth length

	Gestational Age (weeks)		Birth Weight (kgs)		Birth Length (cm)	
	r (95% CI)	p-value	r (95% CI)	p-value	r (95% CI)	p-value
MCL (mm)	−0.06 (−0.17 to 0.06)	0.330	−0.62 (−0.96 to −0.29)	**<0.001**	−0.03 (−0.09 to 0.03)	0.390
MCW (mm)	−0.1 (−0.17 to −0.02)	**0.020**	−0.54 (−0.78 to −0.31)	**<0.001**	−0.04 (−0.08 to 0)	0.070

Linear regression utilized for analysis; r: Coefficient of linear regression
Significant p-values are in bold italics

Riley and Rosenbloom (1980) [13] and Oberfield et al. (1989) [17]; who both reported an upper limit of 6 mm for clitoral width range in newborns. However, the range for clitoral width is not well established as fewer studies have reported clitoral width. In this study, as many as 31 / 612 newborns (5.1%) had a clitoral width greater than 6 mm. These patients were followed up and they remained healthy. Jarrett et al. [19] also reported a clitoral width range of 1–7 mm, and so regional differences in clitoral size may exist. More African data will be needed to clarify this. Our MCW of 4.21 ± 1.1 mm was similar to reports from Jarrett et al. [19] and Yokoya et al. [21] of 4.4 ± 0.89 mm and 4.4 ± 1.2 mm respectively. Oberfield et al. [17] reported a relatively lower mean clitoral width (MCW) of 3.32 ± 0.78 mm in North American term newborns.

Factors that may be responsible for the reported variation in clitoral sizes include differences in study population. Some studies included preterms [13, 19, 20] whereas this study recruited only term newborns. Clitoral size has also been reported to correlate with anthropometric parameters of the study population [10]. Furthermore, differences in tools and techniques of measurement as well as inter observer variability may play a role. This study utilized calipers in the measurement of clitoral length and width while other studies utilized tumorimeters or rulers [19, 23]. MCL have also been reported to vary with ethnicity/race, which may also partly account for the differences in reported values [12, 13].

Only MCW but not MCL in our study was negligibly associated, though inversely, with gestational age. The lack of significant association was not unexpected as all the newborns were full term. The analysis for correlation between maternal herbal intake and clitoral size was done to evaluate for possible hormonal effects of the ingested herbal medicines, since their constituents were largely unknown. There was no significant difference in genital measurements done in the first 24 h and those done afterwards. Oberfield et al. [17] also noted no difference in clitoral sizes when they compared measurements done before and after 24 h in order to evaluate for possible variation from swelling of the genital area due to birth trauma.

Birth weight was inversely associated with both MCL and MCW, implying newborns with a lower birth weight had larger clitoral sizes and vice versa. Similarly, Kutlu and Akbiyik [10] also found a negative correlation between MCL with birth weight. However, unlike this study they also reported a negative correlation between MCL and birth length. Oberfield et al. [17] found no correlation between clitoral size and birth weight or length.

Kutlu and Akbiyik [10] reported that the clitoral length was < 5 mm when it appeared to be covered by the labia majora and concluded that no extra clitoral measurement was clinically indicated in such cases. In our study, the highest recorded MCL and MCW in newborns with completely covered clitoris was 8.3 mm and 6.22 mm respectively. Overall, newborns whose clitoris was completely covered by the labia majora had the lowest mean clitoral size (p < 0.001) and indeed further clitoral measurements may not be indicated in such newborns; as suggested by Kutlu and Akbiyik [10].

One limitation of our study is that measurements were done by two examiners and could have introduced an error due to inter-observer variability. However, an extensive training was done and a subset of study subjects was examined by both 2 examiners to evaluate and control for variability, which remained insignificant throughout the study.

Table 4 Correlation between clitoral appearance and size

ªClitoris	Completely covered number =132 (21.6%)		Partially showing number =188 (30.7%)		Prominent number = 278 (45.4%)		p-value
	Mean (SD)	Median (range)	Mean (SD)	Median (range)	Mean (SD)	Median (range)	
CL (mm)	3.3 (1.2)	3.3 (1.1–8.3)	3.8 (1.4)	3.8 (1.4–10.8)	4.8 (1.6)	4.8 (1.2–10.6)	**<0.001**
CW (mm)	3.5 (1.0)	3.5 (1.3–6.2)	3.8 (0.9)	3.8 (1.8–6.1)	4.8 (1.1)	4.8 (2.0–8.82)	**<0.001**

Analysis of variance utilized for analysis; Significant p-values are in bold italics
ªFourteen missing data

Conclusions

Our study suggests that the mean clitoral size of Ghanaian newborns is similar to results reported by others but regional differences may exist in clitoral size range. Our data will be useful for the assessment of female neonates in Ghana by establishing the norm and thus help promote early recognition of deviation from the norm; such as genital abnormalities in female neonates.

Abbreviations
CAH: Congenital Adrenal Hyperplasia; CI: Confidence Interval; KATH: Komfo Anokye Teaching Hospital; MPL: Mean Penile length; MPW: Mean Penile Width; r: Coefficient of linear regression; SPL: Stretched penile length

Acknowledgements
The authors will like to acknowledge Mr Isaac Appiah, the research team, the staff of KATH Obstetrics and Gynaecology department and the co-ordinators and fellows of the PETCWA programme. This research was jointly funded by Global Pediatric Endocrinology and Diabetes (GPED) and the European Society for Paediatric Endocrinology (ESPE).

Funding
This research was jointly funded by Global Paediatric Endocrinology and Diabetes and the European Society for Paediatric Endocrinology.

Authors' contributions
SBAA participated in the study design, data collection and entry and manuscript writing. EA sought for ethical clearance, participated in the study design, data collection and entry and supervision and completion of final manuscript. JPC and MZ participated in the study design, supervision and completion of final manuscript. SBN participated in the study design, statistical analysis and completion of final manuscript. All authors read and approved the final manuscript.

Competing interests
The authors declare that they have no competing interests.

Author details
[1]Department of Child Health, Komfo Anokye Teaching Hospital, Kumasi, Ghana. [2]Endocrinology and Diabetes Unit, British Columbia Children's Hospital, University of British Columbia, Vancouver, BC, Canada. [3]The Royal Children's Hospital, Murdoch Children's Research Institute and University of Melbourne, Melbourne, Australia.

References
1. Kaiser GL. Symptoms and signs in Pediatric surgery. New York: Springer; 2005. p. 565–79.
2. Hughes IA. Ambiguous genitalia. In: Brook CGD, Clayton PE, Brown RS, editors. Brook's clinical pediatric endocrinology. 5th ed. Oxford: Blackwell Publishing Ltd; 2005. p. 171–82.
3. Pang S, Hotchkiss J, Drash AL, Levine LS, New MI. Microfilter paper method for 17 alpha-hydroxyprogesterone radioimmunoassay: its application for rapid screening for congenital adrenal hyperplasia. J Clin Endocrinol Metab. 1977;45(5):1003–8.
4. Gidlöf S, Falhammar H, Thilén A, Ritzén M, Wedell A, Nordenström A. One hundred years of congenital adrenal hyperplasia in Sweden: a retrospective, population-based cohort study. Lancet Diabetes Endocrinol. 2013;1(1):35–42.
5. Therrell Jr BL, Berenbaum SA, Manter-Kapanke V, Simmank J, Korman K, Prentice L, Gonzalez J, Gunn S. Results of screening 1.9 million Texas newborns for 21-hydroxylase-deficient congenital adrenal hyperplasia. Pediatrics. 1998;101(4 Pt 1):583–90.
6. Tsuji A, Konishi K, Hasegawa S, Anazawa A, Onishi T, Ono M, et al. Newborn screening for congenital adrenal hyperplasia in Tokyo, Japan from 1989 to 2013: a retrospective population-based study. BMC Pediatr. 2015;15:209.
7. White PC. Optimizing newborn screening for congenital adrenal hyperplasia. J Pediatr. 2013;163(1):10–2.
8. Thilén A, Nordenström A, Hagenfeldt L, von Döbeln U, Guthenberg C, Larsson A. Benefits of neonatal screening for congenital adrenal hyperplasia (21-hydroxylase deficiency) in Sweden. Pediatrics. 1998;101:E11.
9. Balsamo A, Cacciari E, Piazzi S, Cassio A, Bozza D, Pirazzoli P, Zappulla F. Congenital adrenal hyperplasia: neonatal mass screening compared with clinical diagnosis only in the Emilia-Romagna region of Italy, 1980–1995. Pediatrics. 1996;98(3 Pt 1):362–7.
10. Kutlu HA, Akbiyik F. Clitoral length in female newborns: a new approach to the assessment of clitoromegaly. Turk J Med Sci. 2011;41(3):495–9.
11. Litwin A, Aitkin I, Merlob P. Clitoral length assessment in newborn infants of 30 to 41 weeks gestational age. Eur J Obstet Gynecol Reprod Biol. 1991; 38(3):209–12.
12. Phillip M, De Boer C, Pilpel D, Karplus M, Sofer S. Clitoral and penile sizes of full term newborns in two different ethnic groups. J Pediatr Endocrinol Metab. 1996;9(2):175–9.
13. Riley WJ, Rosenbloom AC. Clitoral size in infancy. J Pediatr. 1980;96:918–9.
14. Dubowitz LMS, Dubowitz V, Goldberg C. Clinical assessment of gestational age in the newborn infant. J Pediatr. 1970;77:1–10.
15. Verkauf BS, Von Thron J, O'Brien WF. Clitoral Size in Normal Women. Obstet Gynecol. 1992;80(1):41–4.
16. Witchel SF, Lee PA. Ambiguous genitalia. In: Sperling MA, editor. Pediatric endocrinology. 3rd ed. Philadelphia: Elsevier Saunders; 2008. p. 127–64.
17. Oberfield SE, Mondok A, Shahrivar F, Klein JF, Levine LS. Clitoral size in full-term infants. Am J Perinatol. 1989;6:453–5.
18. Jarrett OO, Ayoola OO, Ritzen M. Clitoral and penile sizes in healthy newborn babies in Ibadan, Nigeria. Endocrine Abstracts 2010;24 P15. http://www.endocrine-abstracts.org/ea/0024/ea0024p15.htm. Accessed 10 Jan 2015.
19. Jarrett OO, Ayoola OO, Jonsson B, Albertsson-Wikland K, Ritzen M. Country-based reference values and international comparisons of clitoral size in healthy Nigerian newborn infants. Acta Paediatr. 2015;104(12):1286–90.
20. Mondal R, Chatterjee K, Samanta M, Hazra A, Ray S, Sabui TK, et al. Clitoral length and anogenital ratio in Indian newborn girls. Indian Pediatr. 2016;53: 299–303.
21. Vilain E, Sarafoglou K, Yehya N. Disorders of sex development. In: Sarafoglou K, Hoffmann G, Roth KS, Courtney H, editors. Pediatric Endocrinology and Inborn Errors of Metabolism. New York: The McGraw Hill Companies; 2009. p. 525–55.
22. Yokoya S, Kato K, Suwa S. Penile and clitoral size in premature and normal newborns, infants and children. Horumon To Rinsho. 1983;31(12):1215–20.
23. Park SE, Ahn SY, Shin CH. Penile and Clitoral Sizes of Normal Full-Term Newborns in Korea. MeetingAbstracts. 2012;MON-634. http://press.endocrine.org/doi/abs/10.1210/endo-meetings.2012.PE.6.MON-634. Accessed 13 Mar 2016.

Permissions

All chapters in this book were first published in IJPE, by BioMed Central; hereby published with permission under the Creative Commons Attribution License or equivalent. Every chapter published in this book has been scrutinized by our experts. Their significance has been extensively debated. The topics covered herein carry significant findings which will fuel the growth of the discipline. They may even be implemented as practical applications or may be referred to as a beginning point for another development.

The contributors of this book come from diverse backgrounds, making this book a truly international effort. This book will bring forth new frontiers with its revolutionizing research information and detailed analysis of the nascent developments around the world.

We would like to thank all the contributing authors for lending their expertise to make the book truly unique. They have played a crucial role in the development of this book. Without their invaluable contributions this book wouldn't have been possible. They have made vital efforts to compile up to date information on the varied aspects of this subject to make this book a valuable addition to the collection of many professionals and students.

This book was conceptualized with the vision of imparting up-to-date information and advanced data in this field. To ensure the same, a matchless editorial board was set up. Every individual on the board went through rigorous rounds of assessment to prove their worth. After which they invested a large part of their time researching and compiling the most relevant data for our readers.

The editorial board has been involved in producing this book since its inception. They have spent rigorous hours researching and exploring the diverse topics which have resulted in the successful publishing of this book. They have passed on their knowledge of decades through this book. To expedite this challenging task, the publisher supported the team at every step. A small team of assistant editors was also appointed to further simplify the editing procedure and attain best results for the readers.

Apart from the editorial board, the designing team has also invested a significant amount of their time in understanding the subject and creating the most relevant covers. They scrutinized every image to scout for the most suitable representation of the subject and create an appropriate cover for the book.

The publishing team has been an ardent support to the editorial, designing and production team. Their endless efforts to recruit the best for this project, has resulted in the accomplishment of this book. They are a veteran in the field of academics and their pool of knowledge is as vast as their experience in printing. Their expertise and guidance has proved useful at every step. Their uncompromising quality standards have made this book an exceptional effort. Their encouragement from time to time has been an inspiration for everyone.

The publisher and the editorial board hope that this book will prove to be a valuable piece of knowledge for researchers, students, practitioners and scholars across the globe.

List of Contributors

Ze'ev Hochberg
Division of Pediatric Endocrinology, Meyer Children's Hospital, Rambam Medical Center, and Rappaport Faculty of Medicine and Research Institute, Technion-Israel Institute of Technology, Haifa, Israel

Aneta Gawlik
Division of Pediatric Endocrinology, Meyer Children's Hospital, Rambam Medical Center, and Rappaport Faculty of Medicine and Research Institute, Technion-Israel Institute of Technology, Haifa, Israel
Department of Pediatric Endocrinology and Diabetes, Medical University of Silesia, Katowice, Poland

Robert S Walker
Department of Anthropology, University of Missouri, Columbia MO 65211, USA

Jennifer N Osipoff and Thomas A Wilson
Division of Pediatric Endocrinology, Department of Pediatrics, Stony Brook Children's Hospital, HSC Level 11 Room 080, Stony Brook, NY 11794-8111, USA

Denise Dixon
Suffolk Health Psychology Services, PLLC, 646 Main Street, 2nd floor Suite 203, Port Jefferson, NY 11777, USA

Thomas Preston
Department of Neuropsychology, Stony Brook Medicine, Health Sciences Center, Stony Brook, NY 11794-8511, USA

John A Morrison and Jessica G Woo
From the Division of Cardiology, Children's Hospital of Cincinnati, 3333 Burnet Avenue, 45229, Cincinnati, USA

Ping Wang
From the Cholesterol and Metabolism Center, Jewish Hospital of Cincinnati, Cincinnati, USA

Charles J Glueck
From the Cholesterol and Metabolism Center, Jewish Hospital of Cincinnati, Cincinnati, USA
Cholesterol Center, UC Health Business Center, 3200 Burnet Avenue, Cincinnati, OH 45229, USA

Juan F Sotos
Department of Pediatric, College of Medicine, The Ohio State University, Nationwide Children's Hospital, Section of Pediatric Endocrinology, Metabolism and Diabetes, 700 Children's Drive, Columbus, OH 43205, USA

Naomi J Tokar
Nationwide Children's Hospital, Section of Pediatric Endocrinology, Metabolism and Diabetes, 700 Children's Drive, Columbus, OH 43205, USA

Emily K Sims and Erica A Eugster
Section of Pediatric Endocrinology/Diabetology, Riley Hospital for Children, Indiana University School of Medicine, 705 Riley Hospital Drive, Room 5960, Indianapolis, IN 46202, USA

Sally Garnett
AstraZeneca, Macclesfield, United Kingdom

Franco Guzman
Former-AstraZeneca, Wilmington, Delaware, USA

Françoise Paris and Charles Sultan
Pediatric Gynecology and Endocrinology, University Hospital of Montpellier, Montpellier, France

Mary Cataletto and Moris Angulo
The Prader-Willi Syndrome Center at Winthrop University Hospital, 120 Mineola Blvd.-Suite 210, Mineola, N.Y. 11501, USA

Gila Hertz
Huntington Medical Group, PC, Sleep Disorders Center, 180 East Pulaski Rd., Huntington Station, N.Y. 11746, USA

Barbara Whitman
Saint Louis University School of Medicine, 1465 S. Grand, St. Louis, Mo. 63104, USA

Scott A Clements
Utah Diabetes and Endocrinology Center, University of Utah School of Medicine, 615 Arapeen Dr, Suite 100, Salt Lake City, UT 84108, USA

Matthew D Anger
University of Colorado School of Medicine, 13001 E 17th Place, N4223, Aurora, CO 80045, USA

Franziska K Bishop, Georgeanna J Klingensmith, David M Maahs and R. Paul Wadwa
Barbara Davis Center for Childhood Diabetes, University of Colorado School of Medicine, 1775 Aurora Ct, A140, Aurora, CO 80045, USA

Kim K McFann
University of Colorado School of Public Health, 13001 E 17th Place, B119, Aurora, CO 80045, USA

Parvin Yazdani and Yuezhen Lin
Pediatric Endocrinology, Baylor College of Medicine, Houston 77030, TX, USA

Vandana Raman
University of Utah, Salt Lake City, UT, USA

Morey Haymond
Baylor College of Medicine, Children's Nutritional Research Center, Houston, TX, USA

Ana Colmenares
Department of Pediatrics, Hospital Dr. Patrocinio Peñuela-IVSS, San Cristobal, Táchira 5001, Venezuela

Peter Gunczler and Roberto Lanes
Pediatric Endocrine Unit, Hospital de Clínicas Caracas, Caracas, Venezuela

Nouhad Raissouni, Andrey Kolesnikov, Radhika Purushothaman, Sunil Sinha, Sonal Bhandari, Amrit Bhangoo, Shahid Malik and Svetlana Ten
Division of Pediatric Endocrinology at Infants and Children's Hospital of Brooklyn at Maimonides and SUNY Downstate Medical Center, 1068 48th St, Brooklyn, NY 11219, USA

Revi Mathew
Department of Pediatrics, Division of Pediatric Endocrinology, Vanderbilt University School of Medicine, Monroe Carell Jr. Children's Hospital at Vanderbilt, 11134A Doctors' Office Tower, 2200 Children's Way, Nashville, TN 37232-9170, USA

Jean-Patrice Baillargeon
Department of Medicine, and Physiology and Biophysics, Division of Endocrinology, University of Sherbrooke, 3001, 12e Avenue Nord, Sherbrooke, QC J1H 5N4, Canada

Maria Isabel Hernandez
Departments of Pediatrics, Endocrinologa Infantil, Instituto de Investigaciones Materno Infantil (IDIMI), Universidad de Chile, Clinica Las Condes Santiago, Chile

Michael Rosenbaum
Department of Pediatrics, Division of Pediatric Endocrinology, Children's Hospital of New York-Presbyterian, 622 West 168th Street, PH-5E-522, New York, NY 10032, USA

David Geller
Department of Pediatrics, Division of Pediatric Endocrinology, Cedars-Sinai Medical Center, David Geffen- University of California, Los Angeles School of Medicine, 8700 Beverly Blvd. Room 4220 North Tower, Los Angeles, CA 90048, USA

Halley P Crissman, Lauren Warner, Melissa Gardner, Meagan Carr and David E Sandberg
Department of Pediatrics and Communicable Diseases Division of Child Behavioral Health University of Michigan Medical School 1500 East Medical Center Drive, SPC 5318 Ann Arbor, Michigan 48109-5318 USA

Aileen Schast
Division of Urology The Children's Hospital of Philadelphia Richard D Wood Center, 3rd Floor 34th Street and Civic Center Boulevard Philadelphia, Pennsylvania 19104 USA

Alexandra L Quittner
Departments of Psychology and Pediatrics University of Miami 5665 Ponce de Leon Blvd. Coral Gables, Florida 33146-2070 USA

Barry Kogan
Division of Urology Department of Surgery Albany Medical College 23 Hackett Boulevard Albany, New York 12208 USA

Amalie Bisgaard, Kaspar Sørensen, Trine Holm Johannsen, Anna-Maria Andersson and Anders Juul
Department of Growth and Reproduction, Rigshospitalet, Copenhagen University Hospital, section 5064 Blegdamsvej 9, DK-2100 Copenhagen, Denmark
Faculty of Health and Medical Sciences, University of Copenhagen, Copenhagen, Denmark

Jørn Wulff Helge
Department of Biomedical Sciences, Xlab, Center for Healthy Aging, University of Copenhagen, Copenhagen, Denmark

Debika Nandi-Munshi
Section of Endocrinology and Diabetes, St. Christopher's Hospital for Children, Department of Pediatrics, Drexel University College of Medicine, Philadelphia, PA, USA

Rita Ann Kubicky, Christopher Dunne and Francesco De Luca
Section of Endocrinology and Diabetes, St. Christopher's Hospital for Children, Department of Pediatrics, Drexel University College of Medicine, Philadelphia, PA, USA
St. Christopher's Hospital for Children, Section of Endocrinology and Diabetes, 3601 A Street, Suite 3303, Philadelphia, PA 19134, USA

Nobuhiro Nakatake, Shuji Fukata and Junichi Tajiri
Tajiri Thyroid Clinic, Kumamoto 862-0950, Japan

Vickie Braithwaite
MRC Human Nutrition Research, Elsie Widdowson Laboratory, Cambridge CB1 9NL, United Kingdom

Ann Prentice
MRC Human Nutrition Research, Elsie Widdowson Laboratory, Cambridge CB1 9NL, United Kingdom
MRC Keneba, Keneba, West Kiang, The Gambia

Andrew M Prentice and Conor Doherty
MRC International Nutrition Group, London School of Hygiene and Tropical Medicine, London WC1E 7HT, UK
MRC Keneba, Keneba, West Kiang, The Gambia

Stephanie E Hullmann, David A Fedele and Larry L Mullins
Department of Psychology, Oklahoma State University, Stillwater, Oklahoma, 74078, USA

Cortney Wolfe-Christensen
Department of Pediatric Urology, Children's Hospital of Michigan, Detroit, Michigan, 48201, USA

Amy B Wisniewski
Department of Urology, University of Oklahoma Health Sciences Center, Oklahoma City, Oklahoma, 73104, USA

Darlene E Berrymann
Edison Biotechnology Institute, Ohio University, Konneker Research Laboratories, 1 Water Tower Drive, The Ridges, 45701 Athens, Ohio, USA

Gabriel Á Martos-Moreno
Edison Biotechnology Institute, Ohio University, Konneker Research Laboratories, 1 Water Tower Drive, The Ridges, 45701 Athens, Ohio, USA
Hospital Infantil Universitario Niño Jesús, Department of Endocrinology, Instituto de Investigación la Princesa, Universidad Autónoma de Madrid, Department of Pediatrics, Av. Menéndez Pelayo, 65, E-28009 Madrid, Spain
CIBER Fisiopatología Obesidad y Nutrición (CIBERobn), Instituto de Salud Carlos III, Madrid, Spain

Lucila Sackmann-Sala
Edison Biotechnology Institute, Ohio University, Konneker Research Laboratories, 1 Water Tower Drive, The Ridges, 45701 Athens, Ohio, USA
Department of Biological Sciences, College of Arts and Sciences, Ohio University, Athens, Ohio, USA
Molecular and Cellular Biology Program, Ohio University, Athens, Ohio, USA

John J Kopchick
Edison Biotechnology Institute, Ohio University, Konneker Research Laboratories, 1 Water Tower Drive, The Ridges, 45701 Athens, Ohio, USA

Molecular and Cellular Biology Program, Ohio University, Athens, Ohio, USA
Department of Biomedical Sciences, College of Osteopathic Medicine, Ohio University, Athens, Ohio, USA

Shigeru Okada
Edison Biotechnology Institute, Ohio University, Konneker Research Laboratories, 1 Water Tower Drive, The Ridges, 45701 Athens, Ohio, USA
Department of Biomedical Sciences, College of Osteopathic Medicine, Ohio University, Athens, Ohio, USA

Vicente Barrios and Jesús Argente
Hospital Infantil Universitario Niño Jesús, Department of Endocrinology, Instituto de Investigación la Princesa, Universidad Autónoma de Madrid, Department of Pediatrics, Av. Menéndez Pelayo, 65, E 28009 Madrid, Spain
CIBER Fisiopatología Obesidad y Nutrición (CIBERobn), Instituto de Salud Carlos III, Madrid, Spain

Pierre Bougnères and Claire Bouvattier
Pediatric Endocrinology, Bicêtre Hospital, Paris South University, 78 Avenue du Général Leclerc, Kremin Bicêtre, 94270 Paris, France

Maryse Cartigny
Pediatric Endocrinology, Jeanne de Flandre Hospital, Lille University, Lille, France

Lina Michala
First Department of Obstetrics and Gynaecology, University of Athens, Alexandra Hospital, Athens, Greece

Aaron L Carrel, Jens C Eickhoff and David B Allen
Department of Pediatrics, University of Wisconsin, 600 Highland Avenue, H4-436, Madison, WI 53792-4108, USA

Jeffrey S Sledge and Stephen J Ventura
Land Information and Computer Graphics Facility, University of Wisconsin, 600 Highland Avenue, H4-436, Madison, WI 53792-4108, USA

Janel D. Hunter and Ali S. Calikoglu
Division of Pediatric Endocrinology, University of North Carolina at Chapel Hill, Campus Medical School Wing E, Chapel Hill, NC 27599, USA

A. J. Arcari, M. G. Gryngarten, A. V. Freire, M. G. Ballerini, M. G. Ropelato, I. Bergadá and M. E. Escobar
Centro de Investigaciones Endocrinológicas "Dr. César Bergadá" (CEDIE), CONICET – FEI – División de Endocrinología, Hospital de Niños Ricardo Gutiérrez, Gallo 1330, C1425EFD Buenos Aires, Argentina

Kimberly L Henrichs
University of Wisconsin School of Medicine and
Public Health, 600 Highland Avenue, Madison, WI
53792-4108, USA

Heather L McCauley and Elizabeth Miller
University of Pittsburgh School of Medicine, 3420 Fifth
Avenue, Pittsburgh, PA 15213, USA
Children's Hospital of Pittsburgh, University of
Pittsburgh Medical Center, 3420 Fifth Avenue,
Pittsburgh, PA 15213, USA

Dennis M Styne
University of California Davis, 2516 Stockton Blvd,
Sacramento, CA 95817, USA

Naomi Saito
University of California Davis, 1616 DaVinci Court,
Davis, CA 95618, USA

Joshua Breslau
RAND Corporation, 4570 Fifth Avenue, Suite 600,
Pittsburgh, PA 15213, USA

**Serwah Bonsu Asafo-Agyei, Emmanuel Ameyaw and
Samuel Blay Nguah**
Department of Child Health, Komfo Anokye Teaching
Hospital, Kumasi, Ghana

Jean-Pierre Chanoine
Endocrinology and Diabetes Unit, British Columbia's
Children's Hospital, University of British Columbia,
Vancouver, BC, Canada

**M. Ahmid1, V. Fisher, E. McNeil, M. Donaldson, A.
Mason, S. F. Ahmed and M. G. Shaikh**
Developmental Endocrinology Research Group,
Royal Hospital for Children, School of Medicine,
University of Glasgow, 1345 Govan Road, Glasgow
G51 4TF, UK

A. J. Graveling, S. McGeoch and J. S. Bevan
JJR Macleod Centre for Diabetes, Endocrinology and
Metabolism, Aberdeen Royal Infirmary, Aberdeen, UK

J. Roach and L. Bath
Department of Endocrinology, Royal Hospital for Sick
Children, Edinburgh, UK

G. Leese
Ninewells Hospital and Medical School in Dundee,
Dundee, UK

C. G. Perry
Department of Endocrinology, Queen Elizabeth
University Hospitals, Glasgow, UK

N. N. Zammitt
Royal Infirmary of Edinburgh, Edinburgh, UK

Melinda Chen, Todd Nebesio and Erica Eugster
Department of Pediatrics, Section of Pediatric
Endocrinology, Riley Hospital for Children, Indiana
University School of Medicine, 705 Riley Hospital
Drive, Room # 5960, Indianapolis, IN 46202, USA

Matthew Lash
Department of Pediatrics, Naval Medical Center, 34800
Bob Wilson Dr, San Diego, CA 92134, USA

**Mary Ellen Vajravelu, Jared Tobolski, Vaneeta
Bamba, Steven Willi and Shana E. McCormack**
Division of Endocrinology and Diabetes, The Children's
Hospital of Philadelphia, 3401 Civic Center Blvd, Suite
11NW, Philadelphia, USA

Evanette Burrows and Marianne Chilutti
Center for Biomedical Informatics, The Children's
Hospital of Philadelphia, 3535 Market St, Philadelphia,
PA 19104, USA

Rui Xiao
Department of Biostatistics and Epidemiology,
University of Pennsylvania, 635 Blockley Hall, 423
Guardian Drive, Philadelphia, PA 19104-6021, USA

Andrew Palladino
Global Innovative Pharma, Pfizer, Inc, 500 Arcola
Road, Collegeville, PA 19426, USA

Jon M. Burnham
The Children's Hospital of Philadelphia, Division of
Rheumatology, 10103 Colket Building, 34th and Civic
Center Blvd, Philadelphia, PA 19104, USA

Nicole Nader and Aida Lteif
Division of Pediatric Endocrinology, Mayo Clinic, 200
1st St SW, Rochester, MN 55905, USA

Amy Weaver
Biomedical Statistics and Informatics, Mayo Clinic,
Rochester, MN 55905, USA

Susan Eckert
Division of Endocrinology, Mayo Clinic, Rochester,
MN 55905, USA

Serwah Bonsu Asafo-Agyei, Emmanuel Ameyaw and Samuel Blay Nguah
Department of Child Health, Komfo Anokye Teaching Hospital, Kumasi, Ghana

Jean-Pierre Chanoine
Endocrinology and Diabetes Unit, British Columbia Children's Hospital, University of British Columbia, Vancouver, BC, Canada

Margaret Zacharin
The Royal Children's Hospital, Murdoch Children's Research Institute and University of Melbourne, Melbourne, Australia

Index